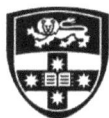

THE UNIVERSITY OF
SYDNEY

THE SYDNEY HANDBOOK OF ANXIETY DISORDERS

A GUIDE TO THE SYMPTOMS, CAUSES AND TREATMENTS OF ANXIETY DISORDERS

EDITED BY

PHILIP BOYCE
ANTHONY HARRIS
JULIETTE DROBNY
LISA LAMPE
VLADAN STARCEVIC
RICHARD BRYANT

sydney.edu.au

First edition published in Australia in 2015
by the University of Sydney
NSW 2006 Australia
sydney.edu.au

For information regarding sales and permissions, write to:

    Richard He
    Discipline of Psychiatry
    Sydney Medical School – Westmead
    Westmead Hospital
    PO Box 533
    Wentworthville NSW 2145 Australia
    F +61 2 9635 7734
    E richard.he@sydney.edu.au

National Library of Australia Cataloguing-in-Publication entry:

The Sydney handbook of anxiety disorders: a guide to the symptoms, causes
    and treatments of anxiety disorders / edited by Philip Boyce, Anthony Harris,
    Juliette Drobny, Lisa Lampe, Vladan Starcevic, Richard Bryant.
    Includes bibliographical references and index.
    ISBN 978-0-9942145-0-8 (pbk.)
    1. Anxiety disorders--Handbooks, manuals, etc. 2. Mental health--Handbooks,
    manuals, etc.
    University of Sydney. Sydney Medical School. Discipline of Psychiatry.
    616.8522

Cover image: Watercolour painting © Julie Goodwin / The Dax Centre
Cover design by Amber Breeze / University Publishing Managed Service

CONTENTS

FOREWORD

I was very pleased when Professor Philip Boyce asked me to write a foreword for his team's new book, *The Sydney Handbook of Anxiety Disorders*. The team at the Discipline of Psychiatry of Sydney Medical School has taken a leadership role in a large educational project funded by an NHMRC Centres of Clinical Research Excellence (CCRE) grant. This grant allowed for leading anxiety and neuroscience researchers to develop, evaluate, and disseminate better treatments of anxiety. They have also been translating their research findings into clinical practice. A key feature of their grant was to develop a state of the art education program *Anxiety Education for Health Professionals*. This book represents a huge collaborative effort from over 10 leading institutions in Australia and New Zealand, drawing from their experience in the development and teaching of the education program.

The editors of this book are clinical academics from the University of Sydney with extensive clinical experience in anxiety disorders with strong track records in clinical research and clinical training. Together with another 15 contributors, they share with the reader their unique expertise, specific insights, and concrete examples for understanding and treating anxiety disorders.

According to Australian Bureau of Statistics (2008), anxiety is the most common mental disorder affecting more than 14% of Australians. Anxiety disorders can have significant effects on patients' quality of life and accounts for considerable disease burden. Unfortunately, anxiety is as misunderstood among patients and health professionals as it is common. Only one in five of those who meet criteria for an anxiety disorder had a consultation with a health professional about their mental health. Of them, only a half received effective treatments. Of those who consulted a health professional three quarters did not believe they needed to.

In light of these statistics, the publication of *The Sydney Handbook of Anxiety Disorders* is timely. It presents the latest and most comprehensive information on the diagnosis and treatment of anxiety, and clearly lays out a biopsychosocial model for understanding anxiety that involves biological activity of the brain, psychological theories on attachment and conditioning, and recognition of social triggers. New and traditional psychological and pharmacological treatment options are meticulously analysed in simple language, while case studies give real-life examples of diagnosis and treatment plans.

There are sections covering the interface between medical illnesses and the anxiety disorders. As an endocrinologist, this is particularly pleasing to me, as they deal with the bidirectional relationship between thyroid disease and anxiety.

Unlike many other research publications, the nature of this book is not overly dry or meant for an academic audience only. It is intended to educate both patients and all health practitioners. It is also suitable for undergraduate and postgraduate students in the health and medical discipline to obtain a comprehensive understanding of anxiety disorders, their symptoms, causes and treatments.

Mental health is a very important subject in Sydney Medical School's curriculum. The Psychiatry and Addiction Medicine (PAAM) rotation is part of our flagship program Doctor of Medicine (MD). It provides our medical students with a wide range of specialised clinical experiences, across our six clinical schools, to give them a deep insight into mental disorders from both patient and professional perspectives. Our Brain and Mind Research Institute (BMRI), one of Australia's leading neuro-psychiatric institutes, recently launched a new postgraduate program Master of Medicine (Psychiatry) to foster the next generation of psychiatrists. This course will help psychiatry trainees develop a sophisticated understanding of the neuro-scientific basis of psychiatry and expertise in critical appraisal and research design. We have other well-established postgraduate coursework such as Master of Medicine (Psychotherapy) to fulfil our mission of creating graduates who will be able to contribute to the mental health and welfare of people, and to contribute to the body of information that we all use every day when we practice psychological medicine. This book will no doubt help us fulfil this mission too. It will play an important role in our teaching of anxiety disorders and become a great addition to our curriculum.

Finally, I hope you will enjoy this book and apply the knowledge in your daily work and life.

Professor Bruce Robinson
Dean, Sydney Medical School
January 2015
Sydney, Australia

PREFACE

Anxiety disorders are more common in Australia than depression; roughly 14.4% of the population suffer from an anxiety disorder, and the disability caused by these disorders is comparable to that caused by physical disorders. Yet less than half of the people who need it get adequate treatment. Over half seek treatment by visiting a doctor but only 60% of those will receive treatment that is known to be beneficial. The rest receive counselling or inadequate advice.

The aim of this handbook is to provide a solid understanding of the biological and psychological theories about the anxiety disorders and the epidemiology and clinical features of various anxiety disorders. It also aims to provide the basis for psychological and pharmacological treatments. The handbook sets out the theoretical models as to why anxiety disorders arise, and show that there is no single cause of an anxiety disorder. Rather, they are best understood through a biopsychosocial model, in which there are biological, psychological and social explanations for their origins.

Along with psychological theories about anxiety disorders, the physiology of anxiety and the roles of the autonomic nervous system are described, as is that of the hypothalamic-pituitary-adrenal axis. The brain networks involved in anxiety – the fear circuitry – are explained, as well as genetic theories that may underlie a propensity to anxiety.

From a psychological perspective, learning theory and the different forms of conditioning are described. But there are also other important psychological theories about anxiety, including disturbances in attachment that underpin many of the psychodynamic theories of anxiety disorders. The way people appraise or think about events has an enormous impact on their response to those events, and this is important to understand in order to comprehend the cognitive theories of anxiety disorders.

Anxiety disorders do not occur in a vacuum, and there are many aspects of the social environment that contribute to their onset. These include the life events that may trigger anxiety, while social support may help buffer against the impact of such stresses.

In understanding anxiety disorders from a biopsychosocial perspective, it is crucial to realise that these different domains interact with each other in contributing to the onset and continuation of an anxiety disorder.

It is important to confirm the type of anxiety disorder from which the individual is suffering, to find out about the context of the disorder, what triggered it, what maintains it and why it has developed. It is also important to ensure, as far as possible, that anxiety is not due to an underlying medical illness.

Given that there are different mechanisms involved in the development of anxiety disorders, it is hardly surprising that there are different approaches to treating anxiety disorders. These approaches include psychological treatments and pharmacological treatments.

There is now a range of evidence-based treatments for the anxiety disorders from a psychological perspective, such as the exposure-based behavioural treatments and cognitive treatments which will challenge cognitive distortions and assist patients to manage worry and rumination, which can be conducted face-to-face or over the Internet.

There are also well-established pharmacological treatments for anxiety disorders; a range of medications that have demonstrated effectiveness in the treatment of the disorders, in particular the serotonin reuptake inhibitors, which are widely used in their treatment, and the benzodiazepines.

This handbook draws on the expertise of specialists from around Australia and New Zealand, who have combined their knowledge to create a comprehensive guide to all aspects of anxiety disorders.

Sincerely,

Professor Philip Boyce
Head, Discipline of Psychiatry at Sydney Medical School
January 2015
Sydney, Australia

ACKNOWLEDGEMENT

This publication was supported by the National Health and Medical Research Council of the Australian Government through the Centres of Clinical Research Excellence (CCRE) Scheme. The Centre for Clinical Research Excellence in Anxiety and Neuroscience, funded by the CCRE Scheme, brought together Australia's leading anxiety and neuroscience researchers to develop, evaluate, and disseminate better treatments of anxiety. This publication is an output of the project entitled "Anxiety Education for Health Professionals".

Thanks to Anne Barrowclough and Laurie Chiko for editorial assistance.

Thanks to Julie Goodwin for the watercolour painting on the front cover. Julie has been diagnosed with bi-polar, anxiety and depression. This work was made in response to her experience of the 2009 Black Saturday bush fires. She has stated, "This work portrays not only the conflicting visuals of the mesmerising beauty and terrifying intensity of what I saw that day, but also the overwhelming anxiety, fear, stress and the ongoing feelings that I had to express in order to return to the work in progress before the fire." This work is part of the Cunningham Dax Collection which is housed at The Dax Centre and consists of over 15,000 artworks created by people with an experience of mental illness and/or psychological trauma. Visit www.daxcentre.org for more information.

CONTRIBUTORS

Gavin Andrews
Professor of Psychiatry at the University of New South Wales at St Vincent's Hospital, Sydney, Australia

Philip Boyce
Professor of Psychiatry at Sydney Medical School, the University of Sydney, Australia

Richard Bryant
Honorary Professor at Sydney Medical School, the University of Sydney, and Scientia Professor at School of Psychology, the University of New South Wales, Australia

Helen Christensen
Professor of Mental Health at the University of New South Wales, and Executive Director at Black Dog Institute, Australia

Rocco Crino
Associate Professor of Clinical Psychology at School of Psychology, Charles Sturt University, Australia

Angela Dixon
Senior Clinical Psychologist at Department of Psychological Medicine, Children's Hospital at Westmead, Australia

Juliette Drobny
Lecturer at Sydney Medical School, the University of Sydney, Australia

Kim Felmingham
Professor and Director of Research at Faculty of Health, University of Tasmania, Australia

Anthony Harris
Associate Professor of Psychiatry at Sydney Medical School, the University of Sydney, Australia

Michael Harris
Respiratory Physician at Sydney Adventist Hospital, Australia

Jennifer Hudson
Professor at Faculty of Human Sciences, Macquarie University, Australia

Caroline Hunt
Associate Professor at Faculty of Science, the University of Sydney, Australia

Kasia Kozlowska
Clinical Associate Professor at Sydney Medical School, the University of Sydney, Australia

Lisa Lampe
Senior Lecturer at Sydney Medical School, the University of Sydney, Australia

Loyola McLean
Associate Professor at Brain and Mind Research Institute, the University of Sydney, Australia

Ross Menzies
Associate Professor at Faculty of Health Sciences, the University of Sydney, Australia

Michelle Moulds
Professor at School of Psychology, the University of New South Wales, Australia

Richie Poulton
Professor at Centre for Genetics Research, the University of Otago, New Zealand

Christopher Ryan
Clinical Senior Lecturer at Sydney Medical School, the University of Sydney, Australia

Vladan Starcevic
Associate Professor at Sydney Medical School, the University of Sydney, Australia

Naomi Wray
Professor at Queensland Brain Institute, the University of Queensland, Australia

PART I   WHAT IS ANXIETY

Anxiety is a universal experience, which at times can actually be helpful. Part I will outline common features of anxiety disorders. It will show how they can interfere with a person's life, and what it might be like to have an anxiety disorder. It will also explain the issues that surround classification of the anxiety disorders.

A key feature of anxiety is that the subjective experience cannot be judged by appearances. The distress related to anxiety derives from not only the physical experience of it, but perhaps more so the individual's cognitive experience. As will become clear in later chapters, it is the "fear of fear" that is most disabling. Individuals worry about the nature and consequences of both the physical and mental symptoms of anxiety, and these worries can fuel further fear and anxiety.

People who feel anxious may experience any of the following symptoms: a racing or pounding heart, shortness of breath, dizziness, nausea or "butterflies in the stomach", shakiness, blushing, sweating, a lump in the throat, a dry mouth or feelings of unreality.

Some of these may be more prominent than others, and typically everyone has their own pattern of anxiety. In the same way, anxiety *disorders* are characterised by somewhat individualised patterns of symptoms.

Usually there is a reason why people are more concerned about some symptoms than others, and this often has to do with what they view as the cause of the symptoms, or the possible consequences of having them. Understanding this is important for treatment.

> A racing or pounding heart, shortness of breath, dizziness, nausea or "butterflies in the stomach", shakiness, blushing, sweating, a lump in the throat, a dry mouth or feelings of unreality are all symptoms of anxiety.

CHAPTER 1   THE NATURE OF ANXIETY

Anthony Harris and Lisa Lampe

WHAT IS ANXIETY

Anxiety is a physical and mental experience. Everyone has experienced anxiety at some time in their life. As a child they may have been afraid of the dark, anxious about learning to ride a bike or sitting exams at school. Most adults would have felt anxious about having to give a speech at a social occasion. Such anxiety would have given rise to a number of physical symptoms, such as feeling hot and sweaty, experiencing butterflies in the stomach, or feeling shaky. Almost certainly on these occasions, individuals worried about the possibility of something going wrong or not working out the way they wanted it to. In other words, they reacted as though there was some threat to them. Nevertheless, anxiety is a normal part of life and can even be helpful.

CASE HISTORY: ANABEL

Anabel is a young woman who suffers from anxiety. When she becomes anxious, her heart starts to race, her hands become sweaty and clammy, she has butterflies in her stomach and she begins to blush.

"I feel that I have not prepared enough for what I am doing. I need to have what I want to talk about in front of me, otherwise I can't get my head around my thoughts."

ANXIETY IS A RESPONSE

Anabel's description is typical of what everyone feels like before a test or in an anxiety-provoking situation. These familiar feelings are a normal response to a perceived threat or challenge. They are an adaptive part of functioning and are essential for survival.

FUNCTION OF ANXIETY: FIGHT OR FLIGHT RESPONSE

Anxiety promotes alertness and primes the body for instant action in the face of danger or challenges by activating the body's "Fight or Flight Response". The fight or flight response involves a cascade of

2

physiological functions that are experienced as physical and mental events.

PERCEIVED THREAT

A person will only become anxious if they feel threatened in some way. Parents worry about their children precisely because they *do not* feel threatened by a lot of things that are actually dangerous, which means that they may put themselves in harm's way – running across roads without looking, for instance, or sticking forks in the electrical sockets to see what will happen. In these cases, people have to *learn* to fear situations so they will be more cautious about them. In other cases, people might be naturally fearful of things. Common examples include phobias of spiders, snakes, heights, and storms.

OBJECTIVE AND SUBJECTIVE RESPONSE

The response of the individual is both objective and subjective. Objectively, some of the somatic symptoms of anxiety may be apparent (for example, blushing, sweating or shaking) as may a person's behavioural response to anxiety (for example, restlessness, pacing or increased motor movements such as hand gesticulations). Subjectively, the person suffers symptoms related to muscular tension, autonomic activity and cognitive aspects of anxiety. Not infrequently, the subjective experience of anxiety is much greater than any objective signs.

SOMATIC SYMPTOMS

The physical symptoms of anxiety are related to muscular tension and autonomic activity. Somatic symptoms of anxiety may be experienced "from head to toe", for example, ranging from feelings of dizziness, to breathlessness, nausea and fatigue.

BEHAVIOURAL RESPONSE

A number of different behaviours may occur as part of the fight or flight response. An individual will take "flight", or run away from the threat, when they can, but if they are cornered, they might "fight". A "freeze" reaction can also be observed. All animals, including humans, experience the fight or flight response when under threat. The manifestations of the fight or flight response may vary with the species, but its purpose is to respond effectively to danger. In this way, anxiety is considered to be "adaptive".

> All animals, including humans, experience the "fight or flight response" when under threat.

AUTONOMIC NERVOUS SYSTEM

The primary system through which the fight or flight response is activated is the autonomic nervous system (ANS). Symptoms related to activation of the ANS may be grouped according to different body systems in which they occur. Within the cardiovascular system, people commonly notice that their heart rate may have increased or they may be aware of a missed beat or a run of strong heartbeats. Symptoms of autonomic arousal within the respiratory system may be experienced as a sense of constriction or tightness of the chest, a feeling of shortness of breath and an increase in breathing rate. This may be so marked as to be considered hyperventilation or over-breathing, which can itself trigger a number of other physiological changes (e.g., dizziness, faintness, tingling in the hands and feet) due to alteration in the acid-base balance.

Symptoms may also occur in the gastrointestinal and genitourinary systems. People often complain of epigastric discomfort including nausea and "butterflies in the stomach"; these are probably related to reduced stomach emptying. Symptoms of intestinal hurry, and feeling a need to go to the toilet are common. Other changes can include an increase in bowel sounds (borborygmi) and wind because of swallowing of air (aerohpagy). A decrease in secretion of saliva due to cholinergic activation can lead to a dry mouth and difficulty in swallowing. Other effects of anxiety on the genitourinary system, besides increasing the frequency and urgency of micturition, include loss of libido and inability to gain an erection. Autonomic activity will also initiate changes to the circulation, causing peripheral vasoconstriction leading to cold hands and pallor, but often vasodilatation of capillaries in the face, leading to blushing. It will activate muscarinic innervation of the sweat glands, causing sweating and adding clamminess to cold hands.

COGNITIVE RESPONSE

The cognitive experience of anxiety can be equally varied. Fear is perhaps the most prominent cognitive response. Feelings of edginess or jumpiness may also occur and are associated with an increased startle reflex. Anxiety about specific threats may result in hypervigilance, and contribute to feelings of uneasiness. Concentration may be impaired, especially if an individual is experiencing worry or anxious ruminations.

The Yerkes-Dodson curve (Figure 1.1) illustrates the interaction of anxiety and performance, and was first described by psychologists Robert Yerkes and John Dodson in 1908. It describes the relationship between anxiety level and cognitive performance. Importantly, the adaptive function of mild to moderate anxiety is shown, as well as the impairing effects of severe anxiety (Yerkes & Dodson, 1908).

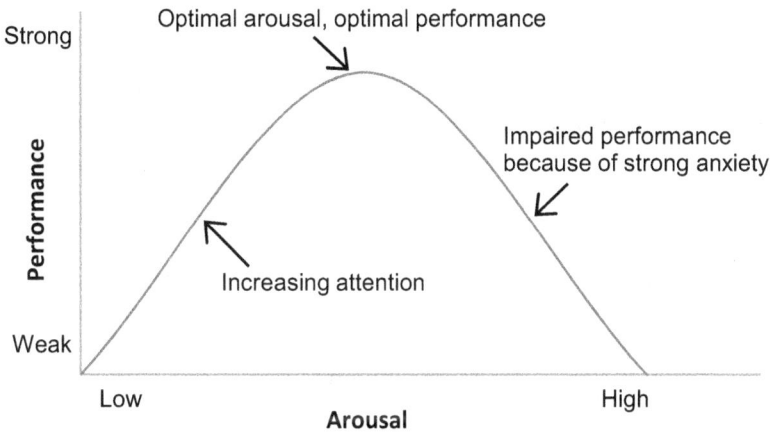

Figure 1.1   Yerkes-Dodson curve

Many patients have come to believe that all anxiety is abnormal and dangerous, so sharing this model that illustrates the dynamic relationship between adaptive and maladaptive aspects of anxiety, can be helpful in treatment. Understanding the role of cognitive factors in anxiety is especially important in treatment, and will be explored further in the following chapters.

CHAPTER 2   MORE ABOUT ANXIETY

Lisa Lampe

A MODEL OF ANXIETY

We have seen that the perception of a threat may trigger the fight or flight response. The sequence of events that underlies the anxiety response is shown diagrammatically on the basic model of anxiety in Figure 2.1.

The trigger will typically be some situation that is perceived as threatening, either instinctively or because it is appraised that way. This in turn triggers the fight or flight response, which involves the release of adrenaline and stress hormones and in turn leads to the autonomic nervous system (ANS) response and physiological changes, and results in behavioural responses of fight, flight or freezing.

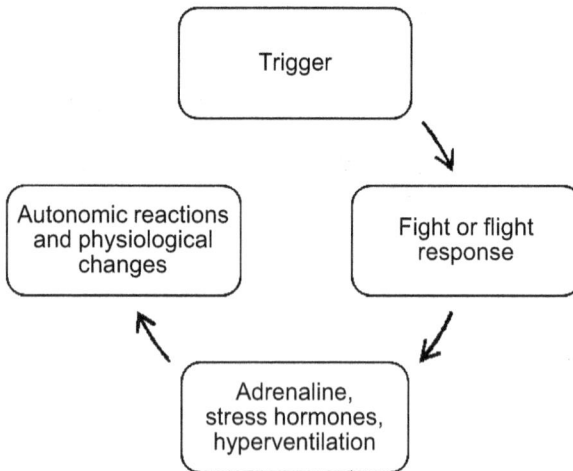

Figure 2.1   Model of anxiety

ANIMALS VERSUS HUMANS

Frequently with animals, the fight or flight response is instinctual – for example when the rabbit becomes aware of the shadow of an eagle. Animals can also learn to associate certain situations with the threat of physical harm. This can be seen in everyday life; for example, a dog that has been mistreated by and comes to fear its owner. For animals, the perceived threat is probably always physical.

However, in humans the fight or flight response is dependent on perception of threat: people have to appraise a situation as potentially dangerous, or fear some harm occurring. Unlike animals, humans have the capacity to think abstractly. People think about the future, create images of how they would like their lives to be; they think about how they appear to others and they want to be liked and accepted.

Humans also have a good imagination, which can make them creative. However, it also means that people can imagine things going wrong, and anticipate how unpleasant this could be; they have the ability to imagine all sorts of scenarios that might threaten the things they care about. Hence, many different types of threat or harm may be apprehended, such as loss of face, embarrassing oneself or feeling that one's reputation is at stake; loss of something important, like a job or a relationship; and loss of one's health, such as developing an illness. Thus, humans may perceive threats beyond the purely physical.

These differences between animals and humans are summarised in the following table:

Table 2.1 Differences in anxiety between animals and humans

	Animals	*Humans*
Response	Instinctual	Dependent on appraisal
Thinking	Concrete	Abstract
Perceived threat	Physical	Physical & non-physical

A HUMAN MODEL OF ANXIETY

The particular role for appraisal in the experience of human anxiety reactions is illustrated in Figure 2.2.

Triggers for anxious appraisal can include situations, thoughts and sensations. Many people also worry about the anxiety itself – for example, they may fear that they will never be free of anxiety or that anxiety may lead to cancer or insanity.

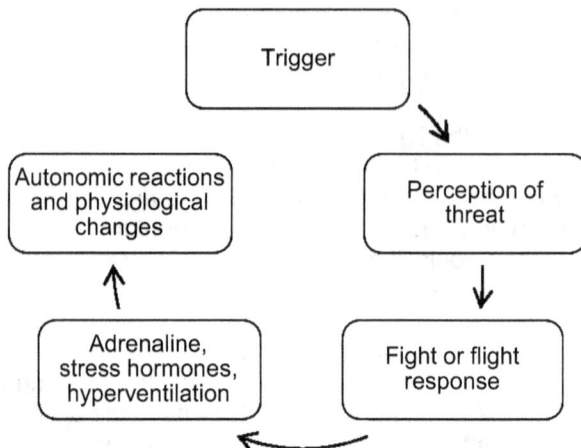

Figure 2.2 A human model of anxiety

PHYSICAL SYMPTOMS AND APPRAISAL: FEEDBACK LOOPS IN ANXIETY

In the previous chapter, a range of physical or somatic symptoms that occur during anxiety were described. These physical symptoms may be very intense and many of them mimic symptoms of serious physical illnesses.

For example, dizziness might be interpreted as a sign of impending stroke. A pounding heart or chest tightness might seem to be a sign of heart attack. Trouble swallowing may be perceived as a sign of imminent choking. Shortness of breath may cause concern about lung cancer or other serious illness. Feelings of unreality may lead to fear of going insane. Numbness or tingling as a result of hyperventilation may be interpreted as a sign of multiple sclerosis or another neurological condition. A tight throat may cause the fear of suffocating.

All these interpretations will intensify the fear and anxiety, forming feedback loops (Figure 2.3).

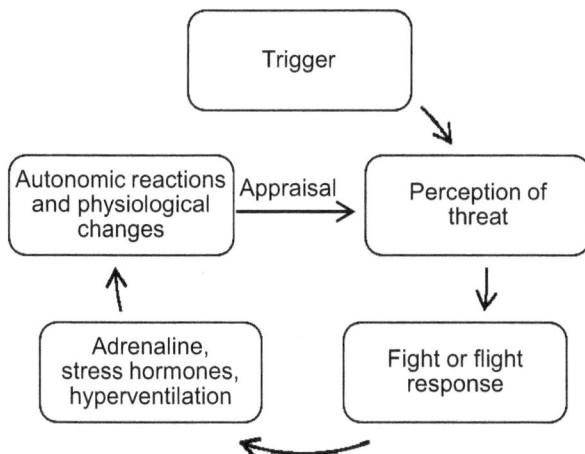

Figure 2.3 Feedback loops in anxiety

CASE STUDY: MARY

Mary has panic disorder and every time her heart beats quickly she worries there must be something wrong with it. Running for the bus triggers anxiety because it makes her heart pound. At the core of her fear is her belief that a pounding heart is linked to the possibility of a serious heart problem. Until she is able to change the way she thinks about a pounding heart, it will continue to be perceived as threatening, and will trigger anxiety.

These catastrophic beliefs about physical sensations occur most commonly in panic disorder with or without agoraphobia. People with social anxiety disorder are more likely to link visible signs of anxiety (e.g., sweating, blushing, shaking) with the belief that others think poorly of them or evaluate them negatively. In just the same way as for Mary, experiencing these symptoms will intensify the anxiety reaction, as the symptom itself (e.g., blushing) is perceived as threatening. Referring back to the model of anxiety in Figure 2.2, this creates a "vicious circle" or a feedback loop for anxiety.

MENTAL/COGNITIVE SYMPTOMS, APPRAISAL AND FEEDBACK LOOPS

The main mental or *cognitive* symptoms of anxiety are fearful thoughts, and emotional reactions of fear, apprehension and impending doom. Symptoms such as derealisation (i.e., a sense that the world around you feels strange or unreal), depersonalisation (i.e., a sense that you do not feel completely in your own body or mind), impaired concentration and trouble thinking clearly can be appraised as signs of serious mental illness and loss of control. It is easy to understand how such experiences might frighten a person into thinking they could be going insane, and therefore make their anxiety even worse. Excessive anxiety can also interfere with task performance – for example, through impaired attention and concentration.

BEHAVIOURAL SYMPTOMS

Basic behavioural responses to threat have been described in the previous section. Typically, individuals also begin to employ behaviours designed to prevent or reduce the severity of anxiety attacks. The most common behavioural response is avoidance of situations that are believed to trigger anxiety. However, more subtle behavioural responses may be employed if the person is unable to avoid the situation, typically safety (seeking) behaviours. Safety seeking behaviours are designed to protect the person from the feared outcome. They may vary according to the anxiety disorder. For example, in panic disorder the individual will often carry a mobile phone, bottle of water and/or medication, all of which it is believed may be able to prevent a panic attack, make it less severe, or summon help in case the panic attack is severe. In social phobia, reducing eye contact and saying very little is often a person's attempt to minimise judgement by others. In OCD, the behavioural symptoms involve compulsions (e.g., hand-washing, checking electrical appliances), which are designed to prevent the person's fear (obsession) from coming true.

CASE STUDY: RICK

Rick is constantly worried, and has lost confidence in his own decision-making. He is so scared of losing his company large sums of money as a result of mistakes he might make, that whenever a superior wants to talk to him, he is convinced he is going to be fired.

"Sometimes I wake up in the middle of the night in a cold sweat, convinced that I have made some terrible mistake.

"Half the time I can't concentrate properly because I'm jumping ahead to other jobs. I feel I have to anticipate every little thing that could go wrong. Sometimes I feel like a loser.

"I worry about how I'm worrying so much. It's almost as if I worry when I'm not worrying. Sometimes, when I'm really tense, I think there's something physically wrong with me. I have a feeling of pressure in my head; I think I might be having a stroke."

In response to his anxiety, Rick tries to check things over and over in order to catch any mistake he may have made. He likes to have reassurance that things are OK. He also tries to be extremely careful about his work, which is time-consuming, so he spends long hours in the office. Rick's behavioural responses relate closely to his specific fears, and contribute to the impairment caused by his anxiety.

PANIC ATTACKS

A panic attack is a very severe, sudden increase in the level of anxiety. Symptoms may include any of the usual physical symptoms of anxiety, but they tend to escalate very quickly (i.e., over five to ten minutes) and reach a high level. These physical symptoms are associated with intense fear, often a sense of impending doom and the desire to flee or escape the situation. Panic attacks do not only occur in panic disorder. They are really an indication that the anxiety has reached very severe levels. The fears that cause the anxiety could be based on any number of issues, as long as they are perceived as threatening in some way. Hence, panic attacks can be seen in any anxiety disorder.

PREDICTABLE OR UNPREDICTABLE?

Panic attacks may occur on a background of increased anxiety and arousal. Panic attacks may also seem to come "out of the blue". *The Diagnostic and Statistical Manual of Mental Disorders*, Fifth edition (DSM-5) places an emphasis on the unpredictability of panic attacks in panic disorder.

However, research does not support the theory that most panic attacks are unpredictable. In most cases, there has probably been a subtle trigger, such as an anxiety-provoking thought or feeling. It is more likely that the triggers for panic attacks in these cases are so subtle that the person is not even consciously aware of them.

Initial panic attacks, however, are usually experienced as out of the blue. Studies suggest that the initial panic attack often occurs at a time of physical stress, such as hangovers, being ill, or recovering from a cold or flu. They also occur for the first time more commonly when a person is a long way from home, for example, on an overseas holiday.

A panic attack is a very severe, sudden increase in the level of anxiety.

PANIC ATTACKS ARE COMMON

As mentioned previously, panic attacks may occur in any anxiety disorder. Having a panic attack does not mean that a person has *panic disorder*. It is estimated that 28% of the general population experience a panic attack at some time in their life, but only a fraction of these people go on to develop panic disorder. Some people are more vulnerable to developing panic disorder with or without agoraphobia, after experiencing an initial panic attack. In such individuals, there may be an underlying predisposition to anxiety. If a person believes the panic attack is dangerous, they may fear having another one and this increased anxiety might predispose them to further panic attacks, especially if they begin to avoid possible triggers or are not able to accept reassurance.

VULNERABILITY FACTORS FOR PANIC ATTACKS

A number of vulnerability factors for panic attacks have been identified. These include a trait known as "negative affectivity". An older name for this trait is "neuroticism". Negative affectivity has a strong heritable component; thus it often runs in families. People with high negative affectivity are more sensitive and reactive to their environment and this appears to be a risk factor for anxiety and depression.

Another trait with a significant genetic contribution is "behavioural inhibition to the unfamiliar". This describes the tendency, observable in infancy and early childhood, for a child to become anxious and cling to its mother when confronted with a stranger. In a baby, an exaggerated startle response (e.g. to loud noises) and difficulty in settling may be a manifestation of this trait. An attribute called "anxiety sensitivity" has also been described in anxious persons, and refers to a heightened sensitivity to physical sensations and the tendency to find these sensations unpleasant or worrying. Persons who experience significant adversity or trauma in childhood also seem to be at increased risk of developing both anxiety and depression later in life.

However, the key factor in determining whether a person goes on to develop panic disorder is their *appraisal* of the panic attack; that is, what they believe the panic attack means. In response to a panic attack, a person who thinks, "I have to go easy on the alcohol", is probably not going to develop panic disorder. However, the person who thinks, "Oh no! There must be something seriously wrong with me! Maybe the flu or the alcohol has caused some damage to my body. I'd better be very careful with myself over the next little while and keep an eye on how I feel", is much more at risk, especially if they also have any of the vulnerability factors described above.

CHAPTER 3   THE ANXIETY DISORDERS

Lisa Lampe and Juliette Drobny

WHEN DOES ANXIETY BECOME A DISORDER

Anyone can be in a state of anxiety, which is a normal part of life. It occurs whenever an individual feels threatened. Symptoms need to be much more persistent and enduring, and to be interfering with a person's work, social and/or home life, before it could be said that someone has an anxiety disorder. Note that in almost all cases, the individuals themselves are aware that their anxiety is excessive and/or unreasonable (at least once they are out of the acute situation).

EXCESSIVE AND UNREASONABLE ANXIETY

The role of perceived threat (threat appraisals) has been discussed. To some degree, there is an association between the intensity of the anxiety an individual feels and the characteristics of the threat, such as how likely it seems and how bad it would be if the fears were realised.

A number of common patterns in fearful thinking in anxiety disorders have been recognised. Firstly, individuals with an anxiety disorder show a tendency to overestimate the likelihood of harm occurring. This is referred to as a "probability" appraisal. Secondly, they overestimate how bad it would be if their fears were realised. This is called the "cost" appraisal. These beliefs are also referred to as "cognitive biases". Another cognitive bias is the belief that one would not cope with or recover from the feared consequence if it happened.

Individuals with an anxiety disorder are generally well aware that they worry more, or are more anxious than the average person. What seems to prevent people from getting help is not a failure to realise they have a problem, but rather that they do not realise that anything can be done to help, or that they prefer to try to manage things themselves. A number of community surveys have confirmed this finding.

PERSISTENCE

An anxiety state is short-lived, and is generally relieved once the triggering stressor has been resolved. To diagnose anxiety at the level of "disorder", the anxiety needs to have been present much of the time over a period of at least four weeks. Hence, it is more than a temporary state of anxiety before an exam, or before giving a speech. In an anxiety disorder, anxiety may be present much of the time, or anxiety reactions occur very frequently, perhaps with relatively minor triggers.

The DSM-5 specifies for some anxiety disorders minimum periods for which the anxiety must be present. This includes four weeks for panic disorder and six months for generalised anxiety disorder and social anxiety disorder.

DISTRESS

For anxiety to be severe enough to meet criteria for a "disorder", it needs to be at least somewhat distressing. Of course, all anxiety states are somewhat unpleasant, but individuals with an anxiety disorder feel distressed and often anxious about their anxiety. An anxiety disorder significantly affects their quality of life. Not only are the symptoms unpleasant, but, as we have seen, they often generate even more anxiety, as the person worries about what the symptoms might mean, or where they might lead. Additionally, some fears may be particularly distressing of themselves, for example fears of harming others in OCD.

A significant aspect of the distress is the "fear of fear", where the person worries about the anxiety itself – for example, thinking, "What if it doesn't go away? What if so much anxiety drives me crazy?" Additionally, the underlying fears and feared consequences (e.g. being seriously ill, going mad, being embarrassed) are very distressing in themselves.

IMPAIRMENT

Anxiety that has reached the level of disorder interferes with a person's ability to function normally. It is hard to perform in your roles of spouse, parent, worker, or teammate when you are consumed with anxiety. Impairment from anxiety can take many forms. Excessive worry and anxiety often make it difficult to concentrate on other tasks at work and at home. When specific situations are feared, a person often begins to avoid them, which in turn makes it difficult to perform normal activities such as going to work, doing the shopping or taking the children to school. Being preoccupied with anxiety may also mean that the person may not be able to devote their time and attention to their relationships. They may be too fearful to participate with their friends or partner in activities that they used to enjoy.

Behaviours adopted in an effort to control anxiety can also cause impairment. Constant monitoring of symptoms can be distracting, and if there are frequent visits to the doctor to check them out, that is time not spent on other tasks. Sometimes, people use alcohol or sedatives to control their anxiety, and this can also interfere with role functioning. In some conditions, most notably OCD and GAD, an affected person might seek frequent reassurance from a partner or friend which can put a strain on the relationship. A relationship can also be adversely affected when anxiety makes a person reluctant to do things they used to enjoy doing together with their partner (e.g., movies, restaurants, holidays), because the activities might cause anxiety. Being preoccupied with anxiety can make a person seem self-centred, and reduce the attention and care they show friends and loved ones. A comprehensive patient assessment for anxiety should include exploration of associated impairment and disability.

The disability and impairment associated with anxiety has tended to be underestimated by health care professionals and health services. Research has demonstrated that anxiety disorders may result in similar levels of disability as many chronic medical conditions. Since effective treatments are available, active intervention to treat anxiety can result in not only reduced personal distress and impairment, but also economic benefits to the community.

THE NATURE AND CLINICAL PRESENTATIONS OF ANXIETY DISORDERS

The DSM-5 classifies panic disorder, agoraphobia, social anxiety disorder, generalised anxiety disorder, specific anxiety disorder and separation anxiety disorder. Other significant anxiety syndromes are classified separately, such as obsessive-compulsive disorder (Obsessive-Compulsive and Related Disorders), posttraumatic stress disorder (Trauma- and Stressor-related disorders), and illness anxiety disorder (Somatic Symptom and Related Disorders).

Although the clinical features differ markedly between the individual anxiety disorders, they share one common theme, namely, each anxiety disorder involves *overestimation of threat*. It is often the nature of the threat that best differentiates the anxiety disorders, and this will be explored below.

PANIC DISORDER

Panic disorder is characterised by recurrent, unexpected panic attacks. While panic attacks can be observed in all anxiety disorders, the hallmark of panic disorder is that the anxiety occurs suddenly, unexpectedly and escalates quickly to severe levels, and the individual develops persistent fear of recurrent panic attacks and their consequences. For example, a person may report sitting on the couch watching TV when suddenly they notice their heart starts racing, they feel hot and sweaty and have difficulty breathing. It can feel as though the panic came on out of the blue, however, on deeper probing, it may often be found that there was a subtle trigger, such as worrying about a future event or monitoring their physical sensations. If they begin to worry about having further panic attacks, or modify their behavior in ways that are designed to prevent future panic attacks or their consequences, they are likely to develop panic *disorder*.

In panic disorder, the panic attacks must be comprised of at least four of the following symptoms:

- increased heart rate, palpitations or pounding heart
- shortness of breath, feeling smothered or unable to take the next breath
- trembling or shaking
- feeling of choking
- chest pain or discomfort
- sweating
- dizziness, lightheadedness or feeling faint
- nausea or abdominal distress
- numbness or tingling sensations (often in the hands, feet or face)
- chills or hot flushes
- feelings of unreality or feeling detached from oneself or one's surroundings
- fear of losing control or going crazy
- fear of dying.

The panic attack also needs to develop quite quickly and peak within 10 minutes. Patients sometimes report that their panic attacks last hours, however for the purposes of diagnosis, this would not be considered a panic attack. In most such cases, patients are in fact experiencing fluctuating levels of anxiety, which at times can be very high and may include recurrent panic attacks.

In addition to experiencing unexpected panic attacks, there must be one month or more of either (1) persistent concern or worry about having additional attacks or their consequences and/or (2) a significant maladaptive change in behaviour related to the attacks – for example, behavior aimed at preventing future attacks.

Underlying Threats

The threats perceived by people with panic disorder typically involve fearing the attack will cause either *physical* harm, such as a heart attack, stroke, fainting, brain tumour, choking or death, or *mental* harm, such as going crazy, losing touch with reality or losing control. Whilst there may be some element of fear of *social* harm such as embarrassing themselves, this is usually not prominent, and is more likely to be associated with loss of control type symptoms – for example, incontinence of bladder or bowels. These catastrophic interpretations of symptoms, particularly concerns about physical safety, are understandable given the intensity of symptoms and their perceived similarity to symptoms of serious physical illnesses.

Behavioural Symptoms

The behavioural symptoms occurring in panic disorder are numerous.

A primary behavioural change is the emergence of agoraphobic avoidance, whereby the person begins to avoid situations or places where a panic attack has previously occurred. These situations have in common that the individual associates them with being far from help or difficult to escape from, and thus they often include shopping centres, motorway driving, lifts, tunnels, enclosed or open spaces or even being at home alone. Many times the individual will be able to enter these situations only if they are accompanied by a trusted companion, such as their spouse, parent, child or friend.

Other behavioural features seen in people with panic disorder include the use of safety seeking behaviours such as carrying a mobile phone, bottle of water, or anti-anxiety medication like alprazolam or diazepam, looking out for exits, keeping windows open and being close to medical attention.

People with panic disorder also often try to avoid experiencing physical sensations similar to panic. This is known as *interoceptive* avoidance and can include avoidance of activities such as exercise or sex. Drinking caffeine or alcohol is also often avoided for fear of inducing rapid heartbeats or feelings of lightheadedness, respectively. Some people will try to avoid experiencing strong emotions such as getting angry or excited, as these emotions trigger similar sensations such as heart palpitations and feeling hot. Other behavioural symptoms include keeping busy or distracted to avoid thinking about having a panic attack, as well as reducing stressful activities.

When making a diagnosis of panic disorder, it is important to determine that the panic attacks are not due to a general medical condition (such as hyperthyroidism) or the physiological effects of a substance (such as a drug of abuse or a medication).

AGORAPHOBIA

Agoraphobia is a term that is frequently misunderstood. Derived from the Greek *"agora"* meaning market place and *"phobos"* meaning fear, agoraphobia is often referred to as 'fear of the marketplace', or, loosely translated, 'fear of open spaces'. However, the name agoraphobia is a misnomer. It is not the *situation* that is actually feared in agoraphobia. Rather, the person fears having a panic attack or panic sensations in such situations and in turn tries to avoid the situation. In short, situations are feared because of their association with anxiety. Very often, the person may have had a panic attack in that situation, or the situation shares similar characteristics to a place where a panic attack previously occurred. If you asked the individual whether they would continue to fear the situation if they could be certain they would not have a panic attack there, they would typically say "no".

In DSM-IV, agoraphobia was only diagnosed in relation to panic disorder, namely panic disorder with agoraphobia, or agoraphobia without a history of panic disorder. However, in DSM-5, agoraphobia may be diagnosed irrespective of the presence of panic disorder. If panic disorder is present, and two or more listed situation types are feared (e.g. open spaces, enclosed spaces), both diagnoses should be given. Alternatively, a person may not experience full panic attacks, but what are referred to as "limited-symptom panic attacks", with fewer than four symptoms of panic present. For example, a patient may only experience dizziness and shortness of breath.

It is also worth noting what agoraphobia is not. It does not relate to avoidance of situations for reasons other than panic attacks or panic symptoms. For example, people with social phobia may avoid many of the same situations as those with agoraphobia – for example, crowded buses. However, the fear in such cases is of negative evaluation, rather than being a fear of panic attacks, and so does not mean such individuals also have agoraphobia. In severe agoraphobia, the individual may be unable to leave the house. However, agoraphobia is not synonymous with being housebound; indeed, many individuals with agoraphobia would be too anxious to be at home alone. For a diagnosis of agoraphobia the avoidance is not limited to specific situations but it *must* be associated with fear of panic. Hence, a patient with severe depression who has not left the house for months would not be considered agoraphobic.

Underlying Threats

The threats perceived by people with agoraphobia are essentially identical to those experienced in panic disorder, namely, fears of physical, mental or social harm. For example, while travelling on a bus, an individual may worry, "What if I had a panic attack on the bus? I could faint and hit my head. No one would help me. What if I had a serious head injury? Plus, I'd be lying there on the floor. The other passengers might think I was a drug addict. That would be embarrassing." In this example, there is a combination of physical and social threats; however, in general, the physical threats in panic disorder and agoraphobia are most compelling for patients.

Behavioural Symptoms

Situational avoidance is the most obvious behavioural symptom in agoraphobia. As mentioned, situations that are commonly avoided or feared include travelling on buses, trains, boats or planes, using motorways, tunnels or bridges, entering open or enclosed spaces, underground car parks, shopping centres, supermarkets, cinemas, theatres, restaurants or churches, visiting the doctor, dentist or hairdresser, standing in line, being in unfamiliar places, being far from home, and being alone. These are the situations where the person believes it would be dangerous or embarrassing to have a panic attack, where it might be hard to get help, or where escape would be difficult in the event of a panic attack. In agoraphobia, the situations are avoided where possible. However, avoidance is not essential. A person can still have agoraphobia if they experience great distress in the situation or are only able to enter the situation with the presence of a trusted companion.

Very often, if the person is unable to avoid the situation outright, they will use a number of safety behaviours designed to protect themselves against the consequences of a panic attack. For example, carrying a bottle of water or lollies in the belief that this will prevent their throat from closing up during a panic attack, or carrying a mobile phone so they can call for help. While these behaviours seem helpful and reduce distress in the short term, as will be explained in later chapters, these behaviours are actually responsible for maintaining the disorder in the long term.

SOCIAL ANXIETY DISORDER

In Social Anxiety Disorder, or Social Phobia as it is also known, the individual has an intense fear of being judged negatively by others. They frequently worry about saying or doing something that will be embarrassing or humiliating, or that others will think badly of them. Social situations that trigger such anxiety vary from person to person but typically include parties, participating in meetings, public speaking, starting a conversation or keeping it going, dating situations, speaking on the phone, writing in public, eating in public, or even using public toilets, for fear of what others may be thinking about them. Some individuals with social anxiety disorder simply fear one specific situation such as having to give a presentation, while others have a more generalised fear of many or almost all social situations. Some will be fearful of the opinions of people they know, such as work colleagues, while others are concerned about being negatively evaluated by everyone, including strangers. Persons with social anxiety disorder are generally not particularly fearful of panic attacks, but worry most about anxiety symptoms that could be obvious to others.

Underlying Threats

As described, the predominant threat underlying social phobia is a fear of negative evaluation from others. Commonly held thoughts include:

- "They'll think I'm boring."
- "They'll think I'm weird."
- "They'll think I'm pathetic."
- "They'll think I'm stupid."
- "They'll think I'm a loser."
- "I'll have nothing to say."
- "Whatever I say isn't good/interesting/intelligent enough."

When the fear of being perceived negatively induces noticeable anxiety symptoms such as a shaky voice, blushing, sweating, trembling or shaking, anxiety is compounded by the worry that others will notice these symptoms, with thoughts such as, "I'll blush and shake. They'll think there's something wrong with me". Predictably, worrying about such symptoms quickly becomes a self-fulfilling prophecy.

Behavioural Symptoms

People with social anxiety disorder usually manage their anxiety by avoiding the feared situation, such as not attending parties, making excuses to get out of giving presentations at work or dropping subjects at university if they are required to give a class presentation. They tend not to participate in meetings and are frequently quiet in social gatherings. As a result of their avoidance, they find it hard to make friends, are often socially isolated and lonely. The anxiety can also impact on a person's career choice or development, seeing them work in areas well beneath their true capabilities. They may choose jobs that don't involve much contact with other people, or refuse promotions if it involves public speaking or managing other people.

When avoidance of the situation is not an option, the person will use a range of safety behaviours such as not speaking or saying very little, rehearsing what they will say before they say it, avoiding eye-contact or wearing sunglasses. Some will avoid wearing clothing that attracts attention, such as bright colours. Drinking alcohol in social situations such as parties is another common safety behaviour used to help the person relax and feel less inhibited about talking. Unfortunately, because this safety behaviour can be so effective within the situation, they may feel unable to function socially without it. Hence it is not uncommon for people with social phobia subsequently to develop a substance abuse problem in an attempt to manage their social anxiety.

One of the main problems in social anxiety disorder is that the safety behaviours the person uses to minimise negative evaluation can actually bring about the consequences the person fears the most. For example, take a person who worries about being perceived as boring. In an attempt to minimise negative evaluation, they will say very little, not make eye contact and have closed body language (e.g., folded arms, looking at the floor), which in turn then may make them appear boring.

GENERALISED ANXIETY DISORDER

Generalised Anxiety Disorder, or GAD, is characterised by excessive anxiety or worry about a range of issues such as health, family, work/study, finances, social relationships, interpersonal situations, or community/world affairs such as crime, the environment, or terrorism. People with GAD find it very difficult to control their worry, often commenting that they cannot stop thinking about their worries even when they want to. Indeed, this is one of the diagnostic criteria. It is not unusual for people with GAD to have difficulty falling asleep as they find themselves worrying for hours while lying in bed. Although many people worry about something when there is a problem, people with GAD worry even when things are going well. For example, worrying about the health of their children even when they are not sick. People with GAD generally identify themselves as worriers, having been that way often since childhood.

The worry results in numerous physical symptoms including feeling restless, keyed up or on edge, feeling easily tired or irritable, having difficulty concentrating, feeling muscle tension and, as previously mentioned, having sleep problems such as difficulty falling asleep, waking frequently or having a restless, unsatisfying sleep.

Underlying Threats

The worries or underlying threats in GAD are typically catastrophic yet in reality unlikely to occur. People with GAD often mistake possibility for probability, believing that if something is possible, then it is likely to occur. Their worries often take the form of "What if…" thoughts such as "What if my husband has a car accident on the way to work?", "What if my daughter gets kidnapped?" or "What if I get breast cancer?" One worry will frequently trigger a cascade of worries, such as "What if I'm late to work and my boss fires me. How will I pay the rent? We could get evicted and end up homeless. They could take my children away." Or, "What if there's a blackout at the shopping centre? People would start to panic. I could get trampled to death."

Typically, individuals with GAD also worry about too much worry, fearing that the worry and anxiety itself may cause mental or physical harm.

Behavioural Symptoms

To reduce their anxiety and worry, people with GAD frequently seek reassurance from others rather than largely avoiding situations as is common in other anxiety disorders: for example, visiting their GP when worrying about their health, calling or texting loved ones when worrying about their safety, calling friends to apologise in case something they said was misinterpreted and caused offence. The constant reassurance seeking can put a strain on relationships.

They may also use other safety behaviours to reduce their worry, such as checking their work very carefully to prevent errors. This may slow them down such that they then stay back late to ensure they finish all their work for the day. Sometimes avoidance is also used to prevent triggering new worries, such as avoiding watching the news on TV or talking about particular topics such as cancer.

OBSESSIVE-COMPULSIVE DISORDER

Obsessions

In OCD, an *obsession* is defined as a thought, image or impulse that is unwanted, intrusive, repetitive and distressing. For example, intrusive thoughts of being contaminated with AIDS after touching door knobs, repetitive blasphemous images of religious figures, or unwanted "impulses" to stab a friend.

Obsessions are *egodystonic*: that is, they are unacceptable or inconsistent with the person's ego or view of themselves. The obsession represents the worst thing they could think about themselves. Another way of looking at it is that it is the opposite of their ideal self-image. It is not surprising, therefore, to find that the specific focus of a person's OCD is frequently linked to their background, upbringing or core values. Hence, religious or blasphemous obsessions are typically experienced by people with a highly religious upbringing, while someone who has been traumatised through being sexually abused as a child may have obsessions about molesting children. Caring, gentle people may be troubled by so-called impulses to harm loved ones. However, the ego-dystonic nature of the experience means that these are probably not true impulses, but more fears of acting in this manner.

It is important to note that people with OCD *never* act on their obsessions. For some people, the content of their obsessions may have similarities with the thoughts of certain antisocial sub-populations such as paedophiles and psychopaths. However, the emotions experienced in response to the obsession are extreme anxiety, disgust and depression rather than enjoyment, excitement or sexual arousal. Similarly, people with OCD lack any desire or motivation to behave in accordance with their thoughts and often attempt to avoid contact with people they fear they will harm.

Compulsions

A *compulsion*, on the other hand, is a repetitive behaviour or mental act that is designed either to reduce the distress associated with the obsession, or to undo or prevent the feared outcome from occurring. Thus, for the previous examples, the associated compulsions might be hand-washing in response to contamination obsessions, praying to neutralise the distress associated with blasphemous images, and keeping hands in pockets in response to obsessive impulses to stab a friend.

Sometimes the compulsion is logically connected with preventing the feared outcome, such as repeatedly checking the rear view mirror in response to obsessions about running over someone while driving, or hand washing in response to contamination obsessions. However, in other instances, the compulsions are not rationally or scientifically linked with preventing the feared outcome. Instead, the compulsion has a "magical" quality that the person typically recognises as irrational, yet still feels compelled to perform. For example, one patient needed to brush her hair a certain number of times to protect her home from burglars, while another needed to eat peanuts in groups of three to prevent her daughter from being harmed. Very often the person will have a range of compulsions, all aimed at preventing the obsession from coming true.

Compulsions can be very time consuming. Routine activities such as checking a lock, hand-washing or showering frequently takes much longer than necessary and the person often feels "stuck" in the activity. This is frequently due to the presence of *pathological doubt* or questioning whether they performed the behaviour properly. If they think they were distracted or doubt whether they completed the task properly, they will have to start again. Such behaviour often causes them to be late for work or appointments, although some people will deliberately allow extra time for their compulsions.

Obsessive-compulsive Subtypes

It is considered that there are five distinct subtypes of obsessive-compulsive disorder. However, individuals with OCD frequently present with more than one subtype at the same time and the nature or focus of symptoms often changes over time.

Contamination obsessions with washing or cleaning compulsions

Here, the person feels anxiety after touching something they believe is contaminated. They fear the contamination may harm themselves or others, although some people deny fearing a consequence of contamination and say they simply do not like the feeling. In response to these fears, the person engages in hand washing or other cleaning behaviours.

Harm obsessions with checking compulsions

The person may fear being robbed and compulsively checks the locks on the doors and windows. They may fear starting a fire and repeatedly checks to make sure they switched off all the electrical appliances or pulled out the plugs. They may worry about knocking down a pedestrian while driving and have to check their rear-view mirror or drive back to the location to make sure no one was hurt.

"Forbidden" obsessions

This subtype consists of unwanted and distressing aggressive, religious or sexual thoughts, images or impulses. Such obsessions are often embarrassing and patients can be reluctant to disclose such thoughts, due to feelings of guilt or shame. Examples include images of having sex with Jesus, or smashing people's heads against telegraph poles. They often perceive such thoughts to be a manifestation of their true, underlying urges and consequently feel they are inherently a very bad person. They usually try to avoid triggers or use mental rituals such as praying or counting to reduce their distress.

Symmetry obsessions with ordering, arranging or counting compulsions

In this subtype, the person experiences a strong urge to arrange and re-arrange objects until it feels "just right". Items may be arranged by colour, size or some other rule. If the item is moved and the individual is unable to move it back, they experience strong anxiety or discomfort. Sometimes the need for symmetry is accompanied with magical thinking – for example, "If all the mugs are aligned with their handles to the right, mum won't die."

Compulsive hoarding

Here there is a compulsive urge to acquire and a difficulty in discarding items, which are often of limited value, such as newspapers, clothes, receipts, toys, etc. The person believes the item may be needed later and typically has excessive emotional attachment to items. There are often problems with planning, organising and categorising. The home becomes so cluttered that furniture and rooms can no longer be used for their intended purpose. In DSM-5, Hoarding Disorder has been given its own diagnostic category within the section of "Obsessive-Compulsive and Related Disorders".

POSTTRAUMATIC STRESS DISORDER (PTSD)

Posttraumatic Stress Disorder (PTSD) can occur after an individual has experienced, witnessed, or in certain cases heard about a traumatic event. The definition of a traumatic event varies, but usually involves actual or threatened death or serious injury, or threat to a person's physical integrity. Examples include experiencing or witnessing a motor vehicle accident, robbery, assault, rape, combat, natural or man made disasters (e.g., fire, flood, earthquake), or hearing that a loved one has been killed.

Underlying Threats

Threats perceived by people with PTSD typically revolve around recurrence of the traumatic event. For example, "If I walk to my car, I could get assaulted again," or, "If I go to the bank, there could be another hold-up." When in public, they often report feeling that something bad will happen to them again or their attacker is still out to harm them.

However, there are a range of other thoughts maintaining the disorder that need to be targeted in treatment. Some of these are more ruminative in nature, such as "Why did this happen to me?" or "What did I do to deserve this?" Some people with PTSD experience extreme guilt, with thoughts such as, "I should have been the one to die, not him," "I should have done something more to prevent it," or, "If only I had left 5 minutes earlier this never would have happened."

Symptom Clusters

There are three symptom clusters associated with PTSD. The first symptom cluster involves *re-experiencing symptoms*. This includes intrusive thoughts, images or perceptions of the traumatic event, having dreams or nightmares associated with the trauma, or experiencing flashbacks where the person feels as if they are reliving the situation (rather than simply remembering it). The person will commonly experience emotional distress or increased physiological arousal such as increased heart rate, sweating and rapid breathing when exposed to reminders of the event. For example, the sound of an ambulance siren can trigger anxiety and heart palpitations in a person who has had a serious car accident.

The second symptom cluster involves *avoidance symptoms*. Here the person tries to avoid thoughts, conversations, places and people associated with the trauma. For example, a patient involved in an armed bank robbery avoids the entire suburb where the robbery occurred, as well as all banks. After a trauma, the person may experience decreased interest or participation in activities such as socialising with friends and family. They often report a sense of detachment from others, a feeling of emotional numbing and the inability to have pleasant or loving feelings. Some people with PTSD develop a sense that their future will be cut short, feeling that life is fleeting and could end at any moment, so that they do not expect to grow old, have a career or see their children grow up.

The third symptom cluster involves *hyperarousal symptoms* including hypervigilance or scanning the environment for related threats. For example, after experiencing an assault, a person will often choose a seat where their back is against the wall and they have a clear view of the entrance so they can see who is coming in at all times. Or, while walking down the street, the person repeatedly checks to see who is behind them. Related to this is the use of other safety behaviours such as carrying a weapon – for example a knife in their sock, or a makeshift weapon such as keys while walking in public – so they can protect themselves in case of a future attack.

There is often an exaggerated startle response, such as becoming jumpy at hearing loud noises like a door slamming, the phone ringing, a car backfiring or people talking loudly. Other symptoms in this category include insomnia, impaired concentration and increased irritability and anger outbursts. The person may turn to alcohol or other drugs to manage these symptoms and develop a secondary substance abuse problem.

The anger outbursts and emotional detachment or numbing seen in people with PTSD can cause profound relationship problems. Physical affection and sexual intimacy are often no longer desired or enjoyed. Romantic partners and other family members often feel hurt and rejected. Patients often report having a shorter fuse, noting they're shouting at their children or other people more frequently. Because of these problems, some people with PTSD prefer to be alone.

SPECIFIC PHOBIA

Specific Phobia, or what was previously referred to as Simple Phobia, as the name suggests, involves persistent and intense fear triggered by a specific object or situation. When a person is exposed to the object or situation (or even anticipates being exposed to it), they experience extreme anxiety or panic attacks. When away from their feared situation, they know their fears are irrational or excessive. Despite this, they will go out of their way to avoid the situation, or else endure it with extreme distress. It is commonly believed that a person's specific phobia was caused by a traumatic experience with the feared object; however, this is not always the case. In fact, humans have a predisposition to many of the common specific phobias, as they represent potential real threats in the environment – for example, snakes, spiders, storms and heights. While everyone has things they fear or hate, such as spiders or cockroaches, it only becomes a specific phobia when the fear interferes with a person's social, occupational or role functioning.

Specific Phobia Subtypes

There are different types of specific phobias. The most common subtype involves *animal phobias*, such as dogs, spiders, snakes, cockroaches and other insects. Safety behaviours may involve requiring others to check rooms, shoes, clothing or beds for the feared object. Some people will board up windows or cover drains to prevent such creatures from entering their home. Others will carry insect spray in their handbag at all times, as well as having numerous additional cans around the house. Thoughts include, "I could get bitten and contract a disease", although some people fear the sensations associated with being touched by the animal or that it will get inside their clothes.

Situational phobias, such as fear of flying, driving, fear of lifts, tunnels or other enclosed spaces, are also common. Usually the person arranges their life to avoid the situation. For example, a person with a fear of flying will avoid travelling overseas for work or holidays, and will drive interstate instead of flying. People with a lift phobia always take the stairs and avoid attending appointments in the upper levels of multi-story buildings. Even in the stairwells, they use safety behaviours such as wedging their shoe in the doorway while checking the door will open at the next level. If forced to use a lift, they will often enlist the support of a friend to accompany them, or make sure they have their mobile phone for help. In situational phobias, the person often fears they will die in the situation, such as, "The plane will crash," "The lift will get stuck and I'll run out of oxygen," or, "I'll crash the car."

Other phobias involve the *natural environment*, such as fear of storms, heights or water. A special type of phobia is the *blood-injection-injury phobia* where there is often a fear of medical procedures such as having injections or blood drawn, or simply a fear of seeing their own or another person's blood. This category of phobia is different from other specific phobias, and indeed the other anxiety disorders, in that the person will often faint when exposed to the stimulus, such as fainting at the sight of blood or a needle. People with this type of phobia can put their health at risk by avoiding medical procedures or delaying contact with health professionals. Thoughts experienced by people with this type of phobia are often around pain associated with the procedure – for example, "It will hurt" – or fear of their anxiety reaction, such as, "I'll look like a baby," or, "I'll faint."

SEPARATION ANXIETY DISORDER

Formerly only considered as a disorder of childhood, Separation Anxiety Disorder was added to the general list of anxiety disorders in DSM-5. Acknowledging that this disorder may also be encountered in adults, DSM-5 quotes a reported prevalence of 1–2 %. The essential feature is excessive fear or anxiety around separation from home or attachment figures, out of proportion to the individual's developmental stage. The person is excessively fearful about events that may result in separation, such as death of the loved one, accidental harm to the individual or the attachment figure, or violent events such as kidnapping. There is often a reluctance to be away from home or the attachment figure overnight. The main differentiation from agoraphobia is that the fear does not relate to being trapped or unable to escape, but purely to separation.

DIFFERENTIATING ANXIETY DISORDERS

This chapter has described the anxiety disorders in detail. In practice, it can sometimes be challenging to differentiate the disorders. There are key features to note that can assist in differentiating. These are:

- the form of the anxiety
- the core fears or perceived threats
- the associated behaviours.

In terms of form, anxiety can be comprised of intrusive thoughts or images, compulsions, worry or panic. Anxiety disorders also vary in terms of the underlying fears or perceived threats. People with social phobia worry about receiving negative evaluation; people with OCD fear causing harm to themselves or others; GAD usually presents with fears of bad or catastrophic outcomes; people with panic disorders often fear the presence of an underlying physical disorder, death, losing control or going crazy.

Table 3.1   Core features of the Anxiety Disorders

Anxiety Disorder	Features
Panic Disorder	Recurrent panic attacks Fear of physical, mental or social harm
Panic Disorder with Agoraphobia	Recurrent panic attacks Fear of physical, mental or social harm Avoidance of situations believed to trigger panic
Social Anxiety Disorder	Fear of negative evaluation Anxiety or panic in social situations
OCD	Intrusive thoughts/images of harm Attempts to neutralise
GAD	Excessive anticipation of harm Worry as effort to control
PTSD	Intrusive images of trauma Efforts to avoid stimuli that provoke memories of the event
Specific Phobia	Fear and avoidance of specific object or situation
Separation Anxiety Disorder	Fear of being away from home or separated from attachment figure

As for the associated behaviours, people who have agoraphobia often avoid situations where escape would be difficult (e.g., trains, crowds), while those with OCD usually have compulsions (e.g., repeated checking, hand washing). The core features of the various anxiety disorders can be summarised succinctly in Table 3.1. This very brief summary does not capture the details of each disorder (refer to the text above), but may be useful as a guide.

CHAPTER 4   CLASSIFICATION OF ANXIETY DISORDERS AND CONCEPTUAL AND DIAGNOSTIC ISSUES

Vladan Starcevic

ANXIETY DISORDERS AS A DIAGNOSTIC GROUP

Anxiety disorders were first recognised as a separate diagnostic group in 1980, with the publication of the American Psychiatric Association's *Diagnostic and Statistical Manual of Mental Disorders*, Third Edition, also known as DSM-III. Prior to 1980, anxiety disorders were classified as neurotic disorders or neuroses, along with several other conditions that were subsequently conceptualised as somatoform and other disorders (e.g., conversion disorder and hypochondriasis). The concept of neurosis was abandoned as a result of the decline of psychoanalysis, the rise of biological psychiatry and increasing need to delineate diagnoses with more precise and reliable criteria, so that clinicians would be more likely to agree when diagnosing mental disorders.

The creation of the separate group of anxiety disorders arose from the need to classify together non-psychotic, non-organic and non-substance misuse-related conditions that are characterised by pathological anxiety. This does not mean that people with anxiety disorders do not have other prominent emotions such as disgust, shame, irritability and even anger and guilt. In fact, the key emotion in most individuals with insect phobia or blood-injection-injury phobia may be disgust rather than fear. Although other emotional states sometimes colour the clinical presentation of people with anxiety disorders, their predominant emotional characteristic is deemed to be pathological anxiety.

The boundaries between anxiety disorders and normality on one hand, and between anxiety disorders and other forms of psychopathology on the other, have not been clearly established. This is related to the issue of the somewhat arbitrary criteria for membership in this group. It is not surprising, therefore, that a number of conditions that "belonged" to the realm of anxiety disorders from DSM-III to DSM-IV are no longer classified as anxiety disorders in DSM-5. This pertains to obsessive-compulsive disorder, acute stress disorder and posttraumatic stress disorder.

ANXIETY DISORDERS IN DSM-5

According to DSM-5, the following conditions are classified as anxiety disorders:

- Separation Anxiety Disorder
- Selective Mutism
- Specific Phobia
- Social Anxiety Disorder (Social Phobia)
- Panic Disorder
- Agoraphobia
- Generalized Anxiety Disorder
- Substance/Medication-induced Anxiety Disorder
- Anxiety Disorder due to Another Medical Condition
- Other Specified Anxiety Disorder
- Unspecified Anxiety Disorder.

Anxiety disorders induced by a substance or a medication or due to another medical condition differ from all other anxiety disorders in terms of their explicit, albeit presumed aetiology. "Other specified anxiety disorder" refers to culture-specific conditions or various diagnostically subthreshold presentations of anxiety disorders (e.g., generalised anxiety disorder that does not occur "more days than not"). "Unspecified anxiety disorder" is a residual diagnostic category, for use in those situations when a diagnosis of the specific anxiety disorder cannot be made.

A number of changes from DSM-IV have been made to this group. Most importantly and as already noted, obsessive-compulsive disorder, acute stress disorder and posttraumatic stress disorder are not considered anxiety disorders in the DSM-5 system and are classified elsewhere. This will be discussed in the text below.

Separation anxiety disorder and selective mutism are new members of the group. They are classified as anxiety disorders because the DSM-IV group of disorders "usually first diagnosed in infancy, childhood or adolescence" no longer exists in DSM-5. In DSM-IV, these conditions were classified there, as their onset is in childhood. However, DSM-5 allows separation anxiety disorder to be diagnosed even if its first manifestations occur after the age of 18.

Another important change in DSM-5 is the separation of agoraphobia from panic disorder. In DSM-IV, agoraphobia was almost always regarded as part of panic disorder. It was defined through panic attacks or symptoms of panic attacks, as the fear of situations in which it would be embarrassing or difficult to escape, or in which help might not be available in case of a panic attack. Thus, when both panic attacks and agoraphobic avoidance were present, agoraphobia was seen as a consequence of panic attacks and the primary and main diagnosis was panic disorder, as embedded in the DSM-IV diagnostic terms "panic disorder with agoraphobia" and "panic disorder without agoraphobia". Although there was a separate category of "agoraphobia without history of panic disorder" in DSM-IV, it was apparently rarely used and considered as a residual diagnosis. The separation of agoraphobia from panic disorder in DSM-5 takes into account findings that the two disorders are conceptually distinct and that there are multiple pathways to agoraphobia – not only via panic disorder and panic attacks. This is also more in line with the way the two disorders are conceptualised in the *International Classification of Diseases,* Tenth Revision (ICD-10), findings of epidemiological studies, and the way other phobic disorders are described.

Obsessive-compulsive and Related Disorders

The following disorders have been classified in this DSM-5 nosological group:

- Obsessive-compulsive disorder
- Body dysmorphic disorder
- Hoarding disorder
- Trichotillomania (hair-pulling disorder)
- Excoriation (skin-picking) disorder
- Substance/medication-induced obsessive-compulsive and related disorder
- Obsessive-compulsive and related disorder due to another medical condition
- Other specified obsessive-compulsive and related disorders
- Unspecified obsessive-compulsive and related disorder.

The group of obsessive-compulsive and related disorders was created because of certain differences between obsessive-compulsive disorder and other anxiety disorders (Table 4.1) and some similarities between obsessive-compulsive disorder and members of this group. Also, the creation of this group was justified on the grounds of its treatment implications: that is, that similar or identical treatment modalities are used for conditions classified here. These include serotonin reuptake inhibitors and psychological therapy techniques of exposure and response prevention and habit reversal.

Table 4.1 Differences between obsessive-compulsive disorder (OCD) and other anxiety disorders

	Obsessive-compulsive disorder	Other anxiety disorders
Female-to-male ratio	No convincing predominance of women	More common in women
Response to biological challenges	No symptom worsening in response to challenges with CO_2, yohimbine, caffeine or cholecystokinin	Frequent symptom worsening in response to challenges with CO_2, yohimbine, caffeine or cholecystokinin
CNS morphometry	Increased bilateral grey matter volume in the basal ganglia (lenticular/caudate nuclei)	Decreased grey matter volume in the basal ganglia (left lenticular nucleus)
Neurocircuitry	Frontostriatal hyperactivity and hyper-responsivity, attenuated amygdala response to disorder-independent threat stimuli	Exaggerated amygdala response to disorder-specific stimuli, insular hyperactivation
Response to pharmacotherapy	Selective response to serotonin reuptake inhibitors	Response to a variety of pharmacological agents, with different mechanisms of action

Some members of the group of obsessive-compulsive and related disorders are new diagnoses (hoarding disorder and excoriation or skin-picking disorder). Others have been moved from various nosological groups in DSM-IV. Thus, body dysmorphic disorder "came" from somatoform disorders, whereas trichotillomania (hair-pulling disorder) was previously classified as an impulse-control disorder.

Trauma- and Stressor-related Disorders

The conditions listed in this DSM-5 diagnostic group include:

- Reactive Attachment Disorder
- Disinhibited Social Engagement Disorder
- Posttraumatic Stress Disorder
- Acute Stress Disorder
- Adjustment Disorders
- Other Specified Trauma- and Stressor-related Disorder
- Unspecified Trauma- and Stressor-related Disorder.

There are several reasons for the creation of the group of trauma- and stressor-related disorders. First, "key members" of this group – posttraumatic stress disorder and acute stress disorder – are often characterised by a variety of emotions instead of, or in addition to, anxiety or fear; these include anger, irritability, shame, guilt or depression. Therefore, it seemed inadequate to classify these disorders as anxiety disorders. The second reason pertains to the complex relationships between posttraumatic stress disorder and mood and personality disorders, which suggested that its link with other anxiety disorders was not unique. Finally, the architects of DSM-5 believed that all psychopathology caused or assumed to be caused by trauma and stress should be brought together in the same diagnostic group.

Besides posttraumatic stress disorder and acute stress disorder, this group includes adjustment disorders, reactive attachment disorder and disinhibited social engagement disorder, as specific diagnostic entities. Adjustment disorders constituted their own group in DSM-IV. Reactive attachment disorder was classified in DSM-IV among disorders "usually first diagnosed in infancy, childhood or adolescence". Disinhibited social engagement disorder was a type of reactive attachment disorder in DSM-IV; hence it is a new diagnostic category in DSM-5. With the elimination from DSM-5 of the group of conditions "usually first diagnosed in infancy, childhood or adolescence", reactive attachment disorder was moved to the group of trauma- and stressor-related disorders because it is conceptualised as a consequence of an inadequate care in childhood.

ANXIETY DISORDERS IN ICD-10

In the ICD-10, anxiety disorders have not been granted a separate, independent status. Instead, they are a part of a large group of disorders labelled "neurotic, stress-related, and somatoform disorders". Within such a group, anxiety disorders, obsessive-compulsive disorder and conditions related to stress and trauma are placed into four subgroups.

The first subgroup is called "phobic anxiety disorders" and comprises agoraphobia with and without panic disorder, social phobias and specific (isolated) phobias. The second subgroup is labelled "other anxiety disorders" and consists of panic disorder (episodic paroxysmal anxiety), generalised anxiety disorder and mixed anxiety and depressive disorder. Obsessive-compulsive disorder is the only condition in the third subgroup. The fourth subgroup, called "reaction to severe stress and adjustment disorders", resembles the DSM-5 grouping of trauma- and stress-related disorders and includes acute stress reaction, posttraumatic stress disorder and adjustment disorders.

The work on the Eleventh Revision of the *International Classification of Diseases* (ICD-11) is well underway. While it is not yet known how anxiety and related disorders will be classified in the ICD-11, it is likely that ICD-11 will be influenced by at least some of the changes introduced by DSM-5. But, it is possible that some of the features specific for ICD-10 will also remain in ICD-11.

DSM-5 VERSUS ICD-10

The DSM-5 and ICD-10 systems differ in some important ways in terms of how they conceptualise anxiety disorders. The ICD-10 espouses a broader conceptualisation of the disorders, whereby anxiety disorders are a part of a larger nosological entity. Moreover, ICD-10 has included, with anxiety and related disorders, conditions that are not present in the DSM system – for example, mixed anxiety and depressive disorder.

At the level of individual anxiety disorders, the most striking difference is in the way the two systems describe generalised anxiety disorder. In DSM-5, generalised anxiety disorder cannot be diagnosed without the presence of pathological worry, whereas pathological worry is not necessary to make the ICD-10 diagnosis of generalised anxiety disorder. On the other hand, symptoms of autonomic hyperactivity are necessary for the ICD-10 diagnosis of generalised anxiety disorder, but they are not necessary to diagnose generalised anxiety disorder according to DSM-5. Thus, generalised anxiety disorder is basically viewed as a worry disorder in DSM-5 and as an autonomic arousal disorder in ICD-10. Also, generalised anxiety disorder is an independent diagnostic category in DSM-5, whereas ICD-10 regards it as a residual disorder that cannot be diagnosed if the criteria for diagnosing other anxiety disorders, depression or hypochondriasis have been met. As a result, although the DSM and ICD definitions of generalised anxiety disorder overlap, they are not identical conditions.

As already noted, changes have been made to DSM-5 which bring its conceptualization of agoraphobia closer to the ICD-10 description of this disorder. The difference remains in terms of how panic attacks are portrayed. While DSM-5 continues to regard panic attack as a qualitatively different type of anxiety, ICD-10 suggests that there is a continuum of severity, from normal fear through phobic fear to panic attacks. In other words, panic attacks are not seen as qualitatively different from other types of anxiety, but only denote a greater severity of anxiety. Therefore, the presence of panic attacks in agoraphobic situations is viewed as an indicator of the severity of phobic anxiety. The main diagnosis in such situations is agoraphobia and hence the ICD-10 diagnostic categories of "agoraphobia with panic disorder" and "agoraphobia without panic disorder".

A CRITICAL LOOK AT THE CLASSIFICATION OF ANXIETY DISORDERS

The two major psychiatric classification systems are only partly compatible, which hampers communication between clinicians and researchers around the world. It would be optimal to use one system that would be adhered to in all countries.

The classification of anxiety disorders seems to suffer from problems similar to those that characterise the classification of other psychiatric disorders. For example, the diagnosis of most anxiety disorders requires exclusion of medical conditions, substance use disorders and, in many cases, other psychiatric disorders, as the cause of, or a better explanation for, pathological anxiety. This exclusion-based status raises questions about the validity of anxiety disorders as a diagnostic group and also represents a challenge to clinical practice.

Still, the key issue is a lack of clear criteria as to how similar two disorders need to be in order to be classified together and likewise, how much they need to be different *not* to be grouped together. If the main criterion for membership in the group of anxiety disorders were the presence of pathological anxiety, this would not be adequate because such a group would be too broad and too heterogeneous. But what is needed in addition to pathological anxiety to classify a psychopathological entity as an anxiety disorder? Also, when patients present with a combination of emotional features, how should their condition be classified? The primacy given to pathological anxiety over some other emotional states (e.g., disgust) for the purpose of conceptualisation and classification does not seem justified.

While conditions that belong to the group of anxiety disorders have many features in common, they also differ in many respects. As already noted, the latter has been the main reason for the changes introduced by DSM-5. It is a matter of controversy, however, whether the nosological groups created by DSM-5 represent a step in the right direction and whether, for example, obsessive-compulsive disorder is more closely related to trichotillomania than to anxiety disorders such as generalised anxiety disorder. A related question is whether forms of obsessive-compulsive disorder with delusional beliefs should be classified separately from psychotic disorders, as is the case in DSM-5.

With regards to similarities, they are numerous among the anxiety disorders. To some extent, this explains their frequent co-occurrence. Many anxiety disorders share a similar genetic risk and are associated with similar neurobiological abnormalities. Except for blood-injection-injury phobia, anxiety disorders are more likely to affect females than males. Most anxiety disorders start in childhood, adolescence or early adulthood. Much less commonly, they manifest themselves for the first time later in life. A notable exception is generalised anxiety disorder, which can commence at any age. Most anxiety disorders have a chronic course and respond to similar psychological and pharmacological treatments.

From the phenomenological point of view, anxiety disorders differ in terms of the object of their anxiety. While this object is quite clear in the case of phobic disorders, it is less clear when it comes to generalised anxiety disorder. Also, the nature of the threat associated with pathological anxiety differs from one disorder to another: while the threat in obsessive-compulsive disorder may be experienced as irrational and alien thoughts, the threat in posttraumatic stress disorder comes from painful memories of the trauma and in panic disorder, it is perceived to result from certain bodily sensations and symptoms. Behaviours in some disorders are a prominent aspect of their clinical presentations – for example, avoidance in phobic disorders and compulsions in obsessive-compulsive disorder. In generalised anxiety disorder, however, anxiety-driven behaviours are subtler. As a result of some differences in their underlying psychopathology and neurobiology, treatment approaches to various anxiety disorders also differ to a certain extent.

When it comes to generalised anxiety disorder, it has been suggested that this condition may be more appropriately classified along with depression because it has an important relationship with depression. Thus, many of the symptoms of generalised anxiety disorder overlap with those of depression, e.g., sleep disturbance, tiredness, poor concentration and restlessness. Of all the anxiety disorders, generalised anxiety disorder is the strongest predictor of subsequent depression. Twin studies suggest that generalised anxiety disorder and major depressive disorder may be genetically indistinguishable.

On the other hand, some symptoms, such as heightened autonomic arousal, are more specific for anxiety (and generalised anxiety disorder) than for depression. Generalised anxiety disorder and major depressive disorder have also been associated with different neuroanatomical, neurotransmitter, neuroendocrinological, and polysomnographic findings. Furthermore, they have relatively few childhood risk factors in common. Therefore, there is a growing agreement that although they are closely related, generalised anxiety disorder and major depressive disorder are not the same. At the level of our current understanding and knowledge, this justifies their separate classification.

CATEGORIES AND DIMENSIONS IN ANXIETY DISORDERS

There is an ongoing debate among mental health professionals and researchers as to whether psychiatric disorders should be conceptualised categorically or dimensionally. This has also been an issue when considering changes to the conceptualisation of anxiety disorders. The two approaches and their advantages and disadvantages are presented in Table 4.2.

Table 4.2   Categorical diagnosis versus dimensional conceptualisation of disorders

Categorical diagnosis	Dimensional conceptualisation
Only 2 values: 1 (meeting criteria for a disorder) and 0 (not meeting criteria for a disorder)	3 or more ordered values on a scale (continuum from the minimum to the maximum value)
"Crude", dichotomous approach to assessment	More precise, numerical approach to assessment
Reliant on (categorical) diagnostic criteria	Reliant on assessment instruments
"User-friendly" in clinical practice	Less suitable for clinical practice

Categorical conceptualisation recognises only two options – the disorder is either present, if the diagnostic criteria have been met, or it is absent, if these criteria have not been met. It is a somewhat "crude", rigidly dichotomous approach to assessment, but it has been popular in clinical practice because it is generally easy to use. After all, categorical conceptualisation is congruent with our general tendency to classify and label phenomena and objects.

Dimensional conceptualisation, on the other hand, takes into account all shades of grey between the extremes of black and white. It posits a number of ordered values on a scale – at least three such values, and usually more – between the minimum and the maximum value. This approach aims to provide a precise, numerical measure, and therefore relies on assessment instruments. Despite its greater precision, dimensional conceptualisation is often perceived as cumbersome for clinical practice. For example, stating that a patient scored fifteen on a measure of anxiety and ten on a measure of depression does not answer the practical question that most clinicians pose: does the patient suffer primarily from an anxiety or depressive disorder?

Instead of portraying categorical and dimensional approaches to assessment and diagnosis as incompatible, it would be more useful to attempt to combine them because both have advantages and disadvantages. Indeed, this has been done in DSM-5, with its alternative conceptualisation of personality disorders. This "hybrid model" might also be useful for anxiety disorders, especially since many features of anxiety disorders are more adequately approached from a dimensional perspective that takes into account a spectrum of manifestations from normality to the most severe forms of anxiety.

Furthermore, categorical and dimensional approaches are mutually convertible and can be combined in a clinically meaningful manner. For example, in a person with a categorical diagnosis of obsessive-compulsive disorder, administration of an instrument such as the Yale-Brown Obsessive Compulsive Scale can help establish the degree of severity of obsessive-compulsive disorder. In turn, this may assist in making treatment decisions. Therefore, the cut-off points in an assessment instrument effectively convert dimensional assessment to a categorical one. Conversely, categorical diagnosis itself incorporates dimensional elements, because it is often based on factors such as the number, duration and severity of symptoms, degree of impairment, and so on. Thus, two persons with the same categorical diagnosis often differ in terms of how the threshold for that diagnosis was reached: a categorical diagnosis that is far above the threshold is substantially, that is, dimensionally different from a categorical diagnosis that is just above that threshold.

The task for the future is to find a way of combining the categorical and dimensional approaches to diagnosis and assessment in a way that would be both practical and scientifically valid.

"LUMPING" AND "SPLITTING" TRENDS IN THE CLASSIFICATION OF ANXIETY DISORDERS

Every classificatory activity reflects the balance between nosologists who advocate the creation of smaller categories – often referred to as "splitters" – and those who are more in favour of broader categories, who are often called "lumpers". The "splitters" and the "lumpers" have fundamentally different approaches to psychiatric diagnosis and classification.

First, "splitters" emphasise the heterogeneity *within* the diagnostic categories and argue that this heterogeneity drives the "splitting" process. "Lumpers", on the other hand, point to the similarities *between* the diagnostic categories, and suggest that these similarities justify the creation of broader entities. Secondly, "splitters" tend to create a large number of small diagnostic entities that differ very little from each other, so their presumed distinctness and validity are questionable. "Lumpers" end up with broad diagnostic categories and overarching concepts. For example, the concept of "general neurotic syndrome" embodies the cross-sectional and temporal links between anxiety disorders, depression, somatoform disorders and some personality disorders, and emphasises that these putatively separate conditions often have a common genetic predisposition and/or common personality traits, such as neuroticism. In this model, the varying cross-sectional symptomatic expression is secondary to the shared underlying features. Finally, "splitting" and "lumping" tendencies have different treatment implications. "Splitters" aim to come up with diagnostic entities that would be responsive to distinct, specific treatments, whereas the categories created by "lumpers" would be amenable to pharmacological and psychological interventions that are effective across various domains of psychopathology and are often referred to as transdiagnostic treatments. Examples of the latter include certain techniques of cognitive-behavioural therapy (e.g., exposure) and selective serotonin reuptake inhibitors.

In recent times, psychiatric classifications have been dominated by "splitters". As a result, the number of psychiatric diagnoses has been increasing with each iteration of the DSM. The trend of splitting the anxiety disorders into smaller diagnostic entities has also been evident. In the era prior to DSM-III, there were four "types" of anxiety disorders:

- anxiety neurosis
- phobic neurosis
- obsessive-compulsive neurosis
- traumatic (or compensation) neurosis.

In DSM-III, anxiety neurosis was divided into panic disorder and generalised anxiety disorder, whereas phobic neurosis was split into agoraphobia, social phobia and simple (specific) phobia. Subsequently, two subtypes of social phobia were recognised (non-generalised and generalised), and several subtypes of specific phobia were conceptualised (animal phobia, blood-injection-injury phobia, situational phobias, etc.). Thus, the proliferation of diagnostic entities has continued through a creation of diagnostic subtypes. As already noted, DSM-5 has also introduced a number of new diagnoses.

The upshot of the dominance of the "splitting" trend is the rarity of "pure" cases of most anxiety disorders in clinical practice and the high likelihood for various anxiety disorders and their subtypes to co-occur. However, high rates of co-occurrence among the anxiety disorders usually represent a consequence of the "splitting" and the subsequent, substantial overlap between the putatively separate disorders, rather than reflecting a genuine co-occurrence of independent disorders.

There have been calls to halt the proliferation of diagnostic categories and to look for what the individual anxiety disorders share, instead of emphasising the ways in which they differ. However, these calls have yet to be taken seriously by the architects of the major classification systems. Neither extreme "splitting" nor extreme "lumping" will advance our understanding of the anxiety disorders and their links with other domains of psychopathology. Therefore, future efforts to classify mental disorders, including anxiety disorders, need to strike the right balance between these trends.

CHAPTER 5   HOW COMMON ARE THE ANXIETY DISORDERS

Lisa Lampe

PREVALENCE AND INCIDENCE

The *prevalence* of an anxiety disorder is an estimate of the percentage of the total population that might have a given disorder at a specified time (e.g. point prevalence is an estimate at the time of the study; one month prevalence is an estimate over the month prior to the study; and lifetime prevalence is over an individual's lifetime). The prevalence of anxiety disorders is most commonly reported as the 12-month or lifetime prevalence.

Prevalence estimates vary because different diagnostic instruments are used to identify whether a person in the study meets the DSM or ICD criteria for the disorder. Usually a large number of people will be interviewed. For example, 5,000 to 10,000 people will be chosen to be representative of the whole population.

Incidence is an estimate of the number of new cases of a disorder that appear in a given time frame. Incidence rates are not commonly reported or measured in the anxiety disorders, probably because it is known that most anxiety disorders start in the second or third decade of life and tend to be chronic.

> The prevalence of an anxiety disorder is an estimate of the percentage of the total population that might have a given disorder at a specified time.
>
> Incidence is an estimate of the number of new cases of a disorder that appear in a given time frame.

ANXIETY: AUSTRALIA'S MOST COMMON MENTAL DISORDER

Although depression is frequently written and spoken about a lot in the public sphere, anxiety disorders are actually more common in the community. The distress and impairment associated with anxiety is under-recognised.

Table 5.1 shows the 12-month prevalence of DSM-IV anxiety disorders in Australia obtained from the two National Mental Health and Wellbeing epidemiological surveys, the first in 1997 and the most recent in 2007. The term "any affective disorder" refers to depression, dysthymia and bipolar disorder. The first survey had 10,640 respondents with a response rate of about 85%; the second survey had 8,841 respondents with a response rate of 60%. These surveys were conducted by trained lay interviewers. This was a household survey in which a random sample of people were approached to participate in the interview process, and were interviewed in their homes with a structured diagnostic instrument assessing a range of psychiatric disorders. They were also asked about their level of impairment and use of health care services.

The importance of this being a household survey is that it gives an idea of how many people are actually experiencing these disorders even though they may not be receiving treatment. Studies that are carried out in clinics and hospitals do not give an accurate estimate of the prevalence of a disorder in the community.

Table 5.1   Twelve-month prevalence of DSM-IV disorders in Australia

Mental disorders	Percentage of sample	
	1997	2007
Any anxiety disorder	9.7	14.4
Substance use disorder	7.7	5.1
Any affective disorder	5.8	6.2
Neurasthenia	1.5	N/A
Psychosis	0.4	N/A
Personality disorder	6.5	N/A
Any disorder	20.3	20.0

Note. Data adapted from Andrews et al. (2001) and Australian Bureau of Statistics (2008).

HOW COMMON IS EACH ANXIETY DISORDER

Table 5.2 displays data from the second National Survey of Mental Health and Wellbeing (NSMHWB), conducted in Australia in 2007. A

World Health Organization (WHO) developed diagnostic interview used criteria from DSM-IV and ICD-10 to determine whether participants had met the criteria for each disorder at some time over the past twelve months. The results can be taken as an estimate for the whole adult Australian population.

Table 5.2 Twelve-month prevalence of anxiety disorders by anxiety disorder type and sex

Anxiety disorder	Percentage of sample		
	Males	Females	Persons
Panic disorder	2.3	2.9	2.6
Agoraphobia	2.1	3.5	2.8
Social phobia	3.8	5.7	4.7
Generalised anxiety disorder	2.0	3.5	2.7
Posttraumatic stress disorder	4.6	8.3	6.4
Obsessive-compulsive disorder	1.6	2.2	1.9
Any anxiety disorder	10.8	17.9	14.4

Note. From Slade et al. (2009). Reproduced under Creative Commons licence.

The ratio between men and women across the different disorders should be noted here; as the table shows, there is a female excess for all the anxiety disorders. However, the female excess is lower for panic disorder and OCD. A female excess in anxiety has been replicated in studies around the world. However, most studies have found that the sex ratio for OCD and social phobia is close to parity, and most have also found a slightly higher female excess for panic disorder (typically about 1.5:1 for panic disorder and about 3:1 for panic disorder with agoraphobia).

AGE AT ONSET

Table 5.3 presents data from the second NSMHWB, from which it can be seen that anxiety disorders typically have their onset relatively early in life, especially social phobia. They also typically start earlier than mood disorders. Because a person can have a traumatic experience at any time of their life, PTSD can develop at any age. The interquartile range for anxiety suggests that developing an anxiety disorder apart from PTSD after the age of about 40 years is uncommon, and so when a person presents with anxiety for the first time after this age, alternative causes of anxiety (such as mood or substance use disorders, or physical illness or its treatment) should be sought and excluded.

Table 5.3   Typical age at onset of anxiety disorders

Disorder	Median age at onset	Interquartile range	Projected lifetime risk
Panic disorder	30	18-42	5.0%
Agoraphobia	22	13-38	2.9%
Social phobia	13	8-19	9.2%
Generalised anxiety disorder	33	20-46	9.1%
Posttraumatic stress disorder	26	15-42	9.7%
Obsessive-compulsive disorder	19	13-35	4.6%
Any anxiety disorder	19	12-39	25.0%
Any affective disorder	34	21-51	23.1%
Any substance use disorder	20	18-26	28.1%

Note. From McEvoy et al. (2011). Reproduced with permission of SAGE Publications.

PREVALENCE BY AGE AND SEX

The prevalence of anxiety declines gradually with age, as is depicted in Figure 5.1. There is a fairly constant prevalence of anxiety amongst women at all ages until late midlife. Men show a peak in the middle years of age.

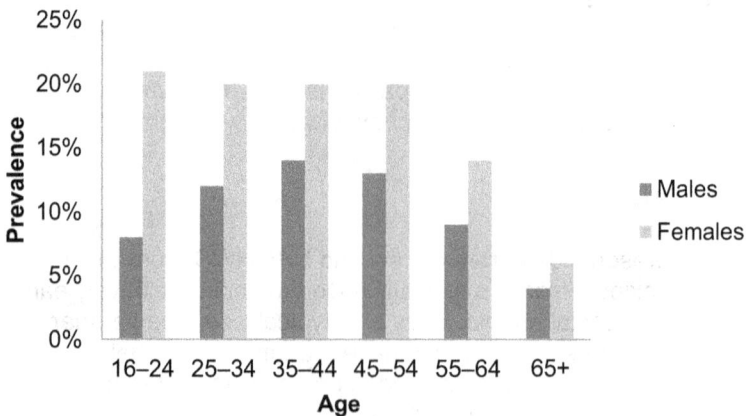

Figure 5.1   Twelve-month prevalence of anxiety disorders by age and sex. From Slade et al. (2009). Reproduced under Creative Commons licence.

Figure 5.2 displays lifetime prevalence results from another large epidemiological study, the National Comorbidity Replication Survey in the United States. The overall pattern of prevalence is similar to Australian 12-month figures, with all anxiety disorders decreasing in prevalence with age. The midlife peak is again seen in this US data.

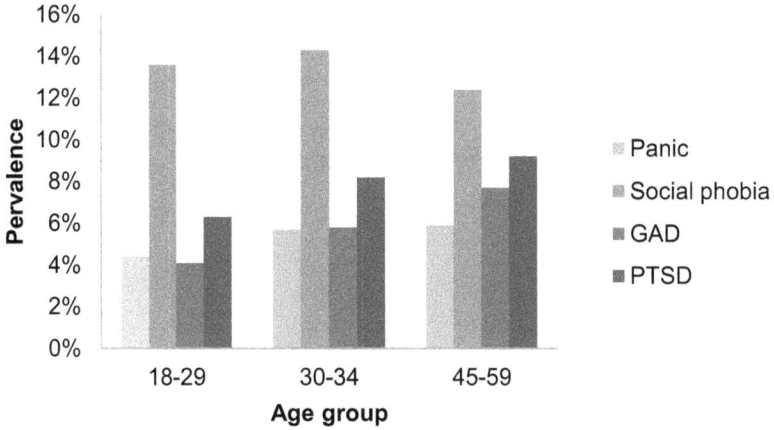

Figure 5.2 Lifetime prevalence of anxiety disorders. Data adapted from Kessler et al. (2005).

PREVALENCE BY SEX AND DEMOGRAPHIC FACTORS

In the NSMHWB, as shown in Table 5.4, the prevalence of anxiety disorders was highest in people who were widowed, separated or divorced (19%), and lowest in those who were married or in de facto relationships (13.3%).

Employment did not appear to be linked to anxiety disorders for men, but women who were employed had lower rates of anxiety disorders than those who were not in the work force. The prevalence of anxiety disorders was associated with level of education, being highest in those who did not complete school and lowest among people with post-school qualifications. However it should be remembered that these are associations, and do not tell us anything about the direction of causation. For example, it could well be that developing an anxiety disorder might prevent a person from completing high school.

There was no association between country of birth and anxiety disorders. However, there was a trend for people from non-English speaking countries to have a lower prevalence of anxiety disorder (9.9%) compared with those born in Australia (15.4%) or other English-speaking countries (14.0%).

Table 5.4 Twelve-month prevalence of anxiety disorders by sex, marital status, labour force status, education and country of birth

	Percentage of sample		
	Males	Females	Persons
Marital status			
• Married/De facto	10.1	16.1	13.3
• Separated/Divorced/Widowed	16.3	20.3	19.0
• Never married	13.4	19.4	16.2
Labour force status			
• Employed	10.7	15.5	13.0
• Unemployed	10.9	22.7	17.3
• Not in the labour force	10.6	23.1	20.9
Education			
• Post-school qualification	10.0	16.5	13.3
• School qualification only	10.8	21.3	15.7
• Did not complete school	14.9	22.5	18.9
Country of birth			
• Australia	11.5	19.2	15.4
• English speaking country	12.7	15.7	14.0
• Non-English speaking country	5.8	13.5	9.9

Note. From Slade et al. (2009). Reproduced under Creative Commons licence.

NATURAL HISTORY OF ANXIETY

The Harvard Brown Anxiety Disorders Research Project is a naturalistic study of outcome in anxiety disorders (Bruce et al., 2005). At the start of the study, 711 patients with a current or past history of anxiety disorder, recruited from eleven different clinical centres, were enrolled and their progress followed over the next twelve years. The authors defined recovery as having experienced eight consecutive weeks without symptoms. Table 5.5 shows the percentage of patients experiencing as few as eight consecutive weeks free of symptoms in a twelve-year period.

These results highlight the fact that anxiety symptoms tend to be chronic and persistent compared with depression, which is more episodic. For example, there was only a 37% chance that a person who had social phobia when they started in the study would experience eight consecutive weeks without symptoms over twelve years. Anxiety also appears to have a slightly worse prognosis than depression, in terms of freedom from symptoms.

Table 5.5 Probability of recovery from an anxiety disorder across 12 years of follow-up

Type of anxiety	Chance of recovery* across 12 years of follow-up (%)
Major depression alone	93
Panic disorder without agoraphobia	82
Recovery from major depression when comorbid with anxiety	73
Panic disorder with agoraphobia	48
Social phobia	37

Note. * Defined as a period of eight consecutive weeks without symptoms. Data adapted from Bruce et al. (2005).

COMORBIDITY

In the NSMHWB, comorbidity between anxiety and affective disorders was the most common mental disorder comorbidity identified. The next most common was between anxiety disorders and substance abuse. These patterns were true for both men and women, although the prevalence rates varied. Having a family history of anxiety disorders, affective disorders or substance use disorder (versus no family history) were all associated with increased odds of meeting criteria for an anxiety disorder (McEvoy et al., 2011). Additionally, comorbid physical conditions, and being a current or ex-smoker, were associated with increased odds of meeting criteria for an anxiety disorder. These important comorbidities highlight the need to screen for these disorders when an individual presents with one of the others.

Anxiety disorders are moderately correlated with each other, but, as reported by Kessler et al. (2005), even more highly correlated with depressive disorders. There are also some patterns of comorbidity for specific anxiety disorders with other mental disorders (Table 5.6). For example, drug abuse is more likely to be comorbid in social phobia and GAD than in other anxiety disorders. Age at onset is relevant in considering these associations; for example, most studies have found that social phobia usually precedes comorbid depression and substance abuse, raising the strong possibility that depression and alcohol abuse may occur secondary to social phobia.

Table 5.6 Correlations among DSM-IV Disorders in the National Comorbidity Survey Replication

	Major depressive episode	Dysthymia	Alcohol abuse	Alcohol dependence	Drug abuse	Drug dependence
Panic disorder	.48	.54	.27	ns	ns	ns
Agoraphobia	.52	.44	ns	ns	ns	ns
Social phobia	.52	.55	.22	.31	.22	.44
Generalised anxiety disorder	.62	.55	.25	.31	.24	.35
Posttraumatic stress disorder	.50	.50	.27	.34	ns	ns
Obsessive-compulsive disorder	.42	ns	.31	ns	ns	ns
Major depressive episode	-	.88	.24	.37	.25	.40
Dysthymia	ns	-	.32	.38	.42	.56

Note. ns = not significant. Data adapted from Kessler et al. (2005).

CHAPTER 6   THE BURDEN OF ANXIETY DISORDERS

Gavin Andrews and Lisa Lampe

BURDEN OF DISEASE

The burden of a disease can be calculated in many ways. For example, the individual may experience distress, and impairment in functioning. They may also incur financial costs in obtaining treatment or through being unable to work to their full capacity. There are also costs to the community – financial costs of treatment, time lost from work and reduced contributions to the community. Hence there may be both direct and easily measurable costs, as well as more indirect costs.

It is important to be aware that the disability caused by anxiety disorders is comparable to that caused by physical disorders. It is also increasingly recognised that anxiety disorders may complicate recovery from other conditions, both physical, such as heart disease, and mental, for example, depression. This represents another indirect burden of disease.

Anxiety disorders tend to be chronic and persist over many years. Studies have shown that distress and impairment in anxiety disorders can be high. However, this fact is often not recognised; most community mental health centres, for example, do not offer treatment for anxiety disorders.

The burden of any disease is calculated in disability-adjusted life years (DALY) lost. That means adding the years of life lost to the disease (YLL) to the years lived with the disability caused by the disease (YLD). That is, DALY = YLL + YLD. The mental disorders overall rank fourth after cancers, cardiovascular diseases and nervous system and sense disorders (Figure 6.1). They account for 13% of the burden of human disease and the largest burden of years lost to disability (Australian Institute of Health and Welfare, 2010). This does not include dementia or suicide, which are grouped elsewhere in the WHO classification.

> The disability caused by anxiety disorders is comparable to that caused by physical disorders.

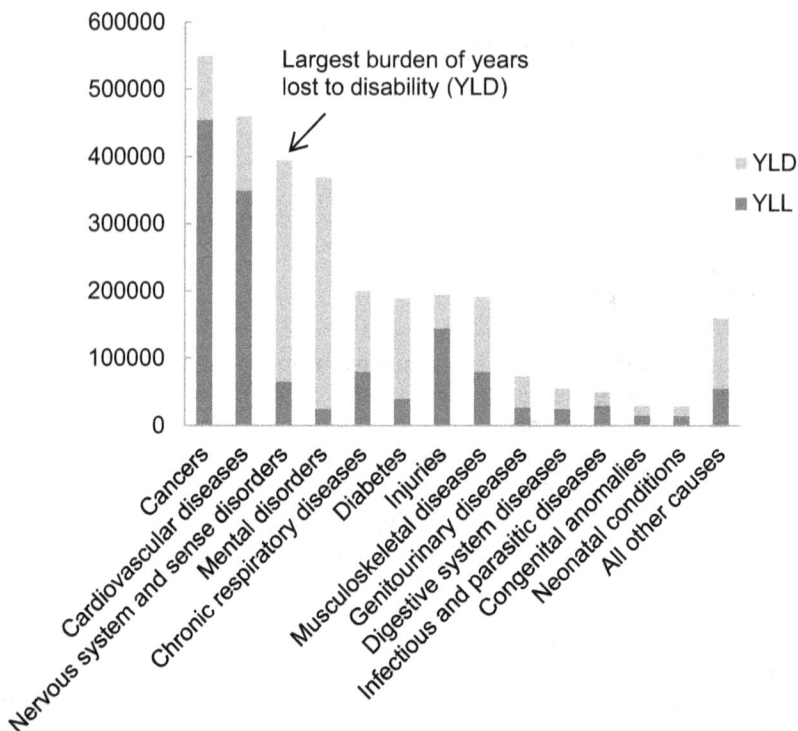

Figure 6.1 Burden of major disease groups, 2010. Data adapted from Australian Institute of Health and Welfare (2010).

In Table 6.1, a more specific example is examined. A random sample of 15,000 telephone numbers in a semi-rural area of Australia were contacted; of those respondents in residential properties, 9,226 completed a telephone screening instrument for mental disorders.

Respondents who were likely to meet criteria for at least one mental disorder were asked to participate in further surveys. Sixty-seven percent completed a computer-assisted personal interview in their home. Respondents were also asked to indicate whether a number of chronic physical disorders were present or absent. Two disability measures were used, one of which was the Short Form Twelve of the Medical Outcomes Study (SF-12). The SF-12 assesses both physical and mental disability on two scales. Scores were added to give a total out of 100. Lower scores indicate greater disablement.

This study shows that anxiety disorders can be as disabling as physical disorders (Andrews et al., 1998).

Table 6.1 SF-12 total scores

Disease	SF-12 total scores
High blood pressure	92.7
Diabetes	88.8
Social anxiety disorder	88.2
Asthma	88.2
"Heart trouble"	86.2
Generalised anxiety disorder	82.4
Kidney disease	80.7
Obsessive-compulsive disorder	77.8

Note. Lower score = more disabled. Data adapted from Andrews et al. (1998).

RECEIVING TREATMENT

Alarmingly, even in Australia, less than half of the people who need it get adequate treatment. Just over half see a health professional, but only 60% of those get any treatment that is known to be beneficial (i.e., evidence-based treatment). The remainder receive general counselling or inadequate treatment advice, such as being told to pick themselves up, or that they will be well soon.

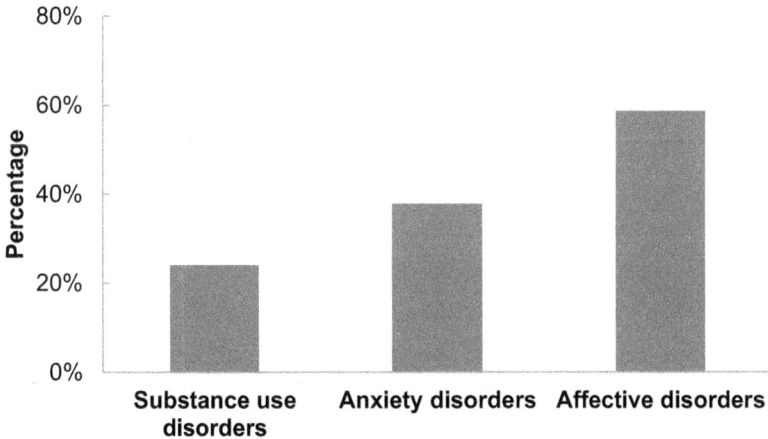

Figure 6.2 Proportion of people using services. From Slade et al. (2009). Reproduced under Creative Commons licence.

SEEKING HELP FOR ANXIETY

In the first National Survey of Mental Health and Wellbeing in Australia, respondents were asked about service utilisation in the 12 months prior to the survey. Potentially effective interventions were defined as cognitive-behavioural therapy, or medication. Other interventions were designated as "unlikely to be effective". In the survey, respondents' perceived need for care was also asked about. This enabled later examination of the match between a person's perceived need for care, whether they sought and received care and the types of care they received. Surprisingly, as shown in Figure 6.3, only 21% of those who would have met criteria for an anxiety disorder in the past twelve months had a consultation with a health care provider about their mental health. Within this group, only 52% received a treatment likely to be effective. Of those who did not consult a health professional, 77% did not perceive a need to do so. Interestingly, males and females appeared equally likely to seek help. Those with panic disorder were the most likely to seek medical attention (Issakidis & Andrews, 2002).

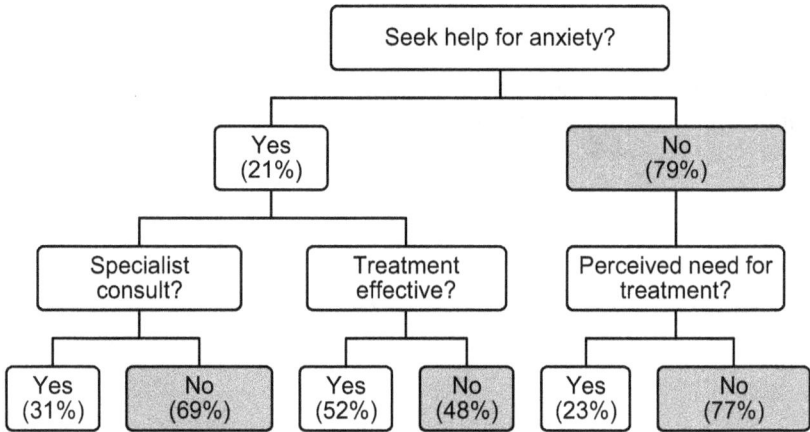

Figure 6.3 Help seeking for anxiety disorders. Data adapted from Issakidis & Andrews (2002).

Close to one-third of people received information about anxiety and its treatment; however, only about half received treatment that was likely to be effective. Many people received more than one type of intervention.

DIFFERENCES BETWEEN ANXIETY DISORDERS

Figure 6.4 shows the proportion of all people in the community who would have met criteria for each anxiety disorder and for whom this was their main mental health problem, who received treatment likely to be effective. The relatively low rates are due to a combination of the high proportion of people who do not seek help, and a low rate of effective treatments for those who do seek help.

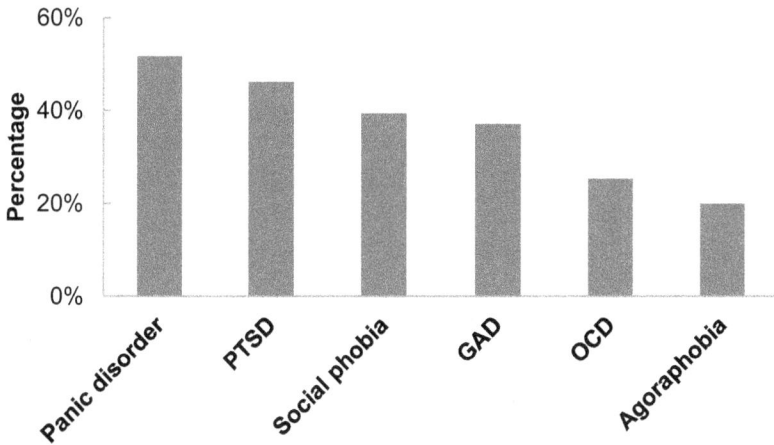

Figure 6.4   Percentage of total with each disorder who received treatment likely to be effective. Data adapted from Issakidis & Andrews (2002).

WHY PEOPLE DO NOT SEEK HELP FOR ANXIETY DISORDERS

When respondents who perceived a need for treatment were asked why they had not sought it, they gave a variety of reasons. Attitudinal reasons, such as that they preferred to manage the problem by themselves or that they did not think anything could help, were given by about 73% of this group. Other reasons, such as financial issues, or reporting that they had found another type of help, were given by about 37% of the group (Table 6.2).

Table 6.2   Reasons for not seeking help

Attitudinal reasons (72.7%)	Other reasons (36.8%)
Preferred to manage myself	I couldn't afford the money
Didn't think anything could help	I asked but didn't get the help
Didn't know where to get help	I got help from another source
Afraid to ask or of what others would think	

Note. Data adapted from Issakidis & Andrews (2002).

ANXIETY AS ONE OF THE INTERNALISING DISORDERS

Anxiety and depression are regarded as "internalising" disorders, meaning that distress tends to be internalised as opposed to being communicated to others through dramatic or dysfunctional behaviour or intense emotional expression ("externalising"). The temperamental trait of "negative affectivity/emotionality", or neuroticism, is a risk factor for anxiety and depression, and has moderate heritability. Thus, both anxiety and depression may be seen at higher rates in families whose members share this vulnerability.

IMPLICATIONS FOR TREATMENT

Most internalising disorders share comorbidity with other disorders in the cluster. Thus, if an individual has an episode of depression, they will more than likely also have a history of anxiety disorder and *vice versa*. Most disorders respond to similar cluster specific treatment: SSRIs, face-to-face cognitive-behavioural therapy, and now internet-based cognitive behaviour therapy. With such effective treatments becoming widely available, the burden of anxiety and depressive disorders must decline.

PART I SUMMARY

Anxiety disorders as a group represent the most common mental disorders occurring in the community. In Part I the key symptoms of anxiety were introduced. It is important to realise that the symptoms of anxiety can be extremely distressing even though they may not be very apparent to an observer.

The concept of anxiety as a spectrum from normal – and even helpful – to distressing and impairing was discussed. Anxiety is often referred to as the "fight or flight" response and is observed in some form in almost every species of mammal. However, the particular role of cognition in the experience of anxiety in humans was stressed. Understanding the role of cognitive factors in triggering anxiety, appraising the symptoms of anxiety and choosing a response is critical in being able to plan effective cognitive-behavioural therapy. Understanding the specific fears and concerns underlying anxiety is also the main way in which anxiety disorders are differentiated from each other.

Given that anxiety is an almost universal experience, it is important to be able to determine when anxiety has reached a level of distress or impairment that meets criteria for a "disorder" according to currently accepted classificatory systems. It is also helpful to understand the advantages and limitations of these classificatory systems. Some people are at greater risk of developing an anxiety disorder than others. Many, but not all, anxiety disorders are more common in women. For many of the anxiety disorders, the risk factors identified by research so far include factors with a moderately strong genetic contribution, such as temperamental factors, and some environmental factors. Anxiety disorders tend to start early in life, are typically chronic, and have important comorbidities with depression and substance abuse.

Finally, the burden of anxiety disorders is considerable and often underestimated by health planners and economists. It is equivalent to that of many physical disorders. Many persons who might benefit from treatment do not seek treatment, and some that do seek treatment do not receive an intervention that evidence has shown is likely to be effective.

PART II   PHYSIOLOGY OF THE NORMAL STRESS RESPONSE

Most people have been in a situation like the following: walking along a track or down a dark city laneway, one is suddenly confronted with a highly threatening situation and their body's automatic survival systems kick in. For example, if you suddenly see a snake while walking in the bush, the snake is likely to trigger an alert. Your reaction is automatic – the pulse races, the individual jumps back quickly, the breathing rate quickens and your body is primed for a rapid retreat.

This "fight or flight" response is also triggered by other stressful events, and is an important component of anxiety. Not everyone confronts snakes in their everyday existence, but the body's automatic response has been developed to save the individual in such a situation. This response can also be triggered by other stresses.

The purpose of this response is not only to help protect one by rapidly mobilising the resources needed to act on the danger, but to help maintain the body's normal homeostatic state if some injury is done. In doing that, the response has both specific characteristics which reflect the nature of the stressor, and general aspects common to the reaction to all stressors.

In Part II, we will examine the response of the body, specific to emotional factors, in the context of the general adaptive response of the body to stress.

Although one's conscious awareness of any threat seems almost instantaneous, even before the individual is consciously aware of a threat, that information is transmitted to their fear processing centres. Thalamo-amygdala and cortico-amygdala circuits channel information into the amygdala, a small region of the brain in the temporal lobe which is part of the limbic system central to the organisation of the body's response to threat.

> Before an individual is consciously aware of a threat, that information is transmitted to their fear processing centres.

Within the amygdala, information is initially channelled into the baso-lateral nucleus of the amygdala, which then feeds forward to the amygdala's central nucleus. From here, information about the threat is dispersed widely, activating the body's defenses. Although the snake was a very obvious external threat, it is important to note that an internally generated threat such as pain would also trigger a similar cascade, the impulse reaching the amygdala via other perceptual pathways.

The information about the perceived or contemplated threat is then dispersed widely via the hypothalamus and the autonomic nervous system, leading to a generalised body response. The major monoaminergic systems of the brain (noradrenaline, acetylcholine, serotonin and dopamine) are also activated. This leads to a generalised increase of arousal across the brain, which in turn feeds back as an increase in the processing of external cues. Changing levels of input from, especially, the prefrontal cortex helps to modulate this response.

These adaptive responses are integrated by the hypothalamus, but activated by the autonomic nervous system and a range of hormonal changes.

In broad terms, the general adaptive response primes the body to be alert to, and respond rapidly to, danger; it activates the "fight or flight" response via the autonomic nervous system.

In doing so, it increases one's cardiac output and respiratory rate, mobilises energy in the form of glucose and fatty acids to fuel the response, and activates renal and cardiac responses to maintain blood volume and blood pressure.

The response of the individual to a stressor is affected by factors inherent to the stressor, such as: the duration of stress (chronic as opposed to acute), the type of stressor (psychological as opposed to physical), and its context (was support available or was the individual in a situation of helplessness?). It is also affected by factors unique to the individual such as: their gender, their developmental stage (childhood trauma as opposed to experiencing a stressor as an adult), and their genetic inheritance.

The stressor elicits a response from overlapping systems of mediators via neurotransmitters, neuropeptides and corticosteroids. These systems effect the eventual response via actions that operate over distinct time periods and, often, in anatomically specific regions.

The response of the body to stress is commonly thought to occur in three waves (Figure II.1). The first is a fast response that is driven by the sympathetic nervous system and corticotropin-releasing hormone (CRH) receptor system, followed by a slower response that is mediated via glucocorticoid activity, the parasympathetic nervous system, corticotropin-releasing hormone 2 (CRH2) receptors and urocortins. A further wave of changes, mediated by transcription factors triggered by the initial wave of monoamines and CRH, can be conceptualised as a third wave, which continues to affect the individual for long periods after the stressor has passed.

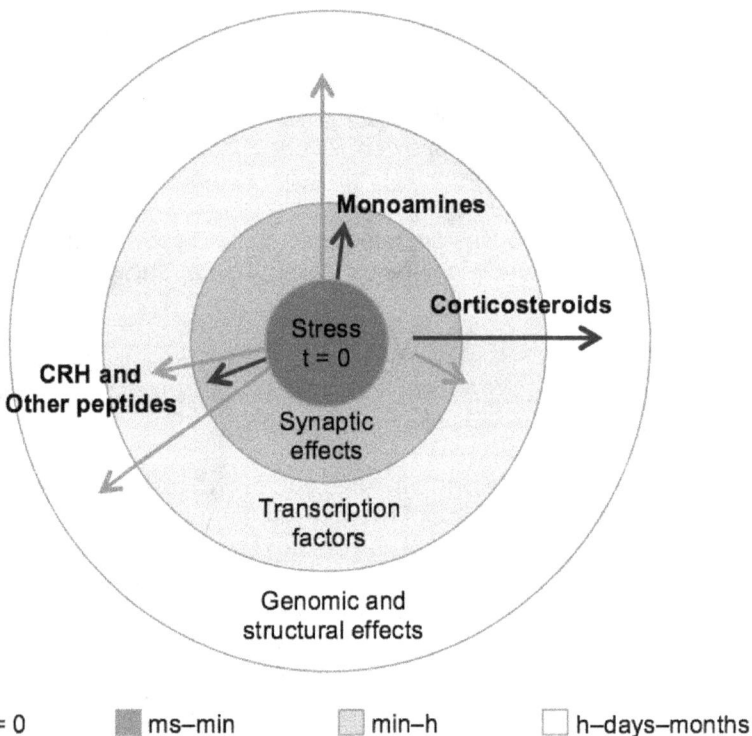

Figure II.1   The three waves of response of the body to stress. From Joels & Baram (2009). Reproduced with permission of Nature Publishing Group.

What is stress? Stress is the general term to describe the response of the body to actual or anticipated disruption of homeostasis or an anticipated threat to wellbeing. This rather abstract definition may include stressors such as infections, physiological factors such as blood loss, chemical factors such as hypoxia or physical factors such as extreme temperature. The response of the body to any particular stress engages a highly evolved and efficient set of systems that are integrated to maximise survival. Which system predominates in that response may alter with the speed of onset of the stress and its nature. Anxiety shares the physiological responses that the body has to all stress.

In Part II, the body's response to stress will be explored in more detail, in particular the autonomic nervous system (ANS), the cardiac and respiratory systems that are both important in the symptomatology associated with anxiety, and finally the hypothalamic-pituitary-adrenal (HPA) axis and the cascade of hormones that is released in the stress response.

Anxiety shares the physiological responses that the body has to all stress.

CHAPTER 7   RESPONSE OF THE AUTONOMIC NERVOUS SYSTEM TO STRESS

Anthony Harris

STRESS RESPONSE VIA INTER-RELATED SYSTEMS

The body responds to stress via multiple interrelated systems. This chapter will consider the effects of the autonomic nervous system, the neuroendocrine system, and the respiratory system. Importantly, all of these systems are interrelated and often tune their function by feedback circuits that modulate the response. This response is also a whole-of-body response and affects other systems such as the immune system; however, only the autonomic nervous system, the hypothalamic pituitary adrenal (HPA) axis and the respiratory system will be considered here.

Autonomic Nervous System (ANS)

The first system is the autonomic nervous system – autonomic because it was originally thought to be outside voluntary control, although this is now known not to be strictly true.

The ANS is, in turn, divided into two complementary systems:

- the sympathetic nervous system. It controls the "fight or flight" response and the parasympathetic nervous system (remembered by the phrase "rest and digest").
- the parasympathetic nervous system. It controls the response to the activation by the sympathetic nervous system, limiting the duration of the response (and hence conserving resources for the body).

The ANS provides the immediate response to a stressor via both neural pathways and via activation of the neuroendocrine systems through innervation of the adrenal medulla.

> The sympathetic nervous system controls the "fight or flight" response.

Hypothalamic Pituitary Adrenal (HPA) Axis

The second system is the hypothalamic pituitary adrenal axis. The HPA axis is a neuroendocrine system, in that it combines central neural responses in the prefrontal and limbic parts of the brain, both with the activation and release from the hypothalamus of a range of hormones – such as corticotrophin releasing hormone (CRH) – that control and modulate the stress response, triggering the release of adrenocorticotropic hormone (ACTH) from the pituitary gland that stimulates release of stress hormones from the adrenal glands.

Respiratory System

The third of the systems considered here is the respiratory system. This system controls our breathing. Increased breathing, or hyperventilation, is a distressing symptom for many people with panic attacks. It has a marked effect on the physiology because of the rapid changes in carbon dioxide concentration in the blood. The respiratory system is sensitive to changes in CO_2 concentration which, in turn, determines blood pH balance. An episode of hyperventilation will result in a respiratory alkalosis and symptoms such as breathlessness and dyspnoea. This system can also react very rapidly.

These systems react to stress by using different mechanisms, and function along different time scales: the ANS and respiratory system react rapidly to the immediate response; the HPA system reacts more slowly and modulates the stress response.

AUTONOMIC NERVOUS SYSTEM

The autonomic nervous system is a basic part of the body's nervous system, but one of which we have little conscious awareness. For the most part it controls the organs that it innervates automatically. The ANS controls the smooth muscles in the abdomen and thorax, as well as secretions from glands throughout the body. It controls the reflexes that govern many of the functions of the body's organs, such as the automatic change in pupil size with changes in light, or the reflex that governs micturition. There are some sensory neurones in this system. The ANS, as is shown in Figure 7.1, is divided into two parts – the sympathetic and the parasympathetic nervous systems. Both of these systems are spread widely across the body and arise from anatomically separate areas. The diagram shows the anatomical spread of the autonomic nervous system and illustrates the extent of its effect on body functions affected by stress. It may also be noted that many of the organs innervated have reciprocal innervations by both sympathetic and parasympathetic systems. The autonomic nervous system in the gut interacts with the enteric nervous system, a separate structure, either directly via connection with both the sympathetic and parasympathetic nervous system, or indirectly via the many neuroendocrinological substances that are active in the enteric nervous system. This system controls aspects of gut motility, endocrine and exocrine secretion and gut microcirculation. It is also important in gut immunological and inflammatory responses. It will not be considered further.

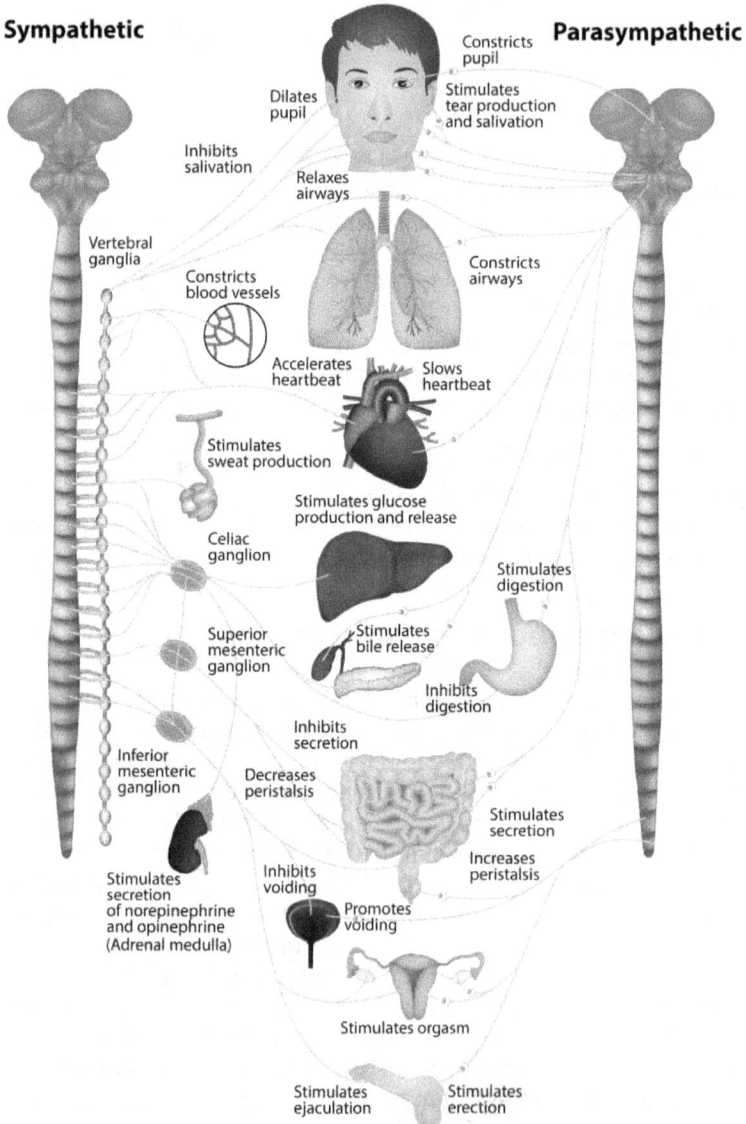

Figure 7.1 Autonomic Nervous System

Sympathetic Nervous System

The sympathetic nervous system, responsible for the "fight or flight" response, originates from preganglionic sympathetic neurons on the intermediolateral cell column, from the level of the first thoracic vertebra to the second lumbar vertebra. These preganglionic neurons then project to a system of pre- and paravertebral ganglia that, in turn, project to a wide range of end-organs. There they release either acetylcholine (in the sweat glands), or noradrenaline (in other postganglionic sympathetic nerve endings) and a range of peptides that modulate the ANS response. The sympathetic NS also projects to the adrenal medulla, which is primarily responsible for releasing adrenaline. The burst of adrenaline released from the chromaffin cells of the adrenal medulla is an important component of the "fight or flight" response; it reinforces the actions of the sympathetic nervous system, circulates to sites not innervated by the sympathetic nervous system and performs tasks such as mobilising fat energy stores. Altogether, the "fight or flight" response is characterised by an increase in the heart rate, vaso-constriction, increased blood pressure, diversion of blood away from the skin and splanchnic vessels, increased pupil size, bronchiolar dilation, increased sweat output and a decrease in gastric secretions and turnover. Sympathetic nerve activity in the kidneys increases renal arteriolar tone, releases renin and increases the reabsorption of sodium, which contributes to the increase in blood pressure. Similar sympathetic activity in the liver increases glycogenolysis and, in the pancreas, decreases the release of insulin and stimulates glucagon release, all of which help to mobilise energy stores and maintain spikes in blood glucose and fatty acids.

Parasympathetic Nervous System

The parasympathetic nervous system opposes many of the actions of the sympathetic nervous system, curtailing the response begun by the sympathetic nervous system and reducing the pulse rate, lowering blood pressure, decreasing sweat output and increasing bowel motility. It arises from preganglionic neurons in the cervical and sacral sections of the spinal cord, and synapse in ganglia which are located near the end organs that they innervate. Most parts of the body that are innervated by the ANS receive both sympathetic and parasympathetic input that provide reciprocal activity. Such balanced feedback helps the body maintain homeostasis of function across a broad range of stresses. This response comes as a second wave of bodily reactions to a stressor, which aims to preserve and build up energy stores.

CARDIOVASCULAR SYSTEM RESPONSE TO STRESS

The effect of ANS stimulation is also seen in the cardiovascular system.

Increased blood pressure and increased heart rate are two responses of the body that occur with the activation of the sympathetic nervous system and the flood of adrenaline.

Direct sympathetic activation of the heart causes an increase in the heart rate and the contractility of the heart muscle. Sympathetic innervations of the smooth muscle in arteriolar walls cause a contraction of those muscles and an increase in the resistance to blood flow, which contributes to an increase in blood pressure. Circulating hormones, such as adrenaline, angiotensin II and vasopressin, secreted as a response to both central and peripheral activation, also act to increase heart rate, increase contraction of arterioles and lessen fluid loss.

Sympathetic nerve activity in the kidneys increases renal arteriolar tone, releases renin and increases the reabsorption of sodium, which contributes to the increase in blood pressure. Changes in blood pH and partial pressures of gases such as carbon dioxide and oxygen, which are controlled by the respiratory system, also feed into this.

Like other parts of the body, the cardiovascular system also has a homeostatic mechanism to help balance the effects of the sympathetic nervous system. One of these responses is mediated through the baroreceptor system located in the arch of the aorta, the heart and in the carotid sinus, which buffers the response of other inputs into the stress response by decreasing blood pressure and heart rate in response to stress. This system feeds back to the nucleus of the solitary tract via the vagus nerve, a part of the parasympathetic nervous system.

EFFECTS OF STRESS ON THE CARDIOVASCULAR SYSTEM

Figures 7.6 and 7.7 chart the body's response to the application of either a physical stressor – in this case, a cold pressor test which required participants to keep their hand in 5°C water for two minutes, or a mental stressor – a test of mental arithmetic – or a combination of both.

The effects of stress on the cardiovascular system can be seen in the following two graphs.

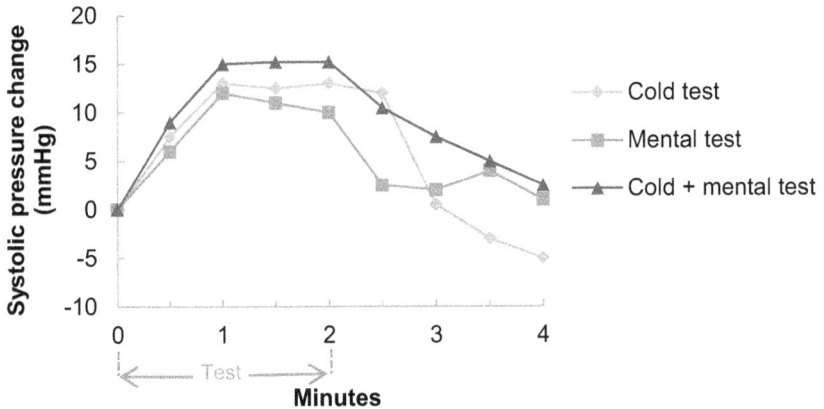

Figure 7.6 Systolic blood pressure change. From LeBlanc et al. (1979). Reproduced with permission of the American Physiological Society.

The application of the physical, mental or combined stressors sees a rapid rise in the blood pressure and pulse rate. With the cessation of the stressor, the systolic blood pressure drops immediately (Figure 7.6). The pulse rate has already peaked and continues to drop rapidly (Figure 7.7).

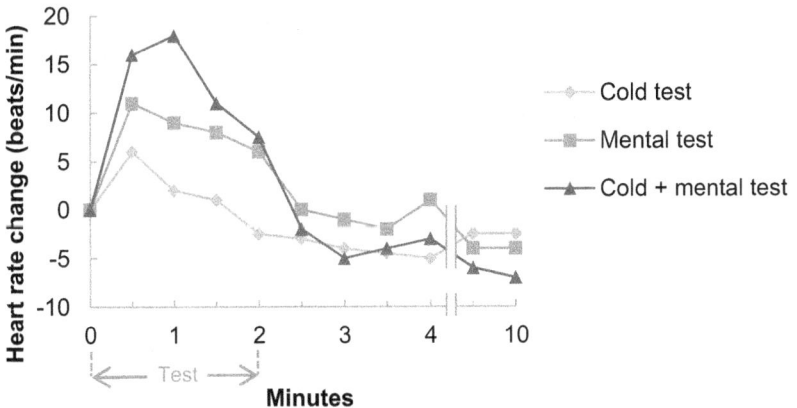

Figure 7.7 Heart rate change. From LeBlanc et al. (1979). Reproduced with permission of the American Physiological Society.

As Figure 7.8 shows, this was mediated by the sympathetic nervous system, as indicated by the plasma adrenaline levels, which only peaked at two minutes, the time at which the stressor stopped. What the individual feels at this point is the racing heart and palpitations of anxiety or a panic attack.

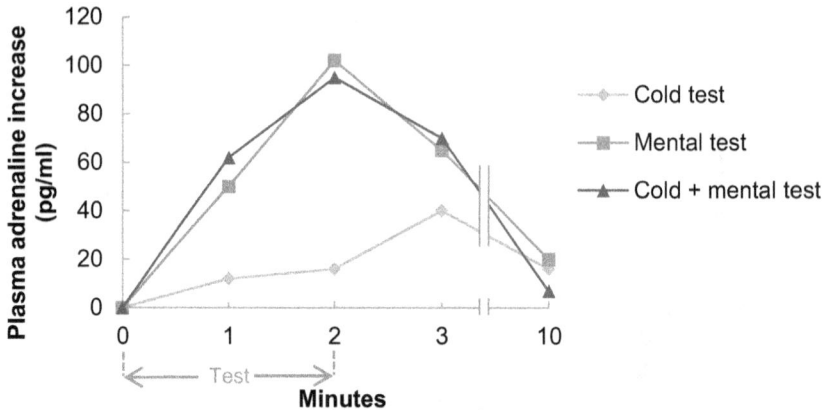

Figure 7.8   Plasma adrenaline increase. From LeBlanc et al. (1979). Reproduced with permission of the American Physiological Society.

CENTRAL REGULATION OF AUTONOMIC OUTPUT

Finally, in the same way that the control of the sympathetic and the parasympathetic nervous systems interact peripherally, the central control of the two systems also overlaps within the nucleus of the solitary tract, which is situated in the brainstem, and the paraventricular nucleus of the hypothalamus, thus integrating input into both systems (Dodd & Role, 1991). The control of the autonomic nervous system is influenced by feedback from many higher cortical centres including the limbic system, thalamus, basal ganglia and reticular formation. The nucleus of the solitary tract acts to integrate, then relay information between upper and lower regions of the nervous system and, with the hypothalamic nuclei, to coordinate responses between the autonomic nervous system and the HPA axis. The nucleus also controls some autonomic functions by way of reflex circuits for autonomic control of the heart, lungs and gastrointestinal tract.

RESPONSE OF THE AUTONOMIC NERVOUS SYSTEM

The response of the autonomic nervous system occurs rapidly and throughout the body, interacting with other body systems to increase cardiovascular tone, mobilise energy stores, and to increase arousal, attention, concentration and vigilance. Many of these responses are the symptoms and signs of anxiety – the heart palpitations, the cold clammy hands and the dry mouth. At the same time as the ANS is doing this, other body systems, such as the respiratory and endocrine system, are also being activated.

CHAPTER 8   PANIC AND HYPERVENTILATION

Michael Harris

CASE STUDY: KATHY

Kathy fears taking a lift alone and occasionally has panic attacks in the lift, the main symptom of which is rapid breathing.

Rapid breathing, or hyperventilation, is a common symptom of anxiety. These episodes frequently occur during panic attacks, but chronic mild hyperventilation is found in many anxious people.

Anxiety causes a number of respiratory symptoms including chest tightness, shortness of breath and a feeling of air hunger or dyspnoea. This can be accompanied by dizziness, faintness and tingling around the mouth, along with a spasm in the hands.

This chapter will explain the underlying physiology of hyperventilation.

NORMAL RESPIRATION

The main function of the respiratory system is to transfer oxygen into the body and to rid the body of carbon dioxide, a product of energy metabolism. In doing this, it also fulfills another important function, in helping balance the acid-based homeostasis of the body. Either increases in breathing rate (hyperventilation) or decreases in breathing rate (hypoventilation) can have marked effects on this balance.

The normal resting respiratory rate is around fourteen breaths per minute, just a fraction more than one breath every five seconds.

> Anxiety causes a number of respiratory symptoms, including chest tightness, shortness of breath and a feeling of air hunger, or dyspnoea.

Obviously, this varies with exercise, increasing with an escalation in energy consumption. Hyperventilation is judged to begin at a resting breathing rate of greater than eighteen breaths per minute.

CONTROL OF RESPIRATION

Most of the time, individuals are not aware that they are breathing. The process is automatic, and tightly regulated by pacemaker neurons that are in the brainstem.

The process is also regulated by chemoreceptor cells in the ventral medulla and in the carotid bodies, which detect changes in carbon dioxide levels and blood pH.

A number of other higher centres in the hypothalamus, cerebellum and cortex also help regulate respiration, in consonance with a wide range of physiological and emotional inputs. These include input from the amygdala, which can stimulate an increase in ventilation via the parabrachial nucleus. Fear or anxiety can affect the respiratory system via a number of pathways, including the sympathetic nervous system, but the stimulus for this is probably orchestrated through the amygdala (Shea & White, 2008).

HYPERVENTILATION (TACHYPNEA)

Hyperventilation, sometimes known as tachypnea, can be caused by illnesses that interfere with the function of the lungs (such as pneumonia or asthma), produce fever, as sepsis or infections do, interfere with the regulation of breathing from higher centres (as seen in a stroke), or change the acid-base balance of the body, as in diabetic ketoacidosis or some drug overdoses. Emotional upset and anxiety can also cause hyperventilation.

Many patients with organic illnesses also feel anxious. This is an important fact to remember, because it can lead to the anxiety being ignored while health professionals concentrate on the physical illness; or the symptoms of the physical illness can be erroneously attributed to the anxiety disorder alone.

BREATHING AND ACID-BASE BALANCE

The body lives within a number of tight physiological boundaries, one of which is the pH or acid-base balance; it also has a number of buffering systems to control this balance and to maintain homeostasis. This is important, because if the body moves out of a narrow range of acid-base balance, physical damage and possibly death may occur.

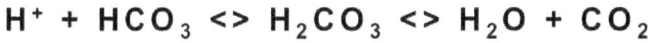

$$H^+ + HCO_3 <> H_2CO_3 <> H_2O + CO_2$$

Hydrogen ion + bicarbonate   carbonic acid   water + carbon dioxide

Respiration allows the body rapidly to change the acid-base balance through the bicarbonate buffering system, which sees carbon dioxide and water dissociating to carbonic acid and to bicarbonate and hydrogen ions. Changes in the concentration of carbon dioxide, controlled by the respiration rate, can rapidly compensate for short-term acid-base problems. Most CO_2 is carried and transported in the blood as bicarbonate (HCO_3).

CONTROL OF BREATHING AND RESPIRATORY FAILURE

However, because of this process, hyperventilation due to anxiety will also change the acid-base balance of the body. Figure 8.1 shows the effects of increased ventilation.

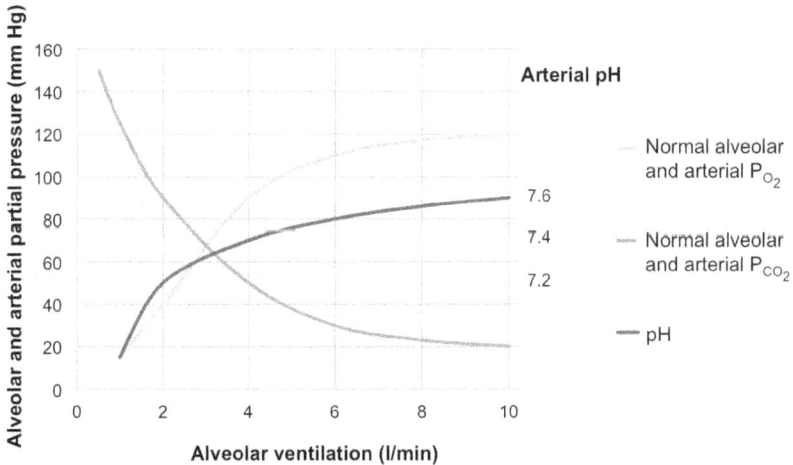

Figure 8.1   Effects of hyperventilation and hypoventilation on arterial Po_2 and Pco_2

As alveolar ventilation increases on the x-axis, the concentration of oxygen (Po_2) and carbon dioxide (Pco_2) on the y-axis rapidly changes. The concentration of carbon dioxide in the alveoli, or air filled sacs in the lungs, are almost in equilibrium with the concentration of carbon dioxide in the blood. With an increase in breathing rate, carbon dioxide levels in the alveoli drop to be more like the concentration in the atmosphere and this rapidly equilibrates with the blood carbon dioxide concentration, causing it to fall. This, in turn, will cause a fall in hydrogen ion concentration in the blood, which will result in a rise in the pH of the blood.

EFFECT OF HYPERVENTILATION

The mild alkalosis that can result from this hyperventilation causes changes that flow on to affect muscle and nerve function. One of these changes will be the increased binding of calcium ions in the blood, which trade places with hydrogen ions that are released from binding sites on albumin, a very common protein in the blood. This change will cause a drop in the amount of free calcium in the blood, causing hypocalcaemia.

Calcium has a number of important functions. The drop in free calcium leads to a constriction of cerebral blood vessels and it affects both nerve and muscle depolarisation. This has effects both centrally and peripherally.

The increase in pH due to the drop in carbon dioxide also has direct effects on muscle contraction, via an increase in myofibril sensitivity and contraction. Together, the decrease in carbon dioxide, or hypocapnia, and the drop in calcium concentration in the blood, can decrease cerebral blood flow by 30%.

SYMPTOMS OF ANXIETY ASSOCIATED WITH HYPERVENTILATION

The drop in cerebral blood flow triggered by the reduction in blood carbon dioxide and calcium levels, can cause light-headedness, fainting and blurred vision. The reduction in free calcium also causes changes in peripheral nerve function, which in turn causes tingling around the mouth, paraesthesia – or pins and needles – in the hands and feet and, in some cases, carpopedal spasms, or muscle spasms, most often in the hands.

OTHER RESPIRATORY SYMPTOMS

A number of other respiratory symptoms are seen with anxiety disorders.

Dyspnoea is a highly unpleasant sensation of air hunger, or suffocation. It is not the same as being "out of breath". At the end of a sprint, an individual might be aware of the effort of breathing but he will expect this, perceive it as normal and understand that it will soon pass, so it should not be associated with anxiety. However, when hyperventilation is a result of anxiety, dyspnoea may be triggered by an alteration in the settings of the chemoreceptors that monitor blood oxygen and pH, and control of oxygen and carbon dioxide levels.

Anxious people frequently complain of a sense of chest constriction, particularly after panic attacks. Most of the time, individuals are unaware of themselves breathing but, during periods of hyperventilation, they become very much aware, both of breathing and of how they control it. There is a disassociation between the muscular effort of hyperventilation and the centrally driven increase in ventilation. This disassociation can trigger a perception that the effort of breathing is not achieving the change in blood gases that is being set by central mechanisms. This perception may also be affected by the feedback from over-stretched muscles in the chest wall, while rapid breathing in itself may fatigue muscle fibres, leading to a sense of being out of breath.

RESPONSE OF THE RESPIRATORY SYSTEM IN PANIC

The response of the respiratory system to anxiety or in a panic attack is rapid and, at least initially, involuntary.

Understanding the effects of rapid breathing on the underlying physiology of acid-base homeostasis helps one appreciate the cause of a number of basic symptoms of panic. It also offers an insight into how people who are hyperventilating may be helped by learning how to control their breathing. This, in turn, can assist in controlling the symptoms of anxiety and panic.

CHAPTER 9   RESPONSE OF THE HYPOTHALAMIC PITUITARY ADRENAL AXIS TO STRESS

Anthony Harris

WHAT IS THE HYPOTHALAMIC-PITUITARY-ADRENAL (HPA) AXIS

When a stressor activates the autonomic nervous system, the amygdala (or other parts of the cortex such as the prefrontal cortex or the hippocampus) simultaneously signals to the body's endocrine system to prepare for the threat. The endocrine system is a series of glands that secrete hormones into the blood stream to help regulate the body (Nemeroff, 1998). The hypothalamic-pituitary-adrenal axis is part of the endocrine system, and works as a system of glands that signal to each other in a cascade which can amplify the signal, but which also feeds back to regulate the signal, in order to help with the homeostasis of the whole system. The HPA axis is distributed across the body. In the brain, its principal sites are the hypothalamus and the anterior pituitary.

Hypothalamus

The hypothalamus is a small part of the brain which is at the "crossroads" between the thalamus, the cerebral cortex (especially the limbic cortex), and the ascending inputs from the brainstem and peripheral nervous system. It is a collection of nuclei located below the thalamus in the ventral part of the diencephalon.

Pituitary Gland

The pituitary gland is a functional and anatomical extension of the hypothalamus and is situated below the hypothalamus, within a small bony cavity of the sphenoid bone called the sella turca. It is connected to the hypothalamus by the median eminence and the infundibular (or pituitary) stalk.

Adrenal Glands

The final part of the HPA axis is the adrenal glands. These are situated on top of the kidneys in the retroperitoneum.

RESPONSE OF THE HYPOTHALAMIC-PITUITARY-ADRENAL AXIS TO STRESS

The signal that switches on the axis originates in the paraventricular nucleus of the hypothalamus. When activated by the amygdala, it secretes corticotopin releasing hormone (CRH) into the portal circulation of the median eminence. A range of additional neuroactive factors such as; neuropeptide Y, glucagon-like peptide-1, inhibin-β, somatostatin and enkephalin also influence HPA activation. This process is also directly affected by feedback from systems such as the sympathetic and parasympathetic nervous systems, via the nucleus of the solitary tract.

The portal circulation takes CRH to the anterior pituitary gland via the median eminence and the pituitary stalk, which then releases adrenocorticotropic hormone (ACTH).

CIRCULATING CORTISOL AND RECEPTORS

ACTH is then transported to the adrenal cortex by the blood stream, where it stimulates the secretion of cortisol into the blood stream. Circulating cortisol interacts with two different receptors – the mineralocorticoid and glucocorticoid receptors – that are found throughout the body.

MINERALOCORTICOID AND GLUCOCORTICOID RECEPTORS

Mineralocorticoid activity causes the reabsorption of sodium and, consequently, an increase in fluid volume and blood pressure, important actions for a body that is preparing for the possibility of threat.

The glucocorticoids have a number of functions. These include the mobilisation of energy stores by an increase in the production of glucose, and the promotion of the breakdown of adipose or other tissues. They are approximately one tenth as sensitive as the mineralocorticoid receptors (MR) and are only activated by the peak levels of cortisol seen in the reaction to acute stress. They also play an important role in modulating the immune system and enhancing arousal and cognition, especially for emotionally salient stimuli.

SECRETION OF VASOPRESSIN

In addition to stimulating the secretion of CRH and thence ACTH from the anterior pituitary, the paraventricular and supraoptic nuclei of the hypothalamus are responsible for the production and secretion of vasopressin (also known as arginine vasopressin or AVP).

Vasopressin is an integral part of the stress response, acting on the kidneys to increase water retention. It also has a lesser action, causing contraction of the arteriolar smooth muscle.

The paraventricular and supraoptic nuclei contain neurosecretory neurons, which communicate with the posterior pituitary via the pituitary stalk. These neurons have axons that terminate on capillaries in the posterior pituitary where they store and secrete vasopressin. This peptide is produced in the neurosecretory neurons in the hypothalamus, packaged into granules which are transported down the axons of the neurons into the posterior pituitary and on into nerve terminals. Vasopressin is then released by a nerve response originating in the hypothalamus, but propagated in the posterior pituitary.

THE RESPONSE OF THE HPA AXIS

The response of the HPA axis to stress does not have the obvious effects on signs and symptoms of anxiety that activation of the autonomic nervous system or the respiratory system may have, but it is essential to the body's overall response to stress.

TIME COURSE OF ACTION OF THE HPA SYSTEM

The response of the HPA axis to a stressor occurs over two time scales.

The initial response is rapid and acts in concert with other fast-acting mediators, such as adrenaline and dopamine, to increase vigilance and concentration. This response is completed in minutes to hours.

In the HPA axis, this is predominately mediated by CRH receptor 1 and mineralocorticoid receptor activity. These receptors not only initiate the cascade described above, but have distinct actions, especially in the limbic system, that maintain the excitability and stability of the system.

The slower mode of response helps the body adapt to stress, commit to memory the lessons it learns from it and prepare for future stress. This happens as a result of the activation, both of urocortins at CRH receptor 2 sites and of corticosteroids at glucocorticoid receptor sites, via their action as regulators of gene transcription, either activating or repressing gene expression. The corticosteroids are also converted to neurosteroids that interact directly with membrane receptors for other neurotransmitters, such as GABA. These responses act to enhance memory, probably via structural change in hippocampal cells.

On the other hand, chronic stress can cause changes in pyramidal cells in the hippocampus, including a loss of dendritic spines and possibly neurogenesis, which may have an effect on cognitive function.

In summary, the initial short-term response to stress contributes to an increase in vigilance and concentration. It also mobilises the body to retain fluids and helps liberate the energy stores that are needed. This assists with cognitive functions such as memory. The slower mode of response helps the body adapt to stress, incorporates the lessons learned into memory and prepare for future stress. As for other parts of the stress response system, these effects of MR and GR, CRH and urocortins overlap and feed back into the response, helping to modulate and control it and thus encouraging homeostasis.

NATURE OF THE RESPONSE OF THE HPA AXIS

The nature of this response differs according to the stressor that elicits it. Thus, psychological stress is thought to be mediated via the areas of the brain that subserve emotion (amygdala and prefrontal cortex), memory (hippocampus) and decision making (prefrontal cortex).

The response of the HPA axis feeds back into other physiological systems that more obviously contribute to the signs and symptoms of anxiety. The threat of being run over by a car elicits a rapid response, predominantly from the brainstem and hypothalamus. However, whatever the stressor, the response is likely to elicit input from all parts of this complex system over the time course of the initial rapid response, and over the secondary slower allostatic response that comes from gene expression and structural alteration within the brain.

THE ACTIONS OF THE ANS AND HPA

The interaction of the autonomic nervous system and the HPA axis are complementary and each feeds back into the functions of the other. The autonomic nervous system can be seen to have an input into structures that are integral to the endocrine response of the HPA to a stressor.

The short-term response to stress contributes to an increase in vigilance and concentration, mobilises the body to retain fluids and helps liberate the energy stores that are needed.

The ANS directly innervates the adrenal cortex, regulating glucocorticoid release. As well as eliciting a response from a range of end organs, the sympathetic nervous system stimulates the chromaffin cells in the adrenal medulla to secrete large amounts of adrenaline and a smaller amount of noradrenaline. It also innervates the adrenal cortex, contributing to the regulation of cortisol secretion.

Feedback by the autonomic nervous system via the nucleus of the solitary tract directly innervates the paraventricular nucleus of the hypothalamus, the structure that initiates HPA axis activity.

Mineralocorticoid and glucocorticoid receptors are found throughout the brain, where activation, particularly in the limbic system (a group of brain structures including the amygdala, the hippocampus and the prefrontal cortex that are involved in emotion and cognition), modulates further brain activity affecting both the ANS and the HPA axis.

PART II SUMMARY

The response of the body to a stressor is complex. It is coordinated via the hypothalamus in response to a wide variety of physiological and emotional stressors and is tailored to the type and severity of each stressor. The stress response activates organs throughout the body in a rapid, integrated reaction that aims to maintain the body's homeostasis against any threat. We have seen how the perception of external cues such as seeing a snake or internal cues such as a fall in blood oxygenation trigger a cascade of neural and endocrine activity, starting with an almost instantaneous response from the sympathetic nervous system in the "fight or flight" reaction driven by the secretion of adrenaline from the adrenal medulla and other sympathetic ganglia. This response drives the cardiovascular activation, the increase in respiration and the mobilisation of energy stores to provide fuel for the body's response. Even within this response by the autonomic nervous system the body strives for balance with the reflex activation of the parasympathetic nervous system to constrain the sympathetic nervous system and conserve the body's reserves. The immediate response of the autonomic nervous system is paralleled by the activation of the HPA axis causing the secretion of CRH, then ACTH, and eventually cortisol from the adrenal cortex. This complements the activity prompted by the autonomic nervous system and prolongs the body's response over hours to days.

The general adaptive response to stress is a normal response of the body. The continuation of the response, its pathological elicitation in normal situations or the development of a chronic stress response, can see these normal functions develop into some of the symptoms of anxiety. Thus an understanding of the normal physiology of the stress response can inform our understanding of the mechanisms underlying the symptomatology of anxiety, helping us to educate people suffering from anxiety as to why they might be feeling the way they do. It can also help in the development of treatment for anxiety disorders.

> An understanding of the normal physiology of the stress response can inform our understanding of the mechanisms underlying the symptomatology of anxiety.

PART III   GENETICS AND GENE-
ENVIRONMENT INTERACTION

In a previous chapter, Anabel described her anxiety symptoms. In a subsequent interview, she discusses her son's debilitating anxiety and wonders if her own anxiety has caused it, or whether the disorder is genetic.

"Does he see me anxious, then he becomes anxious, or is it in his genes and my genes?"

Anabel's observations about her son's anxiety get to the heart of the nature versus nurture debate. It is known that anxiety runs in families, but the fact that a particular disorder is common within a family does not necessarily imply that it is genetic.

There are many things that families will have in common that are related to cultural transmission and have nothing to do with genes. For example, all members of a family may speak English but English-speaking is not under genetic control. Anabel's concern that her son's symptoms could have been learned within the family context is very relevant. Behavioural and psychodynamic theories would suggest that the symptoms of anxiety are learned, or developed, within the family context.

But the fact that symptoms can be learned or developed within the family does not rule out the possibility that there could be a strong genetic component to them as well.

There is a well-defined process in determining the genetics of the anxiety disorders.

The first step is to find out whether it is true that the disorder runs in families. This is done using well-established techniques of family studies, in which the rates of disorders among family members are determined. If high rates of the disorder aggregate in families it suggests, but does not confirm, a genetic component to the disorder.

The next step in determining whether there is a genetic component is to use either adoption studies or twin studies. In adoption studies, the rates of the disorder among the adopted away children of affected probands (who would not have the experience of being raised in an "anxious" family) are studied. In twin studies, the concordance rates among monozygotic (identical) twins and dizygotic (non-identical) twins are compared. Higher concordance rates among monozygotic twins compared to dizygotic twins point to a genetic cause.

Once a genetic link has been established, the next step is to identify the gene – or, more likely, the genes – involved in the anxiety disorders, by using linkage and association studies. In considering the nature versus nurture debate, it is becoming increasingly clear that the answer is not straightforward, as we now recognise that the genes interact with the environment. This is proving to be a very fruitful area of research and is discussed later in Part IV.

CHAPTER 10   GENETIC EPIDEMIOLOGY OF
ANXIETY DISORDERS

Naomi Wray

COMMON COMPLEX GENETIC DISORDERS

Anxiety disorders and other psychiatric disorders are known as "complex genetic disorders". Other examples of complex genetic disorders are: breast cancer, coronary artery disease, and type 2 diabetes. Common complex genetic disorders are common disorders occurring in the population, which tend to run in families. This is the first line of evidence that these disorders may have genetic factors contributing to their aetiology. However, despite the fact that these disorders run in families, there is no clear pattern of inheritance, which implies that they are not controlled by a single gene. Instead, they are caused by multiple genetic and environmental risk factors working together.

However, families share a common home environment as well as genetic material, so it is important to determine whether this shared familiality reflects shared genes or a shared environment.

INCREASED RISK TO RELATIVES

We can measure the familiality of a disorder by measuring the prevalence of the disorder in the population and measuring its prevalence in relatives of affected individuals – for example, in the children of affected people. Figure 10.1 includes schizophrenia and major depressive disorder to allow some comparisons with the anxiety disorders.

It is very difficult to tell which disorder has the highest contribution of genetic factors to its underlying causality, because both the population prevalence and the prevalence in children differ. For example, the population prevalence of OCD and schizophrenia are about the same, yet the prevalence of schizophrenia in the children of those with schizophrenia is higher than the equivalent rates for OCD. This implies, correctly, a higher genetic contribution to schizophrenia than OCD. However, it is hard to draw other conclusions from this graph. For this reason, the genetic contribution to disorders or traits is expressed as the heritability, which is calculated from the prevalence estimates.

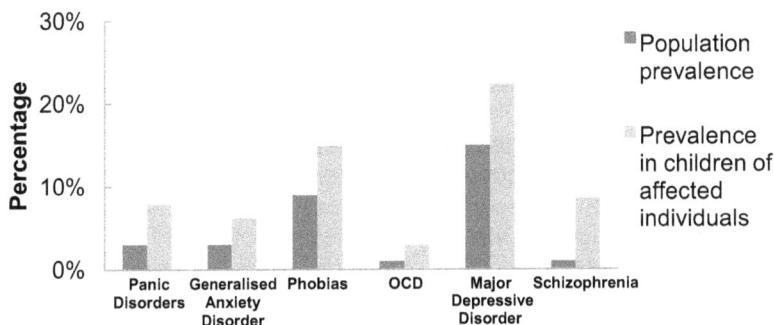

Figure 10.1 Prevalence of mental disorders in population and in children of affected individuals

To make a fair comparison between the prevalence in the population and the prevalence in the children of people with disorders, it is important to ensure that the estimates are drawn from the same demographic region. It is also important to account for the fact that the lifetime prevalence in the children is censored compared to that of their parents, because they are younger and may not yet have reached the age of onset. When disorders are uncommon, large sample sizes are needed in order to estimate these prevalences with certainty. However, it is also important to remember, when interpreting prevalence rates and the estimates of heritability derived from them, that estimates can be inaccurate.

ESTIMATING HERITABILITY

Everyone has an innate awareness of the heritability of human height. It is also commonly known that the distribution of height in the population is approximately normal or bell-shaped and that tall parents tend to have tall children, while short parents tend to have short children. However, there is also a lot of variation in height between the children in a family, which is consistent both with genetic segregation and non-genetic effects. Genetic segregation means that, although each child receives half its genetic material from their mother and half from their father, each child receives a differing sample of genes, which causes variation within the family. When the height difference between the sexes – i.e., that men are taller than women – is corrected for, the heritability of height is 80%, which means that 80% of the variation in height between individuals can be attributed to genetic differences.

HERITABILITY OF LIABILITY

It is more difficult to think about heritability of a binary disease trait. To estimate heritability, it should be assumed that there is an unobserved liability to disease. Liability can be explained thus: hypertension is the medical term given to the condition experienced by people with high blood pressure. Blood pressure can be measured and is normally distributed, so a person's blood pressure represents their liability to hypertension. For many complex genetic disorders like anxiety disorders, there is no liability that can be measured directly, but it is not intuitively unreasonable to imagine that there is an underlying liability – a sort of spectrum – to anxiety. A dimension of personality, for example, might approximate the liability to anxiety.

In estimating heritability, it is assumed that the distribution of that liability in the population is approximately normally distributed. It is reasonable to assume a normal distribution, because experience indicates that most things that are measured have a normal distribution, the key feature of which is that it is unimodal and symmetric. This is consistent with many underlying risk factors. Given a normal distribution of liability, it can be assumed that those individuals ranked at the top of the liability curve have the disease (Figure 10.2), so the proportion of the area under the normal curve – that is in the shaded region on the top graph of Figure 10.2 – is equal to the prevalence of the disease in the population.

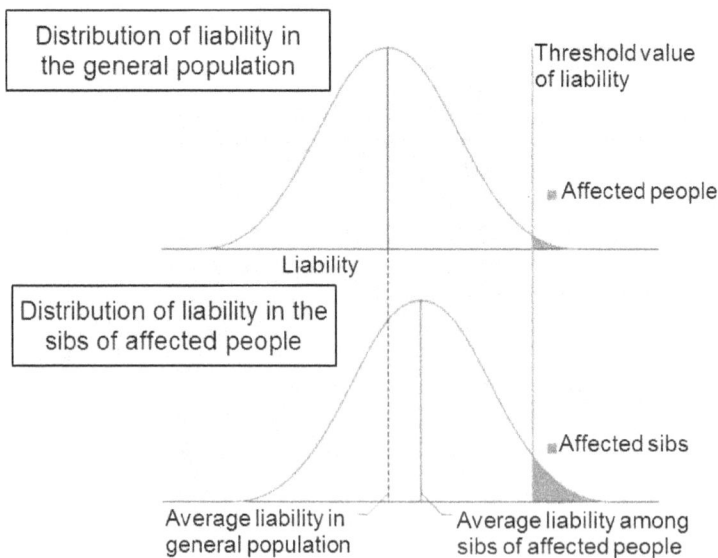

Figure 10.2   Distribution of liability

The distribution of liability in children of affected individuals is also normal. If the bottom graph of Figure 10.2 is moved horizontally until the proportion of the shaded area corresponds to the prevalence of the disease in children of those affected, the difference in the position of the mean of the bottom graph compared to the top graph, and the fact that parents share half of their genetic complement with their children, can be used to calculate what proportion of the variance in liability must be genetic to be consistent with the observed data. That is how heritability and liability are estimated.

HERITABILITY OF LIABILITY TO SCHIZOPHRENIA

Before considering the heritability of liability of anxiety disorders, it is useful to consider the heritability of schizophrenia, which is about 80%, similar to the heritability of height. The prevalence of schizophrenia in the population is about 1%, and about 8–10% of children of schizophrenics have schizophrenia.

One way to understand why these numbers are consistent and make sense is to think of a cohort of 100 people in any sector of the population. The tallest person in that cohort will be the top 1%. Their family members, or first-degree relatives – mothers, fathers, brothers and sisters – are probably all tall, but probably fewer than 10% of them would also qualify as being in the 1% based on height. This observation is also consistent with rates of schizophrenia in first-degree relatives of those affected by schizophrenia.

As more is learned about complex genetic disorders, the empirical evidence is consistent with this analogy. However, the analogy does not claim that schizophrenia and height have the same genetic risk factors. It is about the genetic architecture underpinning the traits, which is an architecture of many genetic and environmental risk factors of small effect.

HERITABILITY OF ANXIETY DISORDERS

In this chapter, the theory of heritability of liability is applied to the observed prevalence rates of anxiety disorders. Figure 10.3 shows the prevalence rates in the general population and in children of affected individuals whereas Figure 10.4 shows the heritability of liability of the same disorders. The graph shows some variation between the estimates for the different anxiety disorders, but the estimates are not statistically different. It is generally recognised that the heritability of both anxiety disorders and major depression is about 40%. In contrast, the estimate of heritability for schizophrenia is much higher, at about 80%.

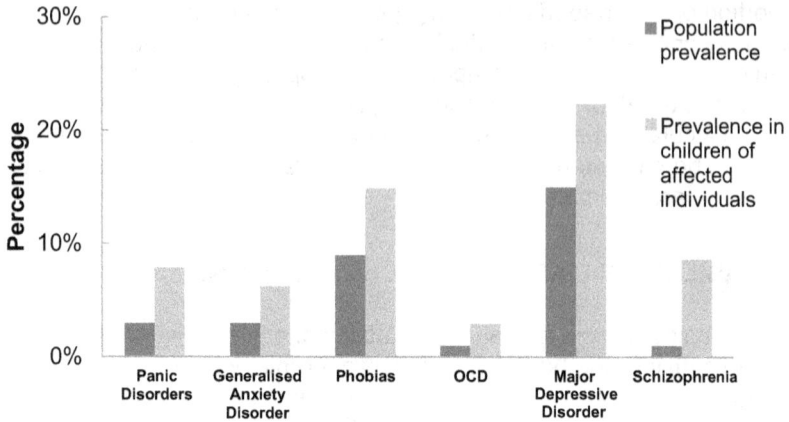

Figure 10.3 Prevalence of liability of mental disorders

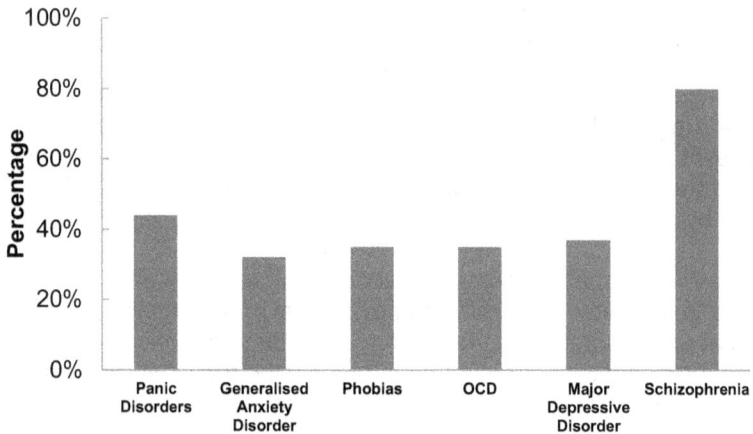

Figure 10.4 Heritability of liability of mental disorders

GENETIC FACTORS VERSUS FAMILY ENVIRONMENT

So far, in estimating heritability, all familiality has been assumed to be a reflection of shared genetic factors only, but family members also share their family environment. One way to separate the genetic factor from the fact of the shared family environment is to compare the rates of disease in adopted children with the rates in their biological and adoptive parents. This is a neat experimental design to separate the effects of genetics and common family environment. But as such data are hard to come by, an experimental design provided by nature can be used.

THE USE OF MONOZYGOTIC AND DIZYGOTIC TWINS

As far back as 1875, the Victorian polymath Sir Francis Galton discussed the use of monozygotic (identical) and dizygotic (non-identical) twins, in order to disentangle the relative contribution of the genetic and common environmental effects to resemblance between relatives.

Monozygotic (MZ) twins receive the same genetic complement from their parents. However, MZ twins are not useful alone, because they also share the same family environment.

In contrast, dizygotic (DZ) twins share half their genetic complement (just like ordinary siblings) and share the same family environment. The comparison of sets of MZ and DZ twins can thus be used to tease apart the genetic and common environment component of familiality.

MZ TWINS VERSUS DZ TWINS

Figures 10.5 and 10.6 below show body postures of MZ and DZ twins. These twin pairs were all adopted at birth, each individual twin to a different family, so that each had a different family environment. The photographs clearly show that the body posture of MZ twins is more similar to that of DZ twins, but even DZ twins are more similar to each other than to the other twin pairs shown here. The similarity between the different types of twins is estimated to quantify the relative importance of genes and environment to any particular characteristic that has been measured.

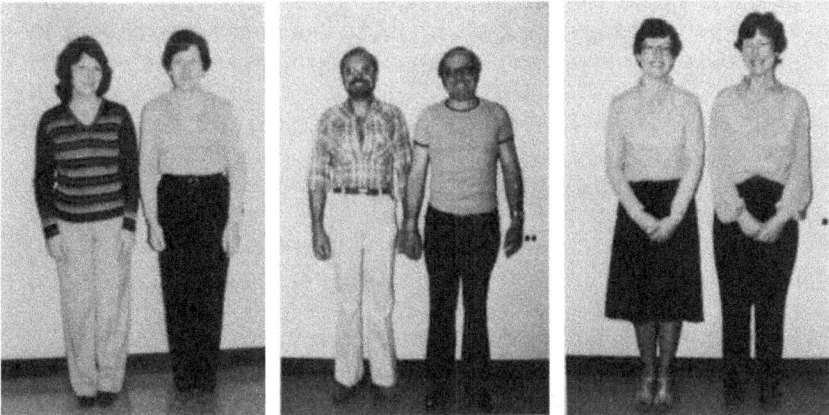

Figure 10.5 Body postures of identical (MZ) twins. From Bouchard (1984). Reproduced with permission of Plenum Press.

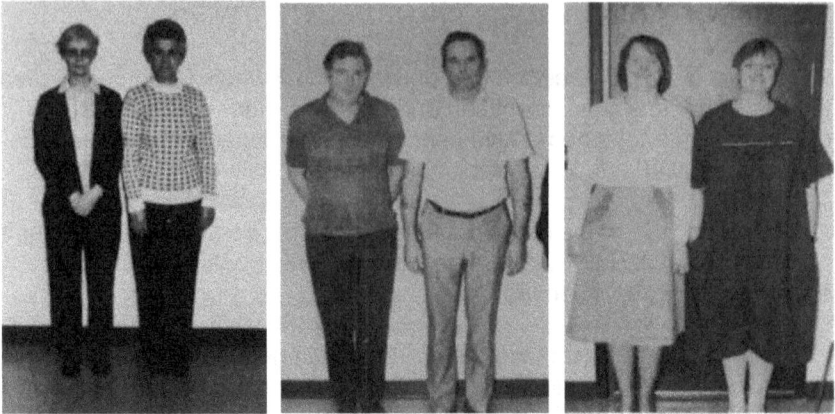

Figure 10.6 Body postures of non-identical (DZ) twins. From Bouchard (1984). Reproduced with permission of Plenum Press.

ASSUMPTIONS UNDERLYING HERITABILITY ESTIMATES FROM TWINS

Estimating heritability from twin pairs requires some assumptions. The two key assumptions are discussed below.

Assumption 1: On average, the impact of the family environment is the same on MZ and DZ twins.

This assumption has been questioned, on the basis that parents provide a more equal environment for MZ than for DZ twins. However, a number of experimental designs have shown that although this may be true, the more equal environment is in response to the more equal behaviour of MZ twins. Other studies have specifically considered families where the children are MZ but the parents consider them to be DZ, and vice versa. Lastly, for some disorders heritability has been estimated from different types of relatives; not just twins, but siblings and second or third degree relatives. With these more distant relatives, the shared environment becomes more diluted, yet the estimates of heritability across the different types of relatives have been about the same.

Modern genetic studies have examined this issue by using variants measured directly in the DNA of affected individuals who are unrelated in the classical sense – that is, they are completely unknown to each other, more distant than third cousins – but who share genetic variants at the DNA level, because of common distant ancestors. These studies also provide estimates of heritability consistent with the estimates from twin studies.

Together, these results support the claim that twin studies provide a valid way to estimate the genetic contribution to traits and disorders. However, these are general findings across a range of disorders and traits, which may not hold for all traits. The number of studies that have estimated heritabilities for anxiety disorders are limited, so the underlying assumptions should always be borne in mind when interpreting these estimates.

Assumption 2: Estimates of heritability can be inflated if there is a correlation between genotype and environment.

For example, it is intuitive to imagine that mothers with high IQ will pass high IQ genes to their children, but may also provide a more stimulating environment to them. In other words, high IQ genes are correlated with high IQ environments, and this may serve to inflate the estimates of heritability.

For many traits and disorders, it can be hard to imagine a genotype-environment correlation, but in relation to anxiety disorders, it is possible to imagine that children growing up in a household with anxious parents may be more aware of anxiety-inducing events than other children.

The existence of a genotype-environment correlation depends on whether genetically anxious parents, exposed to the same environmental stressors as genetically non-anxious parents, would produce a more anxious environment for their children. This is quite a subtle distinction and, once again, there is a dearth of information on it for anxiety disorders, so it is hard to draw any definite conclusions.

Comorbidity between Disorders

Many anxiety disorders co-occur in the same individual. Similarly, anxiety and depression are often diagnosed in the same individual. The general consensus in the field is that it is likely that the same genetic variants are responsible for both anxiety and depression.

> Children growing up in a household with anxious parents may be more aware of anxiety-inducing events than other children.

GENETIC AND PHENOTYPIC CORRELATIONS BETWEEN ANXIETY DISORDERS AND MAJOR DEPRESSION

In Table 10.1, the genetic and environmental relationship between disorders is quantified. The genetic correlations are very high; that between panic disorder and agoraphobia is particularly high at 0.83. The lower environmental correlations between major depression and the anxiety disorders partially result from the differences in prevalence rates. This supports the concept of shared genetic factors between anxiety disorders, and between anxiety disorders and major depression.

Table 10.1 Genetic and environmental relationship between anxiety disorders and major depression

	Major depression	Panic disorder	Agoraphobia	Social phobia
Heritabilities	0.33	0.38	0.48	0.39
Genetic correlations				
Major depression		0.79	0.70	0.76
Panic disorder			0.83	0.60
Agoraphobia				0.53
Environmental correlations				
Major depression		0.22	0.30	0.17
Panic disorder		0.67	0.52	0.67
Agoraphobia				0.71
Phenotypic correlations				
Major depression		0.42	0.45	0.37
Panic disorder			0.73	0.54
Agoraphobia				0.63

Note. From Mosing et at. (2009). Reproduced with permission of Wiley.

Parents affected with a disorder often wish to know whether their children might be affected with the same disorder. There are increased rates of anxiety disorders in children of those affected with the disorders. The heritability of anxiety disorders is about 40%, which means that about 40% of the variation in anxiety traits observed between individuals in the general population can be attributed to genetic risk factors. Environmental risk factors also have an important contribution to anxiety disorders, which means that anxiety symptoms are modifiable through intervention strategies. Children of those with anxiety disorders will have an increased risk of being affected, so it is important that symptoms are picked up earlier, to allow early intervention therapies such as cognitive behaviour therapy (CBT).

CHAPTER 11 IDENTIFICATION OF GENETIC FACTORS CONTRIBUTING TO ANXIETY DISORDERS

Naomi Wray

FROM HERITABILITY OF LIABILITY TO IDENTIFICATION OF SPECIFIC GENETIC RISK VARIANTS

The last chapter explored the results from genetic epidemiology studies. These studies show that the heritability for anxiety disorders is about 40% – that is, 40% of the variation in anxiety between individuals in the general population is of genetic origin.

Notably, the contribution of environmental risk factors is greater for anxiety disorders than for the more severe psychiatric disorders, such as schizophrenia. The studies also provide evidence for an important shared genetic aetiology between different anxiety disorders, and between anxiety disorders and major depression.

For any complex genetic disorder, it is reasonable to seek out the specific genetic variants that contribute to the observed heritability. Those genetic variants are encoded in the DNA that is passed from parent to child. There is a whole range of different types of genetic variant. In fact, 99% of the DNA code is shared between individuals; i.e., it is not polymorphic. This makes sense, because much of the code is tied up with functions central to life. It is the DNA code that differs between individuals – that is, the polymorphisms – that is of interest here. Polymorphisms could be single nucleotide polymorphisms (SNPs) or inversions, deletions or duplications. The purpose of identifying genetic variants is to inform understanding of the causes of anxiety disorders and, ultimately, to inform diagnostic and treatment strategies.

> The contribution of environmental risk factors is greater for anxiety disorders than for the more severe psychiatric disorders, such as schizophrenia.

GENETIC LINKAGE STUDIES

A number of genetic approaches have been considered. The first was genetic linkage studies. These studies require collections of family members with recorded disease status, as well as DNA for measuring genetic markers across the genome. Linkage analysis searches for regions of the genome that are shared by affected members and not shared by unaffected members of the family. This type of study has been highly successful for identifying the genes affecting very rare disorders. However it was not very successful for complex genetic disorders in general, because large pedigrees with multiple affected members of families are not usually available. Another type of linkage study used affected sibling pairs. It was hoped that this type of study would identify regions of the genome shared by affected siblings and also shared across families. These studies could identify only genetic variants of intermediate to large effect and, across all complex genetic disorders, linkage studies generated few replicated results. One of the notable linkage studies for anxiety disorders was by Camp and colleagues using Mormon pedigrees from Utah (Camp et al. 2005).

GENETIC ASSOCIATION STUDIES

Advances in technology allowed genotyping of specific SNPs in association studies – that is, testing for an association between a genetic polymorphism and case-control status. Figure 11.1 shows DNA code in which the dark letters represent bases pairs that do not vary in the population, while the grey letters represent bases that are polymorphic in the population. These are the single nucleotide polymorphisms. The squares represent alleles of a genetic marker in cases and controls. In this example, the shaded allele is more common in cases than controls, so it is associated with disease status.

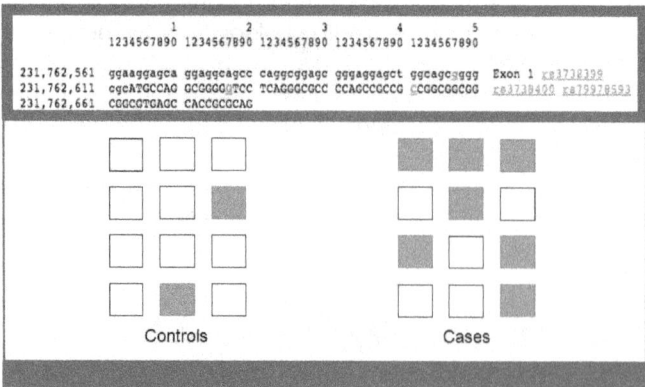

Figure 11.1 Genetic polymorphism and case-control status

CANDIDATE GENES

Candidate genes are genes for which there is some prior evidence that they may contribute to the causes of disease.

When the technology to genotype SNPs first became available, association studies were designed to consider candidate genes only. However, candidate gene studies generated little conclusive evidence about association with common complex genetic disorders in general. Compared to other disorders, relatively few studies were conducted for anxiety disorders. A key result of a review of candidate gene studies for anxiety disorders by Smoller, Block, & Young (2009) was that, in at least two studies, only six candidate variants showed evidence of association, but even for these variants the replication evidence was weak.

A review of molecular genetics studies for panic disorder by Maron et al. (2010) also concluded that candidate gene studies had not been successful in identifying associated genetic variants. The same conclusion has been drawn for candidate gene studies across most complex genetic disorders. This implies either that the choice of genes to study was poor, or that the effect sizes of genetic risk variants were smaller than expected, so the studies were underpowered and the sample sizes were too small to detect the associations.

MOUSE STUDIES

Of all psychiatric disorders, anxiety disorders are the easiest to explore using mouse models. The Oxford psychiatrist Jonathan Flint was a dedicated advocate of using mouse models for the discovery of loci associated with anxiety in mice, in order to guide human studies. In 1995 he wrote in the magazine *Science*: "There are cogent reasons for expecting that the genetic basis of emotionality is similar in other species and that it may underlie the psychological trait of susceptibility to anxiety in humans." (Flint et al., 1995, p. 1434).

Thirteen years later, after carrying out many comprehensive studies to identify genetic loci associated with quantitative traits of anxiety in mice, he concluded differently. In Fullerton et al. (2008), Flint and colleagues concluded that the complexity of the genetic basis of anxiety meant that using the mouse for discovery of disease causing variants in humans had limited utility. However, this does not mean that mouse models can play no role. Indeed, Flint continued to use the mouse model, although in different ways. Mouse models may be useful for investigating the function of genes identified from human studies, and for identifying pathways that might be relevant to human disease.

ADVANCES WHICH HAVE ENABLED GENOME-WIDE ASSOCIATION STUDIES

Since 2007, it has been possible to conduct genome-wide association studies. Three important advances made these studies possible.

Firstly, the Human Genome Project provided a greater understanding of variation in the genome. In a nutshell, although there are three billion base pairs in the DNA that comprise the human genome, only ten million bases commonly vary between individuals in the population. Moreover, many of the variants within chromosomal regions are correlated, which means that about 80% of the common variation can be captured by genotyping only 500,000 markers in the genome. That is, only 5% of variants can be genotyped but 80% of the variation can be captured, which makes a very cost effective study.

The second advance was in genotyping technology. It is now possible to genotype 500,000 positions simultaneously for about AU$700 (and costs are dropping all the time).

Lastly, researchers came together in a spirit of collaboration to pool sample collections, in order to generate very large samples of cases and controls.

These advances have allowed genome-wide association studies, which are no longer dependent on an ad-hoc selection of candidate genes. Instead, the genome can be interrogated in an unbiased way, thus allowing it to tell us which variants are associated with disease.

In a genome-wide association study (GWAS), scientists know that, because they are genotyping only 5% of the polymorphisms, any association they find is unlikely to be the causal variant. However, it flags a relatively small genomic region in which to investigate the association at the functional level.

THE WELLCOME TRUST CASE CONTROL CONSORTIUM

The beginning of the GWAS era was marked by the publication of the Wellcome Trust Case Control Consortium Study, in which 2,000 cases from each of seven diseases and 3,000 common controls were genotyped (The Wellcome Trust Case Control Consortium, 2007). The results are shown in Figure 11.4. The plots are called Manhattan plots, because the associations form towers that look like the Manhattan skyline.

In the plots, each dot represents the p-value of the test of association between a single nucleotide polymorphism (SNP) and the disorder.

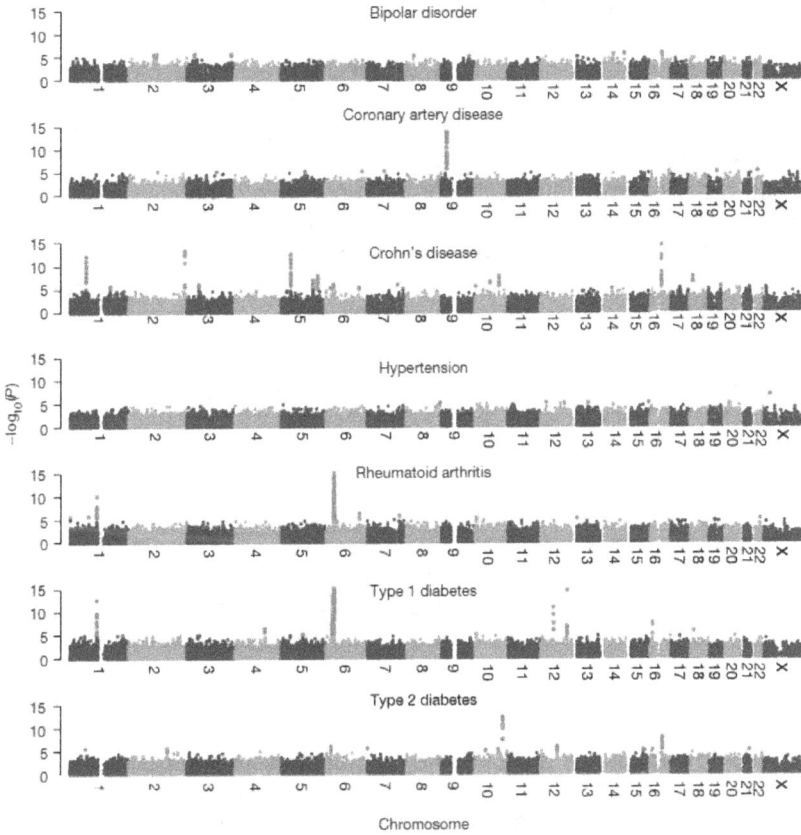

Figure 11.4   Genome-wide scan for seven diseases. From The Wellcome Trust Case Control Consortium (2007). Reproduced with permission of Nature Publishing Group.

The x-axis represents the position of the chromosomes in the genome, from chromosome 1 to chromosome 22, and, lastly, the X chromosome. Dark and grey denote alternate chromosomes. When chromosome numbers were first allocated, they were allocated by size, hence the decreasing length of the chromosome from left to right. The y-axis is on the scale of minus log10 of the p-value of association. That means the bigger values represent more association.

Because 500,000 SNPs are being tested, large sample sizes are needed to demonstrate that the associations detected are not simply chance findings.

GENOME-WIDE ASSOCIATION STUDIES: A SUCCESS FOR COMPLEX GENETIC DISORDERS IN GENERAL

Since 2007, many genome-wide association studies have been conducted for a range of complex genetic disorders. These studies have been considered paradigm shifting, with more progress made in this time period that in the previous 20 years. It has been recognised that "compelling signals have been found, often highlighting previously unsuspected biology" (McCarthy et al., 2008, p. 356). In 2007, very few genetic variants associated with common complex genetic diseases/disorders had been identified, but in the 4-year period since, there has been an unprecedented period of discovery (Visscher et al., 2012). For some complex genetic disorders, results from GWAS have already led to clinical trials for new treatments.

GENOME-WIDE ASSOCIATION STUDIES: A SUCCESS FOR BIPOLAR DISORDER AND SCHIZOPHRENIA

For the first time, genetic studies are generating important new information about genetic contributions to psychiatric disorders. In September 2011, mega-analyses of the genome-wide association studies for bipolar disorder and schizophrenia were published in the magazine *Nature Genetics*. The bipolar study had more than 7,000 cases and 9,000 controls and the schizophrenia study had more than 9,000 cases and 12,000 controls.

It is clear that these studies have only identified a small fraction of contributing genetic variants, but the methodological approach has been validated, opening the way for future discoveries. These studies have demonstrated that many genetic variants contribute to psychiatric disorders, each of small effect.

VISUALISING COMMON COMPLEX GENETIC DISEASES

It is generally accepted that complex genetic disorders, including anxiety disorders, are underpinned by many variants of small effect. It can be difficult to visualise what this means for individual people. A simple way to visualise this is to imagine that the causes of a disease are explained by 100 genetic variants, and the risk allele at each locus has a frequency of 10% in the population. The pie chart in Figure 11.5 represents a person's genetic profile, with each slice of pie representing the genotype at one of the loci. The slice of pie is blank if a person carries two alleles of no effect, grey if they carry one risk allele, and dark if they carry two risk loci. In theory, people could carry between zero and 200 risk alleles, but in actuality, these extremes are impossible (just like tossing 200 heads from a flip of a coin). Most people will carry between 12 and 38 risk alleles. In the case of Figure 11.5, there are 20 risk alleles in that person's genetic profile. If a disease has a prevalence of 1% in the population, then people who are diseased carry more than 30 risk alleles.

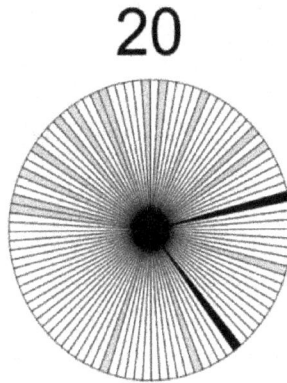

Figure 11.5   A simple model of a person's genetic profile

Unaffected people also carry many risk alleles. This is consistent with a very robust biological system; that is, if an individual carries some risk alleles, they will have back-up systems to compensate for sub-optimal gene products generated from these loci. People who are affected by a disorder carry multiple genetic risk factors, which, in combination with environmental risks, generate a burden of dysfunction for which their system can no longer compensate. This explanation is also consistent with the small effect sizes for each risk allele, because the difference in allele frequency between cases and controls at any locus will be small. The importance of carrying a risk locus depends on the genetic and environmental background that accompanies it.

Each affected person could carry a unique genetic profile of risk alleles that would be consistent with the heterogeneity in symptoms of psychiatric disorders. Some risk profile patterns are more similar to each other than other patterns, which might be consistent with similar symptoms or response to treatment.

GENOME-WIDE ASSOCIATION STUDIES: NOT SUCCESSFUL FOR MAJOR DEPRESSIVE DISORDER OR PERSONALITY TRAIT NEUROTICISM

Six genome-wide association studies have been published for major depression. These studies have been brought together by the Psychiatric GWAS Consortium for major depressive disorder, for a total of nearly

10,000 cases and 10,000 controls. No variants identified as being associated, and this result was replicated in independent samples.

Similarly, a sample of over 17,000 individuals measured for the personality trait neuroticism identified no significant associations.

These results are disappointing but not surprising, given what has been found with other complex genetic disorders. Because major depression is very common in the general population, larger samples are needed, compared to less common disorders. A study of 10,000 cases of major depression has the same power as a study of fewer than 4,000 cases of schizophrenia.

NO GENOME WIDE ASSOCIATION STUDIES CONDUCTED FOR ANXIETY DISORDERS

To date, no GWAS have been published for anxiety disorders. In a recent commentary article, Professor Jordan Smoller of Harvard University gave some explanation as to why this was so. "Compared with the explosion of large-scale genetic research on other mental disorders – autism, attention-deficit/hyperactivity disorder, schizophrenia, bipolar disorder, depression – genetic studies of anxiety disorders have been relatively scarce," he wrote. "Some of this might be due to disparities in funding and advocacy, but a more fundamental reason might have to do with the complexity of the phenotype itself" (Smoller, 2011, p. 506). The complexities of the phenotype might have fostered a "fear of anxiety genetics".

CHAPTER 12   GENE-ENVIRONMENT INTERACTION AND HUMAN BEHAVIOUR

Richie Poulton

GENETIC UNDERPINNINGS OF HUMAN BEHAVIOURS

There is a great deal of interest in understanding the genetic underpinnings of a whole range of human behaviours. Most research in this area has attempted to identify direct linear relationships with the behaviours of interest.

Unfortunately, this approach has not been particularly successful. Most studies have failed to identify genes associated with certain behaviours and the handful that have, often fail to replicate; in other words, they are flimsy. The problem with the very small number that do replicate is that the genes explain very little variation in the phenotype of interest. In other words, the genes are weakly associated with the behavioural outcome.

An alternative way of thinking about this issue is to try to model genes that are interacting with an environment. It is probably reasonable to suggest, *a priori*, that human variation, or behavioural difference, is likely to be a product of multiple genes interacting, which then interact with multiple environments, which again interact with each other. It is this gene-environment interaction, which occurs in a dynamic and at different points in the life course, that gives rise to variability among human beings.

THE CYCLE OF VIOLENCE

The conventional wisdom around the turn of the century was that gene-environment interactions as described above were extremely rare. They were hard to demonstrate and if they did exist, they were probably of little consequence. One paper in particular changed thinking. *Role of Genotype in the Cycle of Violence in Maltreated Children* published in *Science* (Caspi et al., 2002), started with the finding that childhood maltreatment elevates the risk of growing into a maltreater, and of becoming a criminal, by about 50%. The 50% figure indicates that the odds ratio of relative risk is about 1.5.

In other words, there are many people who are exposed but do not progress to become delinquents or criminals.

This is an age-old puzzle. Why is it that some do and some do not progress? Some have posited psychological differences in terms of cognitive personality as the explanation, and behavioural scientists have suggested that it might be due to a difference in genetic endowment. The genetic endowment is related to a gene called the MAOA gene, which will be described later in this chapter.

GENETIC FACTORS AND ENVIRONMENTAL RISK EXPOSURE

Genes can act to increase or decrease environmental risk exposure. This is known as gene-environment correlation. There are two main types of gene-environment correlation: passive and evocative (or active).

An example of passive gene-environment correlation is where two parents who provide genetic material to their offspring, also provide the early, sometimes high-risk, rearing environment.

Evocative, or active gene-environment correlations, are typically seen when, over time, people select certain environmental niches for themselves (such as in social gatherings), then, once in those environmental contexts, behave in a certain way.

A good example of this is the difference between an extrovert and an introvert. The extrovert seeks out social gatherings and behaves in a gregarious fashion whilst in those settings, while the introvert tends to avoid or shun such gatherings. Gene-environment correlation can be a problem when trying to model gene-environment interaction – in this example, how someone behaves in a social gathering – and needs to be ruled out.

GENETIC FACTORS AND THE INFLUENCE OF ENVIRONMENTAL RISKS

Genes also act to determine how we respond to certain environmental risk factors. These days, people get much of their information about health from the media, which leads them to think of genes like time bombs ticking away in their bodies, about to give them a heart attack, cancer, or make them depressed. But from an evolutionary point of view, it makes sense that genes may also have a protective function. For example, some people are resistant or resilient to malaria based on their genotype, while others are not. This idea can be extended to include psychosocial pathogens.

GENETIC SUSCEPTIBILITY TO CHILDHOOD MALTREATMENT

Genetic susceptibility to childhood maltreatment is characterised in terms of individual differences in a functional polymorphism in the promoter of the monoamine oxidase A type (MAOA) gene. The MAOA gene is a functional gene, which regulates three important neurotransmitters in the brain: dopamine, serotonin and/or adrenaline.

A polymorphism is a gene in which there is a naturally occurring variation in the population. For example, everyone has a gene that dictates that they have two eyes; it comes in only one form. But individuals also have a polymorphic gene, a naturally occurring variation in that gene, that determines their eye colour, and which varies across the population. Some people have a set of blue eyes, some green, some hazel and some brown.

This, then, is a polymorphic gene of known function, in this case the MAOA gene.

TESTING GENE-ENVIRONMENT INTERACTION IN A COHORT DESIGN

In one ongoing study begun nearly three decades ago, researchers at Dunedin University obtained genetic information on a longitudinal birth cohort. The study subjects were an unselected group of people representative of the general population, who were born in the early 1970s in Dunedin, New Zealand, and who have been followed and measured repeatedly for over 26 years as they have grown up to become young adults.

DNA was obtained directly from them, and two groups were created from the sample: one was identified as having low MAOA activity, and the other high. Thirty percent of the population will have low MAOA activity, which is known to be the risk variable (the risk allele), and two thirds will have the high version of MAOA activity.

Ethnic stratification – that is, confounding by ethnicity – was ruled out by focusing on those people with four European grandparents. Only the men in this group were looked at because of base rate issues – men are more violent and antisocial.

CHILDHOOD MALTREATMENT

Firstly, in order to characterise the environmental risk variable, five different measures of maltreatment were chosen, which were directly measured in three cases and retrospectively obtained in two (Table 12.1).

Paediatricians observed the mothers' behaviour when they were assessing the children at the age of three. At the first assessment, mothers were deemed to be behaving in an atypical fashion if their treatment or interaction with their child was rough and awkward, and the mother appeared indifferent to the child's needs, e.g. being unconcerned that the child was unkempt.

Table 12.1   Measures of maltreatment

Age	Data collection	Environmental risk variable
3	Directly	Observations of mother's behaviour
7–9	Directly	Parental reports of harsh discipline
11	Directly	Multiple caregiver changes
26	Retrospectively	Physical harm
26	Retrospectively	Unwanted sexual contact

When the children were aged seven and nine, they were asked directly about recent discipline by their parents, then the top 10% in terms of harshness were taken for this particular cohort at the time.

Through to the age of eleven, the child may experience multiple changes in their primary care giver. The children were characterised as having multiple caregivers if they had two or more in their first decade.

When the subjects were aged 26, they were asked to report on having experienced extreme physical violence in their childhood. This would include being beaten, for example with an electric jug cord, to the point where they were left bleeding and bruised, and requiring medical intervention. In addition, they were asked about unwanted sexual contact, ranging from interference with genitalia right through to forced penetrative sex.

All five measures were combined to characterise the first decade of life. When a cumulative exposure was created, 68% of the sample had none of these experiences, 28% had one of those experiences (shown in Figure 12.1 as "some") and 8% had two or more of those experiences in their first decade of life (shown in Figure 12.1 as "severe").

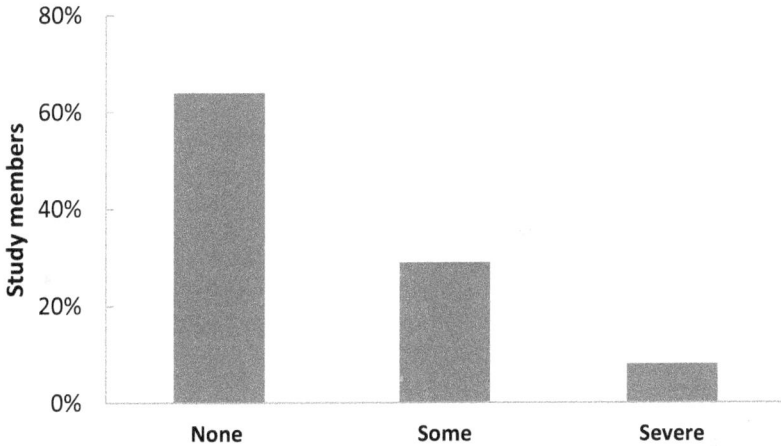

Figure 12.1   Physical violence in childhood

EXPOSURE TO CHILDHOOD MALTREATMENT AS A FUNCTION OF MAOA ACTIVITY

To rule out gene-environment correlation, the relationship between the levels of MAOA gene activity (low and high) and the levels of maltreatment (none, probable and severe) during childhood needed to be examined. Each level of maltreatment shows that there are no appreciable differences based on genotype. In other words, gene-environment correlation can be potentially ruled out.

Next, the high and low MAOA activity of the groups was compared against the severity of childhood maltreatment in the first decade. Evidence for a gene-environment interaction would be found if the MAOA gene modified the influence of maltreatment on the development of severe antisocial behaviour in the children.

CONDUCT DISORDER IN ADOLESCENCE

A diagnosis of conduct disorder during adolescence was considered as an outcome. In other words, those carrying out the study wanted to see if the relationship between childhood maltreatment and a particular version of the MAOA gene predicted a likelihood of being diagnosed with conduct disorder during the adolescent years.

The diagnoses were made according to DSM-IV. They were based on direct interviews at eleven, fifteen and eighteen, and information was augmented via parents and teachers. At each assessment age, the subjects were asked about symptoms during the last twelve months, because it is hard to remember accurately further back than that.

The study found that 28% of the study males were diagnosed with conduct disorder at one or more of those assessment ages.

As shown in Figure 12.2, the findings were consistent with the hypothesis that the relationship between childhood maltreatment and the likelihood of being diagnosed with a conduct disorder was conditional. In other words, it depended on which version of the gene an individual had. This illustrates an interaction. There is a highly significant relationship between levels of maltreatment and the likelihood of conduct disorder diagnosis among those with the low MAOA activity gene hypothesised to be the risk gene, or version of the gene. Among those with the high MAOA activity gene, there is no relationship to speak of, despite high levels of maltreatment.

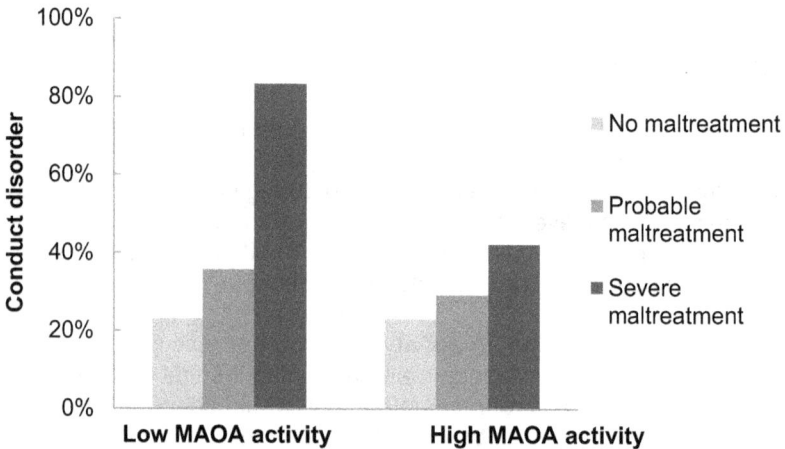

Figure 12.2   Conduct disorder, childhood maltreatment and MAOA activity

After the basic interaction was established, it had to be replicated using an alternative measure of the phenotype; in other words, antisocial behaviour.

PERSONALITY DISPOSITION TOWARD VIOLENCE

The second measure of antisocial behavior was a personality disposition towards violence, via self-report at age 26. This was carried out via the multidimensional personality questionnaire. People who scored highly in the questionnaire endorsed items such as "I daydream about hurting people", "I am quick and hot tempered", "I fly off the handle when I get angry", "I want to smack someone around", or "I enjoy a good brawl".

As shown in Figure 12.3, the study found that the relationship between the MAOA activity gene and a high disposition to violence was conditional. It depended upon which version of the gene the subject had. The relationship was highly significant among those with a low MAOA activity gene and, again, nothing much to speak of for those with a high MAOA activity gene.

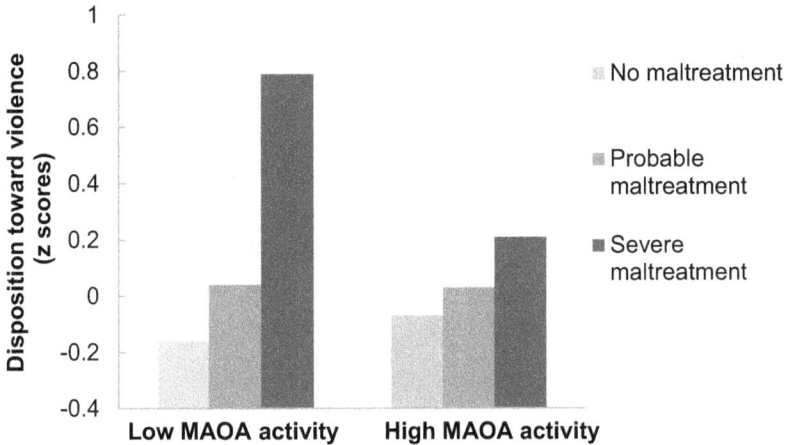

Figure 12.3   Aggressive personality, childhood maltreatment and MAOA activity

ANTISOCIAL PERSONALITY DISORDER SYMPTOMS

The third way that antisocial tendencies were operationalised was to ask people who knew the study members well about their tendency to behave in an antisocial fashion.

With the study members' permission, questionnaires were sent to these people, asking:

- Did our study member have problems controlling their anger?
- Do they blame others for their problems?
- Are they guiltless and remorseless after doing bad things?
- Are they a bad person?
- Do they want to get into a lot of fights?
- Do they break the law?

This was a slightly different approach, in that others were being asked about the study members and their relationship between childhood maltreatment by others.

As shown in Figure 12.4, once more, behaving in an antisocial fashion was conditional, depending upon which version of the gene the individual had: it was strong, clear and highly significant among those with a low MAOA activity gene and, again, was nothing much to speak of among those with a high MAOA activity gene.

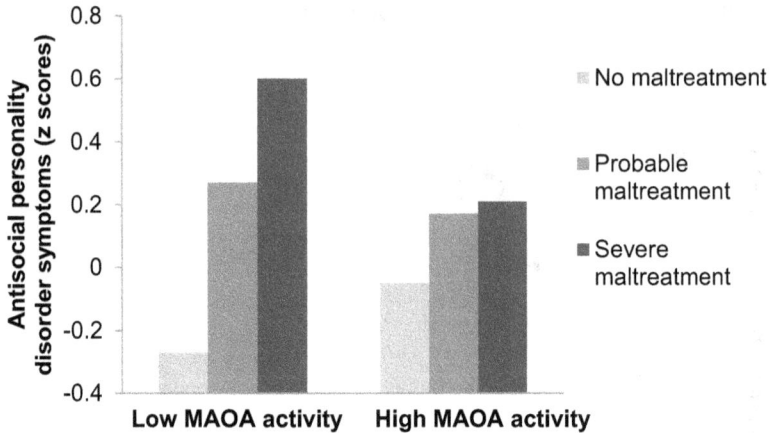

Figure 12.4   Antisocial personality disorder, childhood maltreatment and MAOA activity

CONVICTION FOR VIOLENT CRIME BY AGE 26

Finally, the courts and the New Zealand Police were asked for the court convictions of all the study members up to the age of 26. These showed that 25% of the study males had received just fewer than 1,000 criminal convictions by the age of 26, of which a subset was for violence.

There were about 172 convictions for violence, ranging from a bar room brawl or a common assault conviction, right through to the more severe end of the spectrum of manslaughter and rape.

The study found the relationship between maltreatment as a child and getting a conviction for a violent offence in either New Zealand or Australia was conditional, and depended upon which version of the gene the individual had. Again, the same pattern – a low MAOA activity confers risk in the context of childhood maltreatment and predicts violent offences – was revealed (see Figure 12.5).

There is no prediction from high MAOA activity gene in the context of maltreatment, despite high levels of maltreatment.

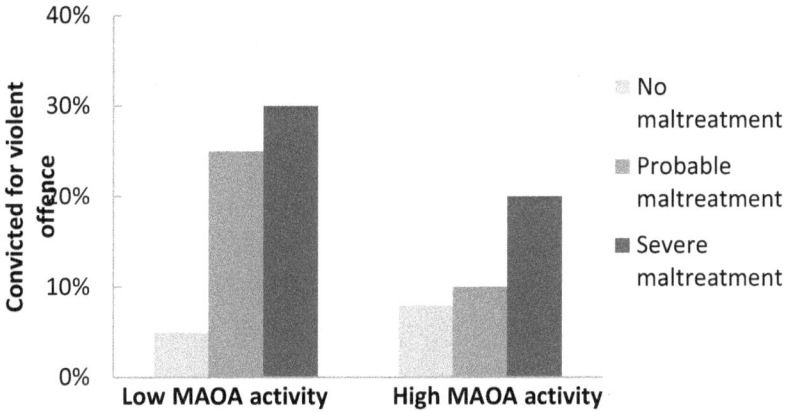

Figure 12.5   Conviction for violent crime by age 26, childhood maltreatment and MAOA activity

THE INTERACTION BETWEEN MAOA AND CHILDHOOD MALTREATMENT

Figure 12.6 shows what a gene-environment interaction looks like when it is plotted on a figure. On the left hand axis is the composite index of antisocial behaviour and on the bottom axis is childhood maltreatment, ranging from none to severe. Low MAOA activity is shown by the grey line and high MAOA by the black line. The graph shows that, despite high levels of maltreatment, the high MAOA activity gene group does not have a significantly elevated score on the composite index of antisocial behaviour. In contrast, the low MAOA activity group has a markedly high score on the antisocial behaviour index.

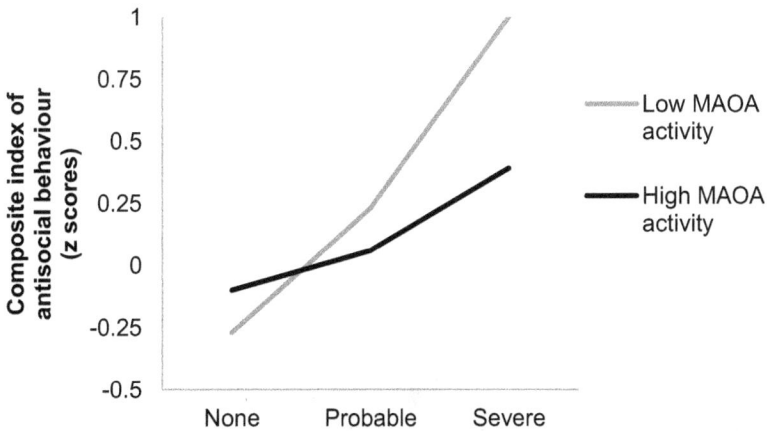

Figure 12.6   Antisocial behaviour, childhood maltreatment and MAOA activity

When the relationship between the gene type and the composite index independent of, or blind to, childhood maltreatment history was examined, no relationship was found. The gene alone could not project antisocial behaviour. It was only when it was placed in the context of childhood maltreatment that prediction could be seen.

PART III SUMMARY

Anxiety disorders and other psychiatric disorders are known as "complex genetic disorders" – common disorders occurring in the population, which tend to run in families. However, despite the fact that these disorders run in families, they are not controlled by a single gene but are caused by multiple genetic and environmental risk factors working together.

As families share a common home environment as well as genetic material, it is important to determine whether this shared familiality reflects shared genes or a shared environment. Part III discussed how to measure the heritability of a disorder by measuring the prevalence of the disorder in the population and estimating its prevalence in relatives of affected individuals.

However, children growing up in a household with anxious parents may be more aware of anxiety-inducing events than other children so the genetic factor has to be separated from the fact of the shared family environment. This can be done using monozygotic and dizygotic twin studies, which provide a valid way to estimate the genetic contribution to traits and disorders.

Part III discussed the various approaches that have sought the specific genetic variants that contribute to the observed heritability. Since 2007, many genome-wide association studies have been conducted for a range of complex genetic disorders. The progress in this area has been paradigm shifting, and for the first time, genetic studies are generating important new information about genetic contributions to psychiatric disorders.

Gene-environment correlation is also an important consideration: for example, where two parents who provide genetic material to their offspring also provide the early, sometimes high risk, rearing environment.

A longitudinal and on-going NZ study into the relationship between childhood maltreatment and the likelihood of being diagnosed with a conduct disorder found that it was linked to a polymorphic gene of known function called the MAOA gene, and depended on which version of the gene an individual had – i.e., whether the individual had high MAOA activity or low MAOA activity.

The study found that there was a highly significant relationship between levels of maltreatment and the likelihood of conduct disorder diagnosis among those with the low MAOA activity gene hypothesised to be the risk gene. Among those with the high MAOA activity gene, there was no relationship to speak of, despite high levels of maltreatment.

However, the study also found that the gene alone could not project antisocial behavior; it was only when it was placed in the context of childhood maltreatment that prediction was seen.

In summary, both genetic and environmental risk factors must be considered in regard to anxiety disorders.

PART IV   DEVELOPMENTAL ANTECEDENTS OF ANXIETY

Everyone can remember, as children, being alone at night, lying afraid in bed, not knowing whether to get up and go to their parents or to stay in bed, not knowing when daylight would finally come. Being frightened is part of growing up for all children.

Unfortunately, for some children, these natural fears will develop into specific anxiety disorders. In fact, many anxiety disorders make themselves known before adulthood. The median age of onset for any anxiety disorder is 11 years of age. Specific phobia, separation anxiety disorder and social anxiety disorder, all have, on average, an onset prior to the age of 18 years old, with all other anxiety disorders having their median age of onset by the end of the third decade of life (Kessler et al., 2005).

The stage is set very early in life for later anxiety by a complex interaction of genes and environment. This has been underlined by work performed in animal models by Feder, Nestler, & Charney (2009).

The maternal behaviour of mice toward their offspring, in turn genetically influenced, has been found not only to affect levels of anxiety in the offspring, but also to change the HPA axis responsiveness and the transcription of nerve growth factor. These changes in the glucocortoid receptor gene expression appear to prime the animal for higher basal levels of corticosteroid production and higher levels of anxiety-like behaviour later in life.

Although this elegant experimental model cannot be repeated in humans, it is clear that the genetic propensity to the development of anxiety disorders is moulded, in turn, by the environment in which a young person is raised and by their interaction with that environment. Evidence from neuroimaging studies of anxiety in humans will be reviewed in a later unit.

An important milestone in the understanding of anxiety and human development was the work on attachment, by John Bowlby, an English psychiatrist and psychoanalyst, and American psychologist Harry Harlow.

The development of emotional links between children and their parents, or primary care givers, is basic to their overall mental and physical health and can be found in many other species.

It is dangerous to ignore these basic needs, as the circle of psychiatrists influenced by John Bowlby has demonstrated with their scientific studies of children brought up in emotionally deprived settings. This was recently shown by the horrific outcomes seen in the children confined to orphanages in Romania during the regime of dictator Nicolae Ceaucescu.

This importance of adequate attachments was explored in a number of animal experiments by Harry Harlow, who observed the effects of maternal deprivation in monkeys.

Harlow developed a paradigm, by which he contrasted the effects of normal attachment between monkey mothers and their infants with surrogate wire "mothers", with or without a towelling cover. Given a choice, infant monkeys invariably preferred surrogate mothers covered with soft terry cloth, and they spent a great deal of time cuddling with them, just as they would have with their real mothers.

Harlow was able to demonstrate a critical period of development during which the effective provision of attachment needs was essential for normal physical and psychological development.

The transgenerational effects of good mothering has recently been extended by Michael Meaney.

This understanding has helped influence public health policies, changed radically such issues as how often parents are allowed to visit their children in hospital, and shifted the care of orphaned or abandoned children from institutional care to fostering.

The first chapter in Part IV will examine anxiety in younger people, in particular, the distinctive factors of anxiety disorders in children. The integration of psychological and pharmacological treatments for anxiety disorders in childhood will also be discussed.

The next chapter will review the genetic and environmental factors underlying the development of anxiety disorders, especially in children, and will examine the interaction of genetic inheritance, along with important and powerful environmental influences on the expression of anxiety.

The final chapter for this part will introduce attachment theory through the work of John Bowlby. Bowlby noted the effect on the infant of separation from the primary carer – usually the mother. This approach has had important implications in a wide range of areas, from public policy regarding child care to a better understanding of the therapist-patient relationship.

CHAPTER 13   DISTINCT DEVELOPMENTAL PRESENTATIONS

Angela Dixon and Kasia Kozlowska

CASE STUDY: REBECCA

"Hi, my name is Rebecca, and I am ten years old. I am in grade one and I have lots of friends. I live with my Mum and my Dad and my cat Mr Tootsie. I have always been a scaredy cat. Mum and Dad don't let me watch scary movies, because I get really scared and I can't stop thinking about them. I'm frightened of the dark. Before going to bed, I check all the doors and windows. I often find it hard to fall asleep because I hear all sorts of noises. I worry that someone may have got into the house or that a monster may be hiding under my bed. I have to have my bedroom door open so that I can check if Mum and Dad are nearby. When it gets really bad, I worry something really bad might happen. I get lots of tummy pains in the morning before I go to school. Sometimes I can't get to school because my tummy is so sore. The doctor said that my tummy was sore because I was worrying and that I am a worrywart like my aunty Jane. "

Rebecca is a 10-year-old girl from an intact, supportive family who was described as "anxious from birth." She had been a cautious, shy pre-schooler, but she adapted well to Grade One, and began making friends and succeeding academically. She presented several times to her GP with chronic, diffuse abdominal pain (tummy aches) that was worst in the morning and never present at night. She had missed about twenty days of school during the previous year because of the pain. She also avoided school field trips, fearing the bus would crash. Her parents reported she had difficulty falling asleep and frequently asked for their reassurance.

She was worried that she and members of her family might die. She was unable to sleep at all when anticipating a test. She could not tolerate having her parents on a different floor of the house from herself, and, fearing intruders, she checked the doors and windows in the evenings. Her clinginess, her need for constant reassurance and school attendance problems were both frustrating and upsetting to her parents. Rebecca had not experienced any traumatic events, although she reacted very strongly to the television images of the Boxing Day tsunami. One of her grandparents had also died the previous year. A maternal aunt had recently been treated with fluoxetine for depression and was described as "a nervous person."

CHILDHOOD AND ADULT ANXIETY DISORDER

Rebecca has symptoms typical of a childhood anxiety disorder. Anxiety disorders affect between 5% and 20% of children. They are among the most prevalent psychiatric conditions in children today. Anxiety does not go away without treatment but worsens over time, and has adverse effects on cardiac, immune and respiratory functioning.

As previously discussed, anxiety disorders are the most prevalent psychiatric conditions in adults. The majority of adults with an anxiety disorder report that their symptoms started in childhood. As well as being more likely to have an anxiety disorder in adulthood, anxiety in childhood also predicts other problems in adulthood including higher rates of depression, drug use and less educational attainment.

TYPICAL FEARS IN CHILDREN

Fears are much more common during childhood and adolescence than in adult life. The focus of fears changes over time, as children develop and encounter new experiences (Table 13.1). The type of fears experienced at each stage of development largely reflects the intellectual and emotional growth of the child at that time.

Table 13.1   Typical fears in children of different ages

Age	Fear
Infancy	Loss of physical support, sudden, intense, unexpected noise, heights
1–2	Strangers, toileting activities, being injured
3–5	Animals (primarily dogs), imaginary creatures, darkness, being alone
6–9	Animals, lightning and thunder, personal safety, school, death
9–12	Tests, personal health
13 and up	Personal injury, social interaction, personal conduct, economic and political catastrophes

The majority of adults with an anxiety disorder report that their symptoms started in childhood.

FEAR AND ANXIETY IN CHILDREN

The boundaries between normal fear and abnormal anxiety are blurred. The best way to distinguish between them is by considering if these emotions produce impairment – that is, if they interfere with the performance of the tasks expected of a child of that age, or if they cause undue distress because of their persistence or intensity.

While the number and variety of fears decrease as the child grows older, the same does not seem to happen with anxiety disorders. These conditions become increasingly prevalent during adolescence.

WHEN DOES FEAR BECOME A PROBLEM

When does fear become a problem? The following questions can be helpful to answer this:

Is the fear out of proportion to the situation?

Some anxiety before an exam is normal; however, if the young person cannot study, vomits in the morning of the exam or forgets all the answers that were so well known the previous night, this would be considered out of proportion to the situation.

Can it be explained or reasoned away?

Despite the best attempts of their parents to explain or demonstrate that there are no monsters under the bed, the child still refuses to sleep in their own room. Reason and logical explanations do not make the fear go away.

Is the fear beyond voluntary control?

Fearful thoughts, as well as associated physiological responses such as crying, rapid heart rate or breathing, cannot be controlled despite reassurances from parents.

Does the fearful reaction persist unchanged for an extended period of time?

Some childhood fears disappear within several months. However, if a fear persists intensely for more than six months, interventions may be required (sooner if the fear involves school refusal or prevents necessary surgery or other medical attention).

Does the fear lead to avoidance of the situation?

The child will avoid doing things such as going to a sleep-over because of the fear of separation

Is the fear connected with a particular age or stage?

It is important to differentiate developmental fears, such as fear of the dark, which are often transient, from anxiety disorders.

Does the fear interfere with social, emotional or academic functioning?

A consequence of the anxiety is that the child does not perform to potential at school, or has difficulty in social relationships.

PREVALENCE OF ANXIETY DISORDERS IN CHILDREN

Estimates of prevalence rates of anxiety disorders in children range from 5% to 20%, with rates increasing with age from childhood to adolescence. There is a dearth of studies examining prevalence rates of specific anxiety disorders in children. As shown in Table 13.2, separation anxiety, specific and social phobias are the most common anxiety disorders seen in childhood. Generalised anxiety symptoms are often seen, although full criteria are rarely met. Panic disorder and agoraphobia are rarely seen. Anxiety disorders occur equally in boys and girls before puberty, with an increase seen in girls after puberty.

Table 13.2 Prevalence rates of anxiety disorders in children

Anxiety disorder	Prevalence rate
Specific Phobia	2–5%
Separation Anxiety	2–5%
Social Phobia	3–5%
Elective Mutism	0.7–0.8%
Generalised Anxiety	<1%
Agoraphobia	<1%
Panic Disorder	<1%
OCD	0.2–1.2%
PTSD	<1%
Developmental Trauma	Not yet in DSM

An important issue in understanding anxiety disorders in childhood is that the disorders rarely occur in isolation. Rather, many children meeting diagnostic criteria for one anxiety disorder will often display symptoms of other anxiety disorders as well. At least one third of children with anxiety disorders meet the criteria for two or more anxiety disorders.

Furthermore, many children may also suffer from a different secondary emotional or behavioural disorder. Up to three quarters of affected young persons will experience a major depressive episode as part of their anxiety syndrome. Attention-deficit/hyperactivity disorder (ADHD) and learning disorders are also highly comorbid with anxiety disorders in children.

Often, it is the depression or disruptive disorders that are presented as the referral problem, which means that, at least initially, the anxiety can often be missed.

It is important to differentiate between children who have two distinct disorders and those who have overlapping symptoms, but only one disorder. For example, if anxious children refuse to do as their parents request because of their fear, their behaviour may appear oppositional. However, in this case, the oppositionality is part of a pattern of avoidance and fear, not an entirely separate disorder. Accurate diagnosis will impact treatment recommendations.

ANXIETY DISORDERS UNIQUE TO CHILDHOOD

Some anxiety disorders are specific to childhood.

Separation anxiety disorder is the classic anxiety disorder of childhood. Its essential feature is excessive anxiety about separation from attachment figures.

Social anxiety disorder in children strongly resembles social anxiety disorder in adults, with the caveat that school settings are commonly the focus of the child's symptoms.

Selective mutism, which is characterised by an inability to speak in specific social situations because of anxiety and humiliation fears, is likely an early childhood variant of social phobia.

A diagnosis of agoraphobia is not made often in children and adolescents. However, there are some similarities between the symptoms of agoraphobia and those of separation anxiety disorder. It is believed that a number of adolescents who suffer from separation anxiety go on to develop agoraphobia in adult life.

DEVELOPMENTAL TRAUMA (COMPLEX PTSD)

Developmental trauma, or complex PTSD, accounts for the sequelae of chronic recurrent trauma - such as abuse, neglect and exposure to domestic violence – that occurs during development. Developmental trauma has a profound impact on many areas of functioning.

Symptoms are pervasive and multifaceted, and often include the full range of anxiety symptoms, depressive symptoms, inattention, impulsive and self-destructive behaviours and an increased incidence of medical illnesses. The symptoms are better conceptualised as reflecting the child's biological and psychological response to chronic trauma.

Current DSM diagnoses fail accurately to capture the pervasive nature of disturbances related to early childhood trauma. Children tend to receive multiple comorbid diagnoses, which are treated as separate conditions and which fail to connect their symptoms and difficulties as representing a self-protective response to past trauma. Clinicians working in the field use the terms "developmental trauma" or "complex trauma" to describe, in a more coherent way, the difficulties manifested by this group of children.

DEVELOPMENTAL DIFFERENCES

Presentations

Anxiety in children is often expressed via somatic complaints (stomach aches, headaches, etc.) compared with adults. Behaviours such as clinginess, tantrums or sudden immobility when facing feared situations, are also more likely to be seen in childhood anxiety disorders than in adult anxiety disorders.

An important difference with psychological problems in children versus adults is that children are still developing on all dimensions. Therefore, in addition to the specific anxiety symptoms pathognomonic of adult disorders, impairment in children can also manifest as deficiencies in positive adaptive behaviours and a failure to progress in the expected fashion along one or more dimensions in development.

Obsessive-compulsive Disorder

Most individuals with OCD, even young ones, are at least intermittently aware that their symptoms do not make logical sense. However, young children are less capable of abstract thought, so their degree of insight may not be as good as that of older people. Young people often have difficulty in reporting their obsessions any more than as a "bad feeling", and that they have to carry out their rituals "until they feel right".

Posttraumatic Stress Disorder

Similarly, due to limited cognitive capacity, young children often have trouble reporting some of the internalising symptoms seen in PTSD, such as depersonalisation, derealisation and restricted range of affect.

Rather than trauma-specific nightmares characteristic of adult PTSD, children's trauma nightmares or flashbacks may be more generalised, such as full of monsters or other scary things. Children may also re-enact their traumatic experience through their play.

ASSESSMENT

To screen quickly for one or more anxiety disorders in children, four questions are often useful.

- Does the child worry or ask for parental reassurance almost every day?
- Does the child consistently avoid certain age-appropriate situations or activities, or avoid doing them without a parent?
- Does the child frequently have stomach aches, headaches or episodes of hyperventilation?
- Does the child have daily repetitive rituals?

These questions address the main thoughts, behaviours and feelings related to anxiety in children. A positive response to any question suggests that diagnostic features for that disorder should be reviewed.

MANAGEMENT

The treatment of anxiety disorders in children and adolescents usually involves a multimodal approach. Comprehensive treatment may include: education of the patient and parents about the disorder, consultation with school personnel and the primary care physician, cognitive-behavioural intervention, family therapy and pharmacotherapy.

Current treatment emphasises correction of distortions in thinking, behaviour therapy, social skills training and, sometimes, the addition of medications to moderate the biological instabilities found in these conditions. Rather than focusing on the child or their family as the problem, such an approach makes the anxiety disorder the problem, and builds on the child's strengths to overcome the adverse effects that the anxiety disorder has on their life.

In some situations, the anxiety symptoms may represent problems in the family system, and family therapy may be indicated. The aim of the therapy with the family is to disrupt the dysfunctional family interactional patterns that promote family insecurity, and to support areas of family competence.

USING MEDICATION FOR CHILDHOOD ANXIETY

Pharmacotherapy can be considered for severe anxiety, or for children with significant cognitive impairment. Selective serotonin reuptake inhibitors are commonly used, and should be started at low doses and increased gradually. They can be continued for six to twelve months while the child is learning other strategies, and then slowly tapered. Medication should always be used as an adjunct to psychological and family work.

COGNITIVE-BEHAVIOURAL THERAPY

The childhood-onset anxiety disorders are remarkably resistant to traditional insight-oriented psychotherapy. In contrast, the benefits of cognitive-behavioural psychotherapy, in the form of anxiety management, graded exposure and response prevention, are well-established, both clinically and in the empirical literature.

Treatment involves a three-stage approach, consisting of information gathering, therapist-assisted CBT and homework assignments. The second element, therapist-assisted exposure, can often be eliminated in favour of patient-directed homework assignments. Because the child's social matrix is critical to the evolution of the symptom picture, family interventions are of prime importance. Praise and rewards to increase the child's interest and motivation to fight the worry, is another important treatment component.

CBT is targeted developmentally, with therapy being delivered via a variety of media (drawings, dolls, pictures, games, etc.), depending on the age and stage of the child.

PARENT AND SCHOOL INVOLVEMENT IN TREATMENT

Most children are unable to take full responsibility for their own treatment program and require parental support, both in terms of implementing the treatment and emotional support.

The child's parent is asked to take on the role of "coach" to help the child take charge of the anxiety in the home setting. In this way, the therapist works with the parents and child, helping them to work together – to form an expert team – in order to combat the anxiety.

In addition, many parents need to address their own levels of stress and anxiety, in order to model good coping behaviour and clear communication, and to facilitate appropriate responses to the child.

School interventions may include implementation of a behavioural program at school, or may include interventions that address bullying, or other contextual issues that perpetuate the child's anxiety.

REBECCA FOLLOW-UP

Rebecca was treated by her family doctor, and then referred to a psychologist at the local Community Health Centre. Because her abdominal pain did not suggest an organic cause, physical examination and blood tests were the only investigations done. Results were all normal. Her parents' report and an interview with Rebecca were used to rule out a grief reaction to her grandparent's death.

Rebecca and her parents were given information and educational materials about childhood anxiety disorders and their treatment. She was started on 5 milligrams of fluoxetine. The dose was incrementally increased to 20 milligrams over a period of two weeks. She got diarrhoea with the last dose increase, so it was maintained at 15 milligrams. She had a noticeable response within one month.

Her parents were encouraged to perform relaxation exercises with her every evening at bedtime and not to discuss worries with her at that time. Her parents charted her school attendance, and offered her a small reward (a chance to watch a favourite television program) if she attended school for an entire day.

Her abdominal pain was acknowledged as real, but was reframed as a temporary result of "tense muscles", as it subsided within half an hour of entering the school building.

Rebecca was encouraged to use "boss back talk", such as telling the anxiety not to bother her and that she was the boss. Although she never became an adventurous child, Rebecca's sleep and school attendance improved dramatically.

CHAPTER 14   DEVELOPMENT OF ANXIETY DISORDERS

Jennifer Hudson

GENETIC AND FAMILY INFLUENCE

A wealth of data has supported the notion that anxiety runs in families. Much of this transmission occurs because of the genetic heritability of anxiety.

The results of twin studies suggest that a moderate degree of variance in anxiety symptoms and disorders is accounted for by genetics. One of the values of twin methodology is that it can be used to estimate, not only the genetic contribution to anxiety, but also aspects of the environment.

Data from twin studies indicate that the majority of variance in anxiety can be attributed to environmental features that are unique to each twin; that is, the non-shared environment, or, put another way, environmental factors that make siblings different from each other.

Adults' twin studies of anxiety show that there is little role for a shared environment (that is, factors that are common to siblings). Yet there is some evidence in twin samples of children that shared environment plays an important role. This makes sense: one would expect that any shared environmental influence, from parenting for example, would be likely to account for the greatest variance in symptoms during childhood, when parents exert their strongest influence on their offspring.

Where does parenting fit into this picture? To some extent, parenting behaviour is likely to be a shared environmental effect. But there are some parenting behaviours that are also likely to exert a non-shared environmental influence. Some parents may also respond differently to a child, depending on the child's temperament.

INHIBITION AND ANXIETY

There is a great deal of similarity between an inhibited, shy temperament style and anxiety disorders in young people. While these are overlapping constructs, most authors have argued that inhibition and anxiety disorders are closely related but separate constructs.

First, a definition of inhibited temperament: children with an inhibited temperament have a long latency period to "warm-up", approach or communicate with strangers, and have a tendency to stay within close proximity of safety figures. These children show signs of distress or withdrawal in the face of novelty, and often exhibit restricted and inhibited social behaviour.

There is fairly consistent evidence to show that children with an inhibited temperament are at greater risk of anxiety disorders in later life.

TEMPERAMENTAL RISK FOR ANXIETY

Figure 14.1 shows data from an ongoing longitudinal study being conducted at the Centre for Emotional Health, Macquarie University. A sample of 200 children aged four was classified as either inhibited or uninhibited, based on parent and observed report. Anxiety disorders were assessed and tracked over time, at age 6 and then age 9.

In the graph, the dark bars represent the inhibited children and the grey bars the uninhibited children. There is a significant drop in anxiety disorders over time in the inhibited group, but the most striking thing in this graph is the significantly higher risk of anxiety disorders over time in the inhibited, compared with the uninhibited group.

It is also clear from this graph that not all children classified as inhibited as an infant have, or will, develop an anxiety disorder.

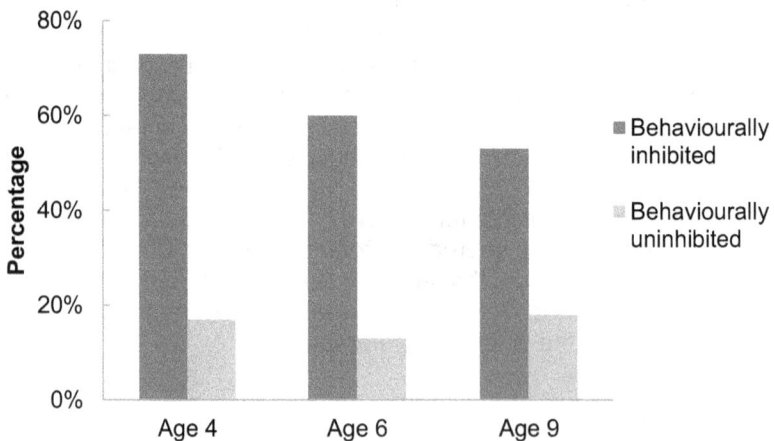

Figure 14.1   Percentage of children with an anxiety disorder

INTERACTIONS BETWEEN TEMPERAMENT AND ENVIRONMENT

As mentioned before, it is also possible that specific environments shape an inhibited child's risk for anxiety disorders. For example, a parent may respond to an inhibited child by "doing things for the child", perhaps because in the short term this reduces distress. But helping too much may in fact help to maintain the child's risk for anxiety.

Conversely, there may be environmental influences in a child's life that shape them away from an anxiety disorder.

Parenting and Anxiety

Two styles of parenting have been associated with anxiety disorders:

- over-protective or over-controlling parenting
- negative or critical parenting.

Several reviews have provided support for these associations: the largest effect sizes and the most consistent results have come from an evaluation of over-protective parenting, whereas negative critical parenting has been more commonly associated with depression. Children with anxiety disorders are more likely to have parents who are over-protective and over-controlling.

There is some preliminary evidence that this is a causal association, and some suggestion that this type of parenting may in fact be elicited by the child's anxiety.

Causally, the construct of over-protection is likely to be important because the behaviour may reduce the child's opportunity to approach novel situations and to experience confidence and independence.

In an observational study of children with and without anxiety disorders carried out at the Centre for Emotional Health, Macquarie University, the parents were observed interacting with their children during a complex puzzle task. Parents were instructed that the task was a test of the child's ability.

Parents of children with an anxiety disorder (represented by the dark bars in Figure 14.2), provided significantly more help and were more critical during the task than parents of non-anxious children (the grey bars). These data provide evidence of the association between certain parenting styles and anxiety disorders.

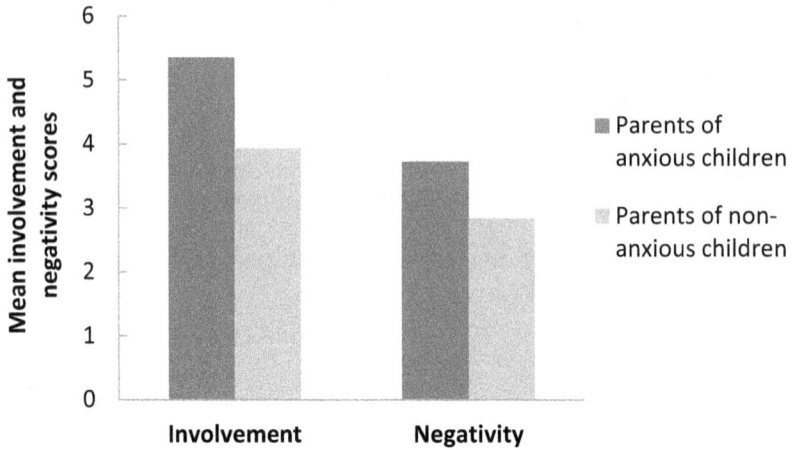

Figure 14.2 Mean involvement and negativity scores. Data adapted from Hudson & Rapee, (2008).

Early aspects of the parent-child relationship may modify a child's risk for anxiety disorders. A parent who is highly involved and over-protective may increase the child's risk. The child's temperamental style may also elicit more protective behaviours from the parent, which in turn may enhance the child's avoidant coping.

LEARNING EXPERIENCES

Anxiety may also develop, at least in part, because of specific learning experiences during development.

Children learn by watching and listening to significant people in their environment.

Parents acting in a fearful or inhibited way can provide their children with information about threat and avoidance. For example, a child whose parent becomes highly fearful when seeing a spider and runs screaming in the opposite direction is likely, not to learn accurate information about spiders, but instead to learn that all spiders are dangerous and should be avoided at all costs.

> Parents acting in a fearful or inhibited way can provide their children with information about threat and avoidance.

Parental expression of anxiety is likely to promote, not only vicarious learning but also transmission of threat information. For example, the parent in the above example may say "Arghh, it is going to jump on me and bite me." Here, the child is provided with specific information about the threat from the spider. The child learns not only by watching, but also by listening to the information given. This will encourage the child to develop cognitive biases towards threat.

The impact of anxious modelling and verbal transmission is not likely to be specific to the parent-child relationship, but may also be true of the relationship with siblings or peers. A child observing a fearful sibling or peer in a new situation may believe that this fearfulness signals real danger, and hence may also learn to avoid this new situation.

Children may also experience aversive events that can precipitate a variety of fears in them. For example, there is some evidence to suggest that children who have had negative experiences, such as falls or injuries, are more likely to have specific fears of heights. This is consistent with conditioning models of the development of anxiety.

LIFE EVENTS

Limited data on the role of negative life events in the development of anxiety in childhood suggests that children with anxiety disorders do experience a greater number of negative life events, compared with children without anxiety disorders. Although the causal nature is not entirely clear, there is some evidence to suggest that acute negative life events and chronic adversities precede the onset of an anxiety disorder.

Being raised within a general environment of family and neighbourhood adversity provides a greater number of negative experiences and further reinforces messages of nonspecific threat.

There is a large body of evidence demonstrating a relationship between children who witness inter-parental conflict and violence, and anxiety symptoms. Children who are repeatedly exposed to conflict that is unresolved, aggressive and hostile, demonstrate increased rates of internalising symptoms (that is, anxiety, depression, withdrawal). The evidence to date suggests that there is an important role played by the child's perceptions of self-blame, the child's perception of threat and the child's emotional security.

Anxious individuals tend to engage in fewer social interactions, are likely to have fewer friends and tend to be less popular than non-anxious individuals. There is some evidence that this is, in part, mediated by poor social skills. Anxiety may lead to poor social skills and it is this lack of social skills that leads to peer rejection. It is also possible that peer rejection leads to increased anxiety. Anxious children, particularly children with social anxiety, are also more likely to experience teasing and bullying. There is longitudinal evidence which shows that bullying and rejection increase anxiety over time.

CHAPTER 15   ATTACHMENT THEORY

Loyola McLean

ATTACHMENT BOND

Mammals and primates give birth to live young that must continue to develop over a long period of time. Attachment begins in infancy, and lasts throughout a lifetime. A newborn baby immediately needs someone to take care of them. This person may be a parent, a sibling or a nanny, but whoever it is, a bond will form between them. The attachment bond between parent and child arises as the result of an evolved motivational system, elaborating with evolution to foster the safe but optimal development of the infant.

ATTACHMENT SYSTEM

The attachment system promotes the help-giving and help-receiving behaviour between parent and child. It plays an organisational role in neurological, psychological and social development, and becomes incorporated into many other relationship systems over development, e.g., the sexual or romantic relationship.

The system is a large determinant in patterns of autonomic regulation, and links with the HPA axis. It is relevant to both a predisposition to anxiety and resilience in the face of stress.

HUMAN INFANTS ARE HELPLESS

In the middle of last century, John Bowlby, an English psychiatrist and psychoanalyst, became interested in his observation that major disruptions to the parent-child bond were precursors of later psychopathology. He began formally to study separation and loss between parents and children.

Bowlby found that infants are inherently motivated to attach to their parents or carers. When the attachment is working well and separation becomes too great, or when other stressors are too severe, the child experiences separation anxiety. The child then tries to increase proximity by crying, calling or reaching out, and eliciting an appropriate response from the parent. The need for the bond is basic. Without sufficient care and holding, an infant may fail to thrive and even die.

Human infants are helpless, because they cannot self-regulate. Feeding, sleeping, temperature and emotion all need to be regulated by another. Their autonomic nervous system is not fully hard-wired. The "soft-wiring" and eventually the "hard" circuitry occur via their own experience and this is mediated, in part, by their attachment experiences.

Babies are programmed at birth to be interested in the social world around them. It is assumed that they learn much about the world through their caregivers, and therefore their caregivers must have much influence on their personality and their sense of others.

EMOTIONS AND ATTACHMENT SYSTEM

Emotions are closely associated with the attachment system and emotional regulation appears to be a target of the system. We can all relate to the joyous formation of a healthy attachment bond, grief at its loss and the threat of loss that arouses anxiety, anger or fear.

The need for attachment relationships extends across the lifespan; literally from the cradle to the grave. When a healthy, secure human being of any age is anxious or distressed beyond their own comfortable capacity, it is normal for them to seek help to manage it from a close other, or a helper.

SECURE BASE AND ANXIETY

Mary Ainsworth, a colleague of Bowlby, pointed out that equilibrium between proximity seeking and the need to explore is synergistically important for development and survival. She termed this the "secure base". When children can smoothly move into care and comfort when they need it and then out again to play and explore, they have the best chance of learning to manage themselves and the world flexibly and calmly. They can develop without the anxiety of being too much on their own, or the anxiety of being too caught up in their caregiver's world.

> Babies learn about the world through their caregivers, therefore their caregivers must have much influence on their personality and their sense of others.

When there are difficulties in either arm of this process, the secure base is compromised and the child will experience anxiety, which they must manage by certain strategies. Instead of a secure attachment, the attachment is then termed insecure. Those who are limiting their attachment needs to cope are down-regulating the system, and termed avoidant or dismissive. Those who heighten their attachment needs to increase the likelihood of having them met are termed ambivalent, preoccupied or resistant.

The most important compromise of the secure base for psychopathology is the situation noted later by Ainsworth and Main, where the child experiences the caregiver as a source of terror or overwhelming anxiety, or experiences the caregiver as terrified or overwhelmingly anxious. This creates a terrible dilemma: *the one who should help me is the source of my fear*. This disorganising state of mind is a disorganiser of cognition, emotions and behaviour.

INTERNAL WORKING MODELS

Bowlby proposed that learned experience of being helped and comforted (or not) within attachment relationships would lead to the development of mental constructs – cognitive templates or schema – composed of mental representations of the attachment figure, the self and the environment. He termed these the internal working models of relationships. These schemas develop out of experience, but similar experience can still result in different schemas for different people. The ways people experience self and others are stored in various memory systems, including the non-verbal and pre-verbal procedural memory, and carried forward into adulthood. They are powerful organisers of social relationships and self-regulation, including habitual stress management.

Security in attachment fosters flexible internal models and flexible self-regulation. Insecure attachments lead to less optimal flexibility in coping. Stress and current attachments will elicit the background internal working model.

MODELS FOR ASSESSMENT PURPOSES

These models have, over time, come to be reliably elicited for assessment purposes by experimental and clinical tasks for various age groups in ways that age-appropriately access them, and that reveal learned beliefs about relationships and self.

For example, in infants, the behaviour is assessed through a task called the Strange Situation, which classifies the attachment of the child according to how the child behaves during test separations from, and then reunions with, the caregiver.

In adults, the gold standard of measurement is the Adult Attachment Interview, where the participant describes early relationships and any experiences of loss and trauma. The ability of the speaker to relate their experience and reflections coherently and collaboratively is analogous to the task of flexible exploration. Patterns during these assessment tasks define attachment classifications.

EARLIER ATTACHMENTS PREDICT LATER ANXIETY

Bowlby proposed that all forms of anxiety disorders, other than discrete animal phobias, are related to anxiety regarding the availability of an attachment figure or absent attachment comforts. He specified that parental control through over-protection or rejection would increase the likelihood of serious separations.

Patterns are now emerging and indicating that earlier attachments are predictors of later anxiety disorders. The risk of agoraphobia in later life is increased by the experience of early separation from the mother, or parental divorce. Adults with agoraphobia had more childhood separation anxiety than controls. Panic disorder and social anxiety have been associated with more traumatic life events and separations.

Attachment style can also contribute to our understanding of how an individual may react when experiencing a distressing event, such as bereavement, when they may experience anxiety symptoms for the first time.

THERAPEUTIC IMPLICATIONS

Understanding attachment has helped frame new treatments, such as the Circle of Security, that offer the possibility of shifting childhood attachment in order to decrease vulnerability to anxiety disorders and increase resilience. Long-term outcomes of these interventions are not yet available. In adults, the containing function of the therapeutic relationship reminds the clinician to "take their own pulse first", in the treatment of anxiety disorders. If the clinician is calm, they are likely to foster calm in the treating relationship and to deal with the expectations the patient brings from any difficult past experiences of care (the transference). Attachment will impact on both illness and treatment processes.

PART IV SUMMARY

Part IV is a reminder that anxiety is common and starts very early in life. The basis for anxiety involves not only a genetic predisposition for the disorders but also important aspects of the environment in which someone grows up. The interaction of that genetic inheritance with the environment is another potent epigenetic cause of anxiety.

The age at which a child or adolescent presents with an anxiety disorder can change the clinical picture of that disorder. However, it is not only the symptoms that may have changed; the presentation, its effects upon the individual and the treatment need to take into account the important place of family and school for the child. The family is an essential resource for the child and must be integrated into any management plans, but in turn, frequently needs to be a focus of intervention in its own right.

The security of early life experiences, in particular the development of strong and secure attachments to key figures about the young child, is essential for optimal development. Factors that may undermine the quality of the relationship need to take into account the general social environment in which the child is brought up, but might also include the temperament of either the child or attachment figure, or the adults' own heightened level of anxiety. All can increase the possibility that the young child will develop an anxiety disorder. Further, the quality of these early relationships will have a continuing effect on the individual, influencing interactions and relationships in later life.

Treatment for anxiety disorders in children may need to embrace both pharmacological and psychological approaches, the latter including the family. Without effective treatment, long-term difficulties for the child can eventuate, impacting on their own ability to form strong, independent relationships and their function in school and in later life.

PART V   NEUROBIOLOGY OF ANXIETY DISORDERS

Part V will set out the most recent developments in the neurobiology of anxiety. It will explain that providing the best therapy possible for patients requires an understanding of the fundamental neurobiology of anxiety. Every therapy session with an anxious patient directly impacts on the neuro-circuitry of anxiety, and in this sense, every clinician influences how the patient's brain manages their anxiety.

Understanding how the therapy impacts on the patient's brain is important, because it can assist the clinician to optimise therapeutic interventions in ways that enhance neural factors which can reduce a patient's anxiety.

Whether one adopts a pharmacological or a psychotherapeutic approach, neural processes will always underpin how the clinical intervention is working.

The individual's behaviour in response to threatening events can be described in terms of fear conditioning. This is a process that has been extensively researched since classical conditioning was first studied. It is important to understand fully the role of fear conditioning in the development and maintenance of anxiety disorders, because this is, without doubt, the most influential model available today in shaping the understanding of anxiety and the recent developments in its treatment. Extinction learning also needs to be understood, because it is the basis of the most effective treatments for anxiety disorders today.

Exposure to a traumatic or aversive event, such as being on a battlefield or experiencing one of many other potential aversive events in life, can form the basis for the development of a subsequent anxiety disorder, such as posttraumatic stress disorder (PTSD). An understanding of fear conditioning has allowed for exploration of many of the neural processes underpinning anxiety disorders.

Part V will start with a description of classical conditioning and fear conditioning. The second chapter will then focus on PTSD to explore how fear conditioning, extinction and a process called "fear reinstatement", enter the clinical manifestation of anxiety.

Annette is a 28-year-old woman living in Australia. Annette has never had any mental health problems, but she has experienced something which many Australians fear – her house was burnt down in a bushfire.

"We had to evacuate. The flames were really close. Then when we came back, our home was just a heap of ashes. There was nothing left. We lost everything. Ever since, I haven't been the same. My whole world has changed and I am not the same person.

"I keep getting images of it all happening; sometimes it's as if I'm back there – I smell the smoke, feel the heat on my face again. It happens out of the blue, at home and at work, and I can't go on with what I'm doing. I'm in tears. There are certain triggers – a barbecue, or a siren going past.

"I find myself constantly worrying that we are going to have another fire and that we'll lose our house or, worse, I will lose my family.

"I'm on guard the whole time in fear that something is going to go wrong. I don't feel that I can ever relax anymore; I can't even concentrate on the things I like doing and I get really irritable really easily.

"There are times when I don't feel anything. I just feel really numb. I feel so cut off from my family, so detached from the world."

Annette suffers from many of the symptoms that are associated with PTSD.

There are other PTSD symptoms that Annette could also have, including: nightmares, avoidance of thinking about the event, problems with memory, loss of interest in life and sleeping problems.

In Chapter 18, *The Neural Circuitry of Anxiety*, the neural structures underlying the fear response, will be identified. The amygdala is central to response for most anxiety disorders but it is important to remember that not all anxiety disorders have the same profile. As we will see, some disorders, such as obsessive-compulsive disorder for example, have a distinct pattern of cortical activation, as shown in most neuroimaging studies. The chapter will also examine how the neuro-circuitry changes over time, especially as people receive treatment.

The disturbances in neural-circuitry are accompanied by changes in the neurotransmission in key monoaminergic, glutamatergic and GABAergic pathways. These changes have been associated with the fear-conditioning model that is so important to anxiety.

Neurotransmitter alterations also underpin the therapeutic action of both pharmacological agents and psychotherapeutic strategies.

In summary, Part V will cover the major topics underpinning the neurobiology of anxiety disorders. Parts I and II showed that anxiety is not just a feeling, but is associated with a range of physiological changes that are, in turn, controlled directly by brain activity and, more distally, by epigenetic and genetic factors.

Greater understanding of the neurobiology of anxiety has meant that the early classical conditioning and fear conditioning models can be extended to an understanding of the underlying neural circuitry and neurochemistry of anxiety disorders generally.

Part V will reveal some of the most important developments in the way neurobiological processes lead to development of anxiety disorders, how they underpin the maintenance of these conditions and, most importantly, how they can facilitate effective pharmacology and psychotherapy treatment.

CHAPTER 16   FEAR CONDITIONING AND ANXIETY

Richard Bryant

CLASSICAL CONDITIONING

Classical conditioning is popularly known from early experiments in Russia by Ivan Pavlov.

In 1903, Pavlov was studying digestive processes in dogs when he stumbled on an interesting phenomenon he termed "psychic reflexes". He noticed that dogs, understandably, began salivating when meat powder was presented to them. Interestingly, he noticed that the dogs also began salivating when the meat powder was not presented but when other events occurred – events that were also present when the meat powder was originally present. These events included seeing the dog handler, or hearing a particular noise, both of which the dog experienced originally in conjunction with the presentation of meat powder. Pavlov then conducted experiments where he paired the meat powder with the ringing of a bell, and demonstrated that subsequent bell ringing reliably triggered salivation.

FEAR CONDITIONING MODELS

One of the most influential theories of anxiety involves fear conditioning. No single model can account for every feature of anxiety, and different models have different strengths. It is fair to say that over the past 100 years, the fear conditioning models have influenced the understanding of behavioural and biological processes of anxiety disorders more than any other paradigm. Fear conditioning is an example of classical conditioning, one of the oldest principles in psychology.

Building on the principles of classical conditioning, subsequent researchers addressed the question of how humans develop anxiety. In the 1920s, the famous case of "Little Albert" set the stage for understanding how anxiety disorders develop. The case of Little Albert remains a seminal case in shaping fear conditioning models and behaviour therapy of anxiety disorders.

LITTLE ALBERT

The Little Albert experiment was carried out by John Watson and his assistant Rosalie Rayner at John Hopkins University. Watson was interested in the idea that when children heard a loud noise, their reaction was prompted by fear. He believed that he could condition a child to fear another stimulus of which he would not normally be afraid.

Before the experiment, Little Albert, a baby of eleven months old, was shown a number of items including a white rabbit, a dog and a monkey, to which he showed no fear.

A laboratory rat was then placed near him, and he was allowed to play with it. Initially, that is before conditioning, Little Albert showed no signs of fear when he was presented with the rat.

However, the rat was subsequently placed near Albert and at the same time a steel bar was struck with a hammer just behind Albert, producing a very loud noise. Understandably, little Albert was very frightened.

On subsequent trials, when the rat was placed near Albert, he also became very frightened even though there was no loud noise. Little Albert generalised this fear to all sorts of furry objects, including rabbits and small dogs.

This case was one of the first demonstrations of fear conditioning, which demonstrated that a previously neutral stimulus could acquire fearful qualities after being paired with an aversive experience.

Today, such an experiment would never be allowed because it is likely that this type of conditioning may have had an adverse effect on Little Albert. It is unknown if Little Albert had persistent anxiety as a result of this experiment, as he died at the age of 6 from acquired hydrocephalus.

DEVELOPING FEAR CONDITIONING

In the years after the Little Albert experiment, much research was conducted with animals and humans, to see how previously neutral things could acquire a fearful quality, and how this might explain anxiety development.

Since the case of Little Albert, the vast majority of knowledge about fear conditioning comes from studies into how animals react to fearful events. The advantage of learning about anxiety disorders by studying animals in laboratory conditions, is that we can control factors and study processes, such as neuroanatomy, which cannot be so readily studied in humans.

In animal studies, a rat is often given an electric shock (this is the unconditioned stimulus) and at the same time presented with a light. The shock understandably leads to strong fear reactions (this is the unconditioned response). The rat learns that the light is a signal of danger, so when it is presented with the light alone (the conditioned stimulus), it responds with fear (the conditioned response).

FEAR CONDITIONING IN HUMANS

Similar patterns can be observed in anxious humans. When people are exposed to a fearful event (the unconditioned stimulus), they will typically respond with fear (the unconditioned response). The various events and situations present at the time of the event can be strongly associated with the fear. They can serve as the conditioned stimuli, because they acquire the fearful properties that were present at the initial aversive experience. Subsequent exposure to any of these associated events can elicit fear, because they signal threat (the conditioned response). For example, a patient may have a severe car accident, which provokes much fear. As a result, all sorts of stimuli that are associated with the event are now conditioned with fear, so they signal danger for this patient. It is possible that being in traffic, the sound of car horns or the sight of an ambulance triggers anxiety because the person fears that another accident will happen.

Although this model has been supported by many animal studies, it is important to remember differences between humans and animals. Most importantly, these studies cannot explain the role of cognition in anxiety.

CONDITIONING AND ANXIETY DISORDERS

Interviewing anxious patients about the onset of their anxiety often reveals that the disorder commenced after they experienced a fearful event that was somehow related to their current anxiety. For example, a socially anxious patient may fear negative evaluation by others after being ridiculed in public at a young age. Or a specific phobia patient may report fearing heights after being on a plane during severe turbulence when they feared the plane would crash.

When people are exposed to a fearful event (the unconditioned stimulus), they will typically respond with fear (the unconditioned response).

The triggers that elicit fear in different disorders relate to the specific stimuli that were conditioned at the onset of the disorder. This is why anxiety is triggered in panic disorder patients by somatic cues, in social phobia by public evaluation cues, and in phobia of cockroaches by any small insects.

CHAPTER 17   EXTINCTION AND FEAR INHIBITION

Richard Bryant

EXTINCTION LEARNING

A central feature of fear conditioning models is extinction learning. As was explained in Chapter 16, in fear conditioning, when a rat is repeatedly shown a light as it simultaneously receives a shock, the animal learns to fear the light alone. However, in extinction learning, the rat will learn that a previously conditioned association is no longer dangerous. When the rat is repeatedly shown a light, but no longer receives the shock, it learns that the light is now signalling safety, rather than danger. This new learning overrides the initial fear conditioning, and results in reduced fear of the conditioned stimulus, the light.

EXTINCTION LEARNING IN ANXIETY

In the case of the anxious patient after the car accident, each time the driver experiences traffic or hears car horns and realises that these events do not result in a car accident, they enjoy extinction learning - that the reminders are no longer signalling danger. The repeated trials of being exposed to reminders that do not lead to any aversive outcomes gradually teaches the person that these situations are not threatening, and this reduces the anxiety.

PERCENTAGE OF VICTIMS WITH PTSD

A good example of extinction learning is that most women suffer PTSD symptoms in the initial period following a sexual assault, but the rates of PTSD subside as the time passes. As women are exposed to reminders such as men, loud voices and sex, they learn that there is no danger involved. This leads to new learning that these reminders are no longer signalling danger, so rape victims suffer less and less anxiety with each new learning trial.

ANXIETY = FAILED EXTINCTION

Fear conditioning models argue that the reason some people develop persistent anxiety disorders is that they fail to achieve adequate extinction learning. That is, whereas many people will initially experience some level of fear conditioning after an aversive experience, most people will successfully adapt by learning that the reminders are no longer harmful. In contrast, a small proportion of people will fail to learn this, and an anxiety disorder persists.

EXTINCTION LEARNING IS *NEW* LEARNING

For many years, it was believed that extinction learning after fear conditioning involved an unlearning of the initial association. In this sense, it was thought that conditioning could be erased from memory by repeatedly breaking the association. However, research on fear reinstatement challenged this notion.

If a rat, or a person, was exposed to the initial shock again after successful extinction learning, the conditioned fear resurfaced. This suggests that the original learning was never erased.

Currently, the research suggests extinction learning does not erase original memories but, instead, overrides it by new learning that different stimuli signal safety rather than danger.

FEAR REINSTATEMENT AND RELAPSE

There is much evidence that people with anxiety disorders can have periods of remission from anxiety, followed by subsequent episodes of the disorder. Often, people may experience renewed anxiety after a stressful or traumatic event.

For example, a person who developed PTSD after an assault may be successfully treated, and be symptom-free for years. They may then experience a severe car accident, and anxiety concerning the initial assault may return. One possible explanation for this pattern may be that the car accident reinstated the initial conditioning.

EXTINCTION AND EXPOSURE THERAPY

One of the most effective treatments for anxiety is exposure therapy. This strategy involves asking the patient to remain in close proximity to items that they fear unrealistically. For example, the height phobic may be asked to remain on a bridge until the anxiety begins to subside. These approaches are based on extinction learning, and presume that the patient is enjoying new learning that being on a high bridge is not hurting them, which inhibits the initial conditioning that high situations are dangerous.

There has been a lot of research into conditioning and extinction learning, and a lot of evidence to support the role that fear conditioning plays in anxiety.

However, the real question is whether fear conditioning can be used to explain the various aspects of anxiety disorders, including onset, maintenance and recovery. It is often easier to study fear-conditioning processes in the onset of a disorder like PTSD because it involves such a salient traumatic event. Many studies have assessed people's heart rate in the hours following a trauma. This can reflect the strength of the unconditioned response to the event, which, in turn, can influence the strength of fear conditioning. These studies reveal a strong pattern, which shows that trauma survivors who eventually develop PTSD have much higher heart rates than those who do not develop PTSD.

CONDITIONED RESPONSES

Many studies have been conducted with anxious patients to assess whether they display conditioned responses to stimuli that are related to their fear. A common paradigm is to present the patient with neutral or fear-related stimuli while they are being assessed for heart rate, skin conductance or muscle tension. These are all indices of arousal, which would be expected to increase if a conditioned response to a certain trigger is present.

For example, in PTSD literature, there are many studies of war veterans with PTSD who show very high physiological responses to reminders of war (such as pictures of combat or even their own memories of the war), compared with war veterans without PTSD. Similar patterns have been found in other anxiety disorders.

UNCONDITIONED RESPONSES

A major study of over 1,000 trauma survivors by Bryant et al. (2008) shows that people who eventually developed PTSD had much higher heart rates immediately after trauma than those who did not develop PTSD.

Another index of the strength of the unconditioned response is the rate at which we breathe. Breathing quickly is necessary for us to engage in the fight or flight response when we feel we are exposed to a threat.

Bryant et al. (2008) found that trauma survivors who were breathing at least 22 breaths per minute on the initial day after the traumatic experience were more than twice as likely to develop PTSD three months later, than people who were not breathing this quickly. This pattern is consistent with the notion that the strength of the unconditioned response is linked to subsequent development of an anxiety disorder.

AVERSIVE EVENTS

One underlying premise of fear conditioning models is that anxiety disorders are precipitated by a fearful event. Overall, the evidence is mixed on this question. By definition, all cases of PTSD are triggered by an initial threatening experience.

There is evidence that stressful events can precede cases of panic disorder, agoraphobia, social anxiety disorder, specific phobia, GAD and OCD. In terms of panic disorder, several studies indicate that panic disorder patients suffer increased stressful life events in the year prior to panic onset. There is also evidence that anxiety in children and adolescents is preceded by stressful events.

However, many cases of these disorders develop without any evidence of an aversive event preceding the initial episode.

This pattern suggests that, while fear conditioning can explain a proportion of anxiety disorders, it is does not adequately account for the onset of all anxiety disorders.

IMMEDIATE ONSET

Fear conditioning not only presumes that stressful events precede the onset of anxiety disorders, but also that this is immediate.

However, the role of stress in precipitating anxiety disorders has been difficult to determine, because most research on life events is retrospective.

This is a problem, because the onset of most anxiety disorders is gradual and insidious. PTSD and panic disorder are the exceptions, as they typically have sudden onsets.

Stressful events can precede cases of panic disorder, agoraphobia, social anxiety disorder, specific phobia, GAD and OCD.

ROLE OF SPECIFIC STRESSORS

Some research has focused on whether anxiety disorders are preceded by specific types of stressors. Whereas depression is often preceded by stressors characterised by loss, anxiety is more often linked to threatening experiences.

The link between specific types of stressors and different anxiety disorders is limited, apart from PTSD, which is typically preceded by direct threats to one's safety.

In evaluating this evidence, it is important to remember that there is increasing evidence that the contribution of stressful events to the onset of anxiety disorders is moderated by genetic factors. It is too simplistic to expect a linear relationship between an event and onset of anxiety, because this link will be influenced by genetic factors that shape how people respond to the event.

CHAPTER 18   NEURAL CIRCUITRY OF ANXIETY

Kim Felmingham

NEUROBIOLOGY OF ANXIETY

This chapter will review the neural structures and processes underpinning anxiety disorders.

In recent years, there have been many advances in our understanding of neural bases of fear and anxiety. This is largely thanks to the convergence between studies of animals and humans experiencing fear states.

This chapter will focus on recent developments in neuroimaging, in particular, to help explain how brain functions contribute to anxiety disorders.

KEY NEURAL REGIONS INVOLVED IN ANXIETY

The major brain structures involved in anxiety are: the prefrontal cortex, the amygdala and the hippocampus.

NEUROBIOLOGY OF CONDITIONED FEAR

The amygdala is central for conditioning fearful states, forming an association between internal and external stimuli that occur at the time of a fearful experience. Specifically, these associations are formed in the basolateral nucleus of the amygdala while the conditioned response, that is, fear and anxiety, is generated in the central nucleus of the amygdala. It is from here that fear responses are expressed.

AMYGDALA HYPERACTIVITY IN ANXIETY

A meta-analysis of forty neuroimaging studies found consistent hyperactivity in the amygdala in PTSD, social anxiety, and specific phobia. This was similar to activations observed during fear conditioning paradigms. In panic disorder, recent studies reveal amygdala activation during a panic attack. Coactivations in the insula are also commonly seen concurrently with amygdala activation. Therefore, amygdala hyperactivity is thought to reflect a common engagement of fear circuitry amongst the anxiety disorders. There are fewer imaging studies in generalised anxiety disorder, but there is some recent evidence of amygdala hyperactivity in GAD. Imaging studies in OCD reveal a distinctive neural circuitry that does not involve the amygdala, but centres on a dysregulation in the frontal lobes, ventral striatum and thalamus (Etkin & Wager, 2007).

NEURAL NETWORKS OF FEAR EXTINCTION

Many models of anxiety suggest that the regulation of amygdala fear networks is impaired in anxiety disorders.

Recent animal and human neuroimaging studies indicate that neural circuits for fear extinction are in the prefrontal cortex and the hippocampus. Activity in these regions works together to inhibit nuclei in the amygdala that are responsible for coordinating a conditioned fear response.

NEUROBIOLOGICAL MODEL OF ANXIETY

Put very simply, the major neurobiological model of anxiety disorders suggests that there is reduced inhibition by medial prefrontal networks onto the amygdala. This means that in anxiety, the amygdala shows increased levels of activity because it is not being inhibited by the prefrontal cortex as much as it should be.

REDUCED PREFRONTAL ACTIVITY IN ANXIETY

Most evidence supporting reduced activity in the ventral prefrontal cortex comes from neuroimaging studies of PTSD. These show reduced activity in the anterior cingulate regions, or ventral medial prefrontal regions.

This is thought to reflect an impairment of inhibitory networks onto the amygdala fear processing circuits, and this reduced inhibition results in ongoing fear and anxiety symptoms. There is also evidence of reduced medial prefrontal activity in social anxiety and panic disorder, although this evidence is not as strong or consistent.

NEUROBIOLOGY OF GAD

Fewer neuroimaging studies have investigated the neurobiology of GAD. However, recent evidence suggests that GAD is associated with a similar dysregulation in the amygdala, hippocampus and prefrontal regions to that of most of the anxiety disorders. In addition, it is also associated with dysregulation in the basal ganglia and cerebellum.

NEUROBIOLOGY OF OCD

The neurobiology of obsessive-compulsive disorder is quite distinct. Unlike the other anxiety disorders, the neurocircuitry in OCD does not appear to involve the amygdala. Rather, the core neural disturbance in OCD lies in a cortico-striatal-thalamic network, with specific dysregulation in the basal ganglia, orbital frontal cortex and thalamus.

EXPOSURE TREATMENTS FOR ANXIETY

Exposure treatments are the first-line treatments for most anxiety disorders (PTSD, social anxiety, panic disorder, specific phobia).

The primary aim of exposure treatments is to facilitate fear extinction.

FEAR FACE PARADIGM

Although there is a convergence of animal and human neuroscience in anxiety disorders, if the neurobiological model of deficient medial prefrontal inhibition on the amygdala is correct, a key question is: can exposure therapy enhance extinction networks in the prefrontal cortex?

Felmingham et al. (2007) investigated the effects of exposure therapy on PTSD symptoms, and amygdala and prefrontal function. Using the fear face paradigm, participants with PTSD viewed fearful faces to test amygdala and prefrontal function. Participants then had eight sessions of exposure therapy.

Six months after completing the exposure therapy, they were retested on the same fear face paradigm. Changes in their PTSD symptoms from pre- to post-exposure therapy were correlated with neural changes in the prefrontal cortex and amygdala activity on exposure to fearful faces.

> Exposure treatments are the first-line treatments for PTSD, social anxiety, panic disorder and specific phobia, and aim to facilitate fear extinction.

AMYGDALA REDUCES AND VMPFC INCREASES WITH SUCCESSFUL EXPOSURE THERAPY

Studies showed that PTSD symptoms reduced with successful exposure treatment. There was an increase in the activity of networks that govern fear extinction (namely, the anterior cingulate cortex), and a reduction in the activity of amygdala-based fear-processing networks.

There was a significant negative correlation between change in total CAPS score and right rostral ACC (anterior cingulate cortex) activity from pre to post-treatment (r = -0.8, p < 0.01). This suggests that as PTSD reduces, rostral ACC activity increases. A significant positive correlation between change in PTSD symptoms and amygdala activity from pre- to post-treatment was found. This suggests that as PTSD reduces, amygdala activity reduces on exposure to fearful faces. The graph in Figure 18.1 shows the change scores from pre- to post-treatment on the CAPS. As the change score increases (moving along the x-axis towards the right), this reflects greater symptom improvement (Felmingham et al., 2007).

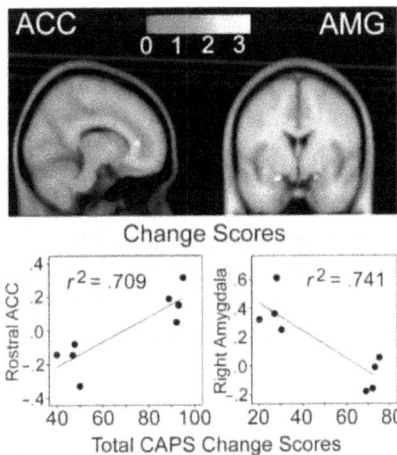

Figure 18.1 Correlation between changes in blood-oxygenation-level-dependent (BOLD) activity and changes in total severity of posttraumatic stress disorder

CHAPTER 19   NEUROCHEMISTRY AND ANXIETY

Kim Felmingham

NEUROBIOLOGY OF ANXIETY

Several neurotransmitters are implicated in the anxiety disorders, including:

- serotonin
- noradrenaline
- glutamate
- GABA
- dopamine.

The HPA axis is also critically involved in the release of cortisol and adrenaline.

ACTION OF NEUROTRANSMITTERS AT THE SYNAPSE

Neurotransmitters are packed and stored in synaptic vesicles in the presynaptic terminals. When the presynaptic neuron is stimulated, they are then released into the synaptic cleft. From here, the neurotransmitters attach to the appropriate postsynaptic receptors. If the neurotransmitter signal is strong enough, this triggers an electrical action potential in the postsynaptic neuron, leading to further activity at the next synapse.

Neurotransmitters have several modes of action, which vary between and within different neurotransmitters. Neurotransmitters may act to increase the sensitivity of presynaptic receptors, they may block postsynaptic receptors or they may stimulate the reuptake of the neurotransmitter from the synapse. These processes may lead to upregulation or downregulation of postsynaptic receptors.

NEUROTRANSMITTER NETWORKS IN THE BRAIN

The noradrenergic system, dopaminergic system, serotonergic system and the HPA axis affect specific neural regions and networks that are involved in fear and anxiety, including the amygdala, prefrontal cortex, hippocampus, hypothalamus and brainstem.

GLUTAMATE AND GABA

Glutamate is the main excitatory neurotransmitter in the brain and GABA is the main inhibitory neurotransmitter in the brain. A dysregulation between glutamate and GABA, via interneurons in cortical pyramidal cells, is also implicated in anxiety.

Regions that are extensively implicated in the mediation of fear and anxiety in animals and humans are richly innervated by glutamatergic pyramidal cells. These include limbic and associated paralimbic brain structures – the amygdala, hippocampus, anterior cingulate cortex, orbitofrontal cortex, medial prefrontal cortex and insular cortex.

Specifically, there is thought to be excessive activity of glutamate in NMDA receptors. This can result in neurotoxicity in brain regions that are important for fear, such as the hippocampus, as well as dysregulation of the HPA system.

Glutamate also exerts its actions in the brain by affecting the release of other neurotransmitters, including monoamines and GABA. There is also some evidence for reduced activity in GABA receptors and neurons in anxiety, as many anti-anxiety medications are GABAergic (e.g. benzodiazepines).

THE HPA AXIS

The HPA axis is responsible for the release of stress hormones, and interacts closely with other neurotransmitters implicated in anxiety. The HPA axis is a feedback loop that includes the hypothalamus and the pituitary and adrenal glands. Cells in the hypothalamus produce corticotrophin releasing factor (CRF) in response to stress, which in turn binds to specific receptors in pituitary cells, which produce adrenocorticotropic hormone (ACTH). ACTH then stimulates the release of stress hormones from the adrenal glands (cortisol, adrenaline) to promote autonomic arousal. The loop is completed by negative feedback inhibition by cortisol on the hypothalamus and pituitary, which prevents further release of ACTH. Evidence suggests that this negative feedback inhibition in the HPA axis is impaired in anxiety, and that levels of CRF are increased in anxiety disorders (see Chapter 7).

Animal and human evidence reveals that interactions of noradrenaline and glucocorticoids in the amygdala mediate the consolidation of emotional memories, a key pathogenic process in anxiety. Glucocorticoid receptors are also particularly dense in the hippocampus, and activation of these receptors also leads to negative feedback inhibition on the HPA axis.

NEUROCHEMISTRY OF FEAR EXTINCTION

Animal studies reveal that fear extinction is mediated via glutamatergic NMDA receptors in the amygdala.

Recently, there have been revolutionary advances in treating anxiety disorders, identifying neurochemical enhancers of exposure therapy, and neurochemical preventive interventions.

D-CYCLOSERINE (DCS)

D-cycloserine (DCS) is an NMDA receptor partial agonist. Animal neuroscience reveals that it facilitates fear extinction (Ledgerwood, Richardson, & Cranney, 2003). This study reveals that injecting D-cycloserine facilitates the extinction of conditioned freezing responses in rats. Figure 19.1 reveals that conditioned freezing reduces in a linear fashion as the DCS injection is moved closer to the actual extinction learning.

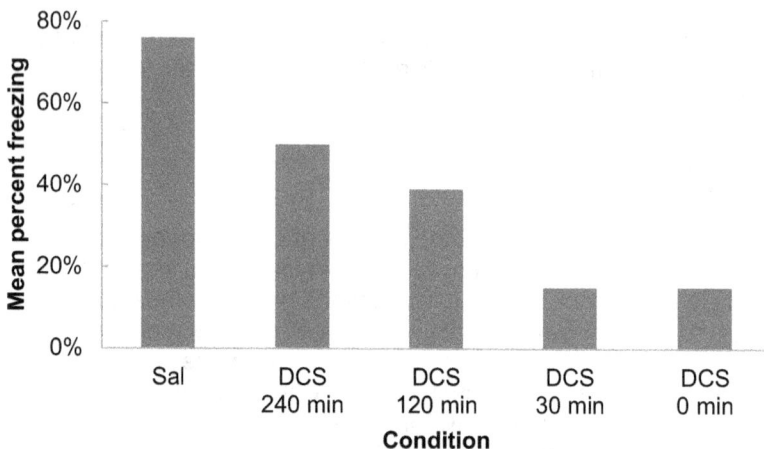

Figure 19.1   Conditioned freezing and DCS injection. From Ledgerwood, Richardson, & Cranney (2003). Reproduced with permission of American Psychological Association.

Specific Phobia

A revolutionary study by Ressler et al. (2004) examined the impact of combining exposure therapy (via virtual reality) with d-cycloserine in height phobics. Height phobic patients were randomly assigned to a DCS plus exposure, or a placebo plus exposure group, and patients underwent several weeks of virtual floor exposure. Results revealed that patients who had exposure combined with 50mg of DCS experienced faster extinction of their fear responses compared with the group who had exposure combined with placebo.

Social Anxiety Disorder

This facilitatory effect of DCS, when combined with exposure to feared stimuli, has also been shown in social anxiety disorder. In a large randomised controlled trial by Guastella et al. (2008), socially anxious patients underwent exposure therapy for public speaking. Half were randomised to a DCS plus public speaking exposure group, and the other half to a placebo plus public speaking exposure group. Again, the DCS group displayed faster extinction of their fear responses compared to the placebo group (Figure 19.2).

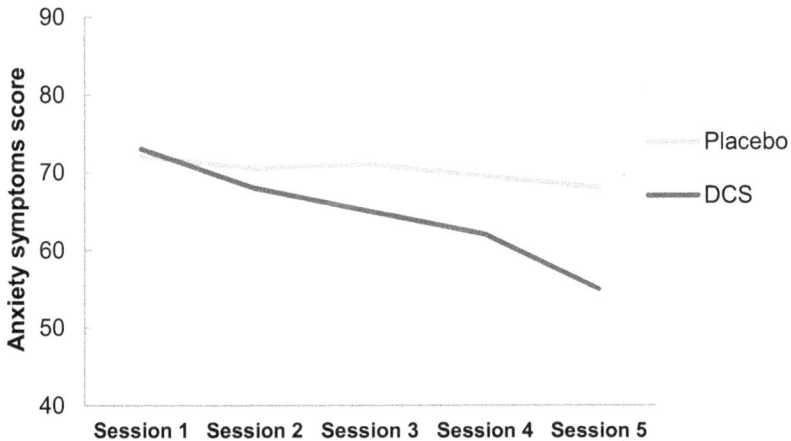

Figure 19.2 DCS in treating social anxiety disorder. From Guastella et al. (2008). Reproduced with permission of Elsevier.

Obsessive-compulsive Disorder

The facilitatory effect of DCS on extinction learning during exposure to feared situations has also been shown in OCD. Kushner et al. (2007) reported that over four exposure sessions, obsession-related fear ratings declined more rapidly in the DCS group compared with the placebo group (see Figure 19.3).

OTHER PHARMACOLOGICAL ENHANCERS TO CBT

Currently, studies are examining the potential preventative effect of propanolol, morphine, cortisol and oestrogen on the development of PTSD following traumatic events.

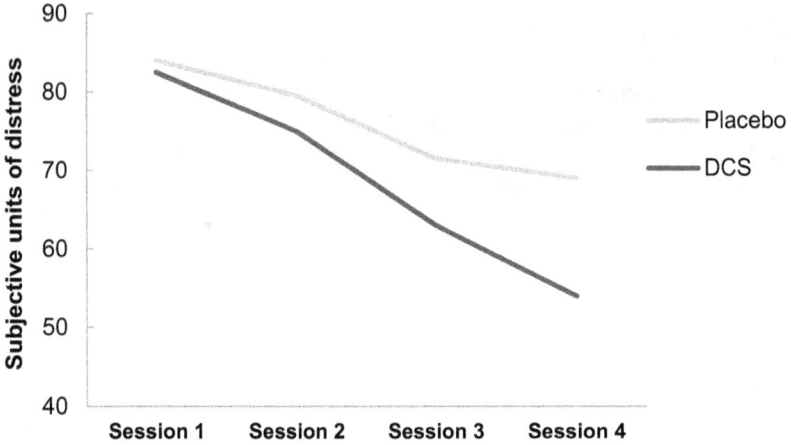

Figure 19.3   DCS in treating OCD. From Kushner et al. (2007). Reproduced with permission of Elsevier.

PART V SUMMARY

Research in the development of anxiety disorders has demonstrated the important role of neurobiological processes. These processes underpin the maintenance of these conditions and can facilitate effective pharmacology and psychotherapy treatment. Understanding of the neurobiology of anxiety has meant that the early classical conditioning and fear conditioning theories of anxiety can be expanded. In turn this serves to increase understanding of the underlying neural circuitry and neurochemistry of anxiety disorders.

The first chapter of Part V describes how seminal studies on fear conditioning, such as the case of "Little Albert", are very important in developing an understanding of the development of anxiety disorders. Essentially, in a patient's life, when a neutral stimulus (e.g., driving a car) is paired with an aversive experience (e.g., a car accident), fear to the neutral stimulus may develop. Conditioned responses have been investigated by assessing a client's physiological arousal in response to a reminder of the feared event. For example, in PTSD literature there are many studies of war veterans with PTSD showing very high physiological responses to reminders of war (such as pictures of combat or even recalling their own memories of the war) compared to war veterans without PTSD. Similar patterns of arousal have been found in other anxiety disorders. The underlying principle of fear conditioning models – that fear is precipitated by a fearful event – may not apply to all anxiety disorders. However, PTSD, by definition, is an anxiety disorder which is always triggered by an initial threatening experience.

Evidence shows that stressful events may precede cases of panic disorder, agoraphobia, social phobia, specific phobia, GAD and obsessive-compulsive disorder. In panic disorder, several studies indicate that panic disorder patients suffer increased stressful life events in the year prior to panic onset. There is also evidence that stressful events precede anxiety in children and adolescents. However, in many instances, anxiety disorders develop without any evidence of an aversive event preceding the initial episode. This pattern suggests that while fear conditioning can explain a proportion of anxiety disorders, it is does not adequately account for the onset of all anxiety disorders.

Extinction learning, aimed to reduce one's fear to a stimulus, works on similar principles. When an anxious person is exposed to feared situations on repeated occasions without any aversive outcomes, they gradually learn that these situations are not threatening and this reduces anxiety. Currently, the research suggests extinction learning does not erase original memories, but overrides it by new learning that different stimuli signal safety rather than danger.

Part V reviews the major brain structures that are implicated in anxiety disorders: the prefrontal cortex, the amygdala and the hippocampus. The amygdala is central to the process of conditioning fearful states, forming an association between internal and external stimuli that occur at the time of a fearful experience. Specifically, these associations are formed in the basolateral nucleus of the amygdala. The conditioned response of fear and anxiety, is generated in the central nucleus of the amygdala. It is from here that fear responses are expressed. Neuroimaging studies have found consistent hyperactivity in the amygdala in most anxiety disorders. Obsessive-compulsive disorder is distinctive, in that a dysregulation has been demonstrated in the frontal lobes, ventral striatum and thalamus. Changes in these neural structures have been observed in pre- and post- exposure therapy, reflecting changes in clients' anxiety levels.

Finally, as well as neural structures, neurotransmitters are also involved in anxiety disorders. Examples include serotonin, noradrenaline, glutamate, and GABA dopamine. The noradrenergic systems, as well as the HPA axis, affect specific neural regions and networks involved in fear and anxiety. Moreover, animal studies have revealed that fear extinction is mediated via glutamatergic NMDA receptors in the amygdala. In attempts to exploit this process, studies have revealed that injecting an NMDA receptor partial agonist, D-cycloserine, facilitates the extinction of conditioned freezing responses in rats. When used in adults, in combination with exposure therapy, anxious clients achieved faster extinction of their fear responses compared to anxious clients who were not given D-cycloserine.

PART VI   COGNITIVE THEORY

Peter is a 44-year-old man who has presented repeatedly to his doctor with physical concerns. He has had many tests and seen a number of medical specialists without any abnormalities being found.

Peter has a history of panic attacks, although he has not had any recently. He also has physical symptoms such as nausea, which his GP feels are being caused by too much anxiety.

"I've always been a worrier and I've always been a bit careful about my health. We were brought up that way. Mum was always taking us off to the doctor for one thing or another and I used to get a lot of unexplained stomach aches.

"I worry about things other than my health, too. My wife tells me I blow things out of proportion and I worry too much, but she doesn't understand the potential for things to go wrong.

"I worry about the kids a lot. I worry about them having an accident or getting sick and I'm not there to help them. I worry about someone in the family dying – I've worried about those sorts of things since I was a kid.

"Last week the car rego and the electricity bill came in at the same time and I really started to stress. All of a sudden, I thought, 'What if some big unexpected bill comes in, then we're going to be short and we won't be able to make the mortgage repayments and the bank will foreclose and we'll be out on the street?' It's stupid, because the money was there – I know because I plan and check things all the time."

Peter describes often being worried, and says he has always been a worrier. This may indicate an underlying predisposition to anxiety. He seems to feel that he may have learned to be concerned about his health because his mother frequently took the children to the doctor, suggesting that she also worried about their health, perhaps excessively. If this were the case, then this could have contributed to Peter's own attitudes towards health and the risk of illness. Peter also describes having had a lot of "unexplained stomach aches" in childhood, and we know that this is a common presentation of anxiety in children. That Peter refers to them as "unexplained" suggests that no medical cause was found.

Peter is using coping strategies such as detailed planning and repeated checking to try to reduce his worry. It may also be an attempt to feel more in control and less uncertain – these are some of the cognitive aspects of anxiety that will be addressed in more detail in Part VI. Peter also demonstrates some underlying schemas (or core beliefs), and some unhelpful patterns of thinking about risks, that are often referred to as *cognitive errors*.

Part VI will cover the development of cognitive theory and current thinking about the role of cognitive factors in anxiety. Cognitive factors refer to the thought processes both within and outside of conscious awareness (although cognitive theory holds that such thought processes can usually be discovered, even if they were initially outside of awareness). These may form some identifiable pattern or theme which frequently recurs, or may arise spontaneously in response to some stimulus such as an event or situation.

Theories about the importance of thought processes in contributing to and perpetuating emotional distress are relatively new, first appearing in the 1950s. Before then, Freud's theories about unconscious drives had great influence.

Information processing models have informed the current understanding of cognitive factors, and research using high and low anxious individuals has helped to identify specific cognitive factors associated with anxiety disorders in general, as well as individual anxiety disorder categories.

In helping individuals to overcome persistent problems with anxiety, it is important to identify patterns of information processing about the self and environments that unrealistically heighten anxiety. The case formulation represents a hypothesis about why anxiety developed in an individual at a particular time, why symptoms have persisted, and how cognitive, behavioural and somatic factors interact. It provides a basis for developing a treatment plan that is comprehensive and tailored to the individual. Treatment focuses particularly on factors contributing to the maintenance or persistence of anxiety. Cognitive, behavioural and environmental maintaining factors are identified, and their interactions postulated, to develop a cognitive model of illness. The model is often represented diagrammatically and it can also be used as the basis for psycho-education around the rationale for the proposed treatment interventions.

CHAPTER 20   COGNITIVE MODELS

Lisa Lampe

THE COGNITIVE MODEL

Although described as a "cognitive" model, this is, in fact, an attempt to link together and understand the possible relationships between identifiable factors that appear to be of relevance in triggering, but especially maintaining, ongoing problems for the individual. In other words, the hypothesised relationship can be between cognitive, behavioural, somatic, environmental and other factors. It is not purely "cognitive".

Generic models have been developed, to provide some guidance about factors that should be looked for. However, the model should always be tailored to the individual. The model can be developed out of the "case formulation", an important part of modern CBT.

The case formulation represents a hypothesis about why symptoms developed and persisted, including predisposing and precipitating factors, but is particularly focused on modifiable aspects of an individual's problems – that is, on the maintaining factors. It is often easier to appreciate the identified "feedback loops" (maintenance cycles) when these are presented diagrammatically. Hence diagrams similar to flow charts are often developed for this purpose.

THE CASE FORMULATION IN ANXIETY

The case formulation represents a synthesis of information obtained from a patient's history, to generate hypotheses about the reasons for the symptoms that they are presenting. The clinician asks questions based on current knowledge about risk factors for anxiety disorders, and cognitive and behavioural perpetuating factors. The patient's own ideas about the causes and consequences of their symptoms are also sought.

A MODEL OF SOCIAL PHOBIA

Central to social phobia are fears of being negatively evaluated by others (Figure 20.1). Individuals may believe that this could happen in a number of ways – for example, by saying something foolish, by appearing anxious or socially inept or by doing something embarrassing. Typically, the symptoms of the fight or flight response that are most likely to be appraised as being inherently threatening are those that the individual fears may make their anxiety visible to others – that is, blushing, sweating and shaking. Note once again the role of cognitive factors in maintaining anxiety (i.e., the anxiety symptoms are appraised as threatening in themselves, thus further increasing anxiety).

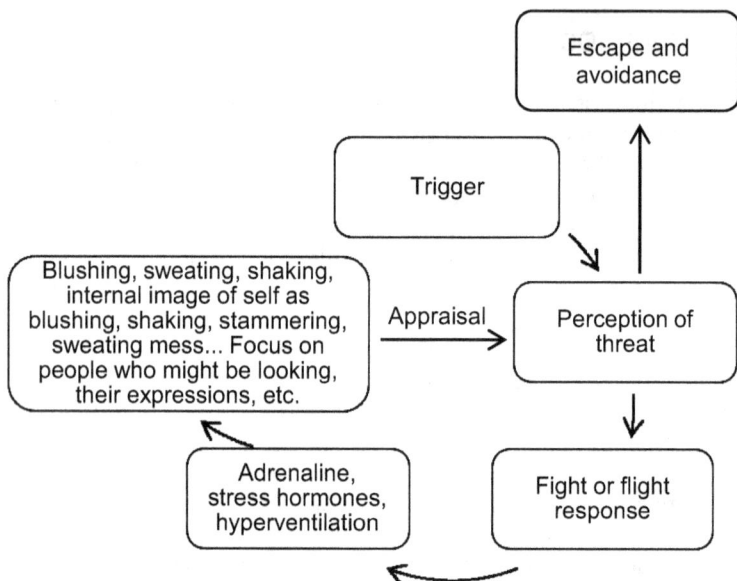

Figure 20.1 Model of social phobia

A number of other maintaining factors have also been identified in social phobia. These include the tendency for the individual to monitor their own performance carefully, and to focus on what they feel are negative aspects. There is also a tendency for some people to be hypervigilant to any possible signs of a critical reaction in others – and it is also known that there is a tendency to think the worst. For example, if someone glances away, this is seen as a sign of disapproval or disinterest, when the action might be entirely coincidental.

Finally, a person may also decide to flee or escape the situation as soon as they feel threatened (or even avoid the situation completely). In this case, they may avoid triggering the fight or flight response. However, in the long run, avoidance itself tends to act as a maintaining factor for anxiety.

THE ROLE OF AVOIDANCE

Avoidance of anxiety prevents the person from learning that the feared outcome may not be as likely as they thought. It also prevents the person from learning that the feared outcome may not be as bad as they expected, and stops the person from developing skills to manage the feared situations better.

However, it continues to be employed as a coping strategy because escaping anxiety acts as powerful negative reinforcement.

A MODEL OF PTSD

In PTSD, the triggers are typically reminders of the traumatic situation experienced by the individual. In an attempt to avoid anxiety being triggered, the person often tries to avoid as many triggers as they can. But if anxiety is triggered (e.g. by thoughts or images), the resulting symptoms may themselves be appraised as threatening, or may contribute to increased arousal and threat detection – for example, through hypervigilance.

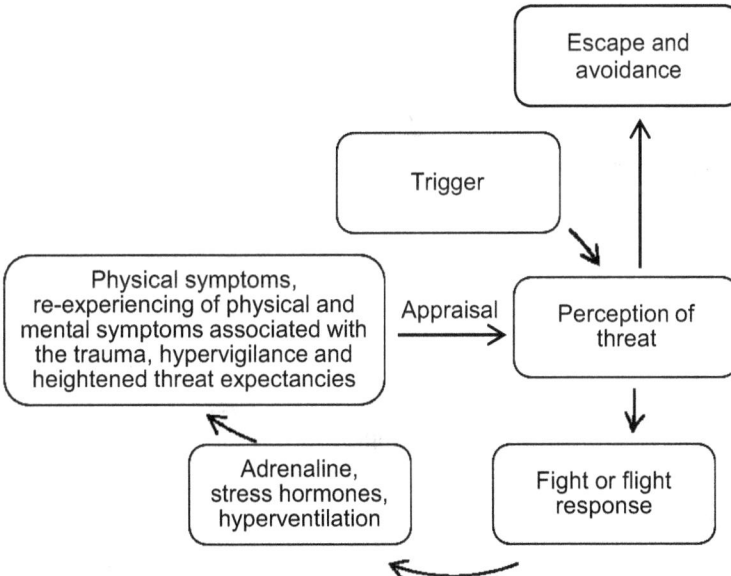

Figure 20.2 Model of PTSD

Overall, in PTSD the specific role of appraisal of anxiety symptoms may not be as great as for phobic disorders.

A MODEL OF OCD

In OCD, an additional feature is added to the model to show the role of compulsions (Figure 20.3). The individual often attempts to avoid triggers in the first place, and compulsions are an attempt to reduce anxiety that has already been triggered. Appraisal of physical symptoms may also be important in some types of OCD – for example, the signs of anxiety may be misinterpreted as those of injury or the result of contamination; the increase in arousal may be misinterpreted as sexual arousal in someone with sexual obsessions. Also, the hypervigilance that results from the fight or flight response may mean that many more "suspicious looking" signs are picked up and appraised in a manner that seems to reinforce fears – for example, a red spot is taken to represent blood, a flash of something shiny is appraised as a needle.

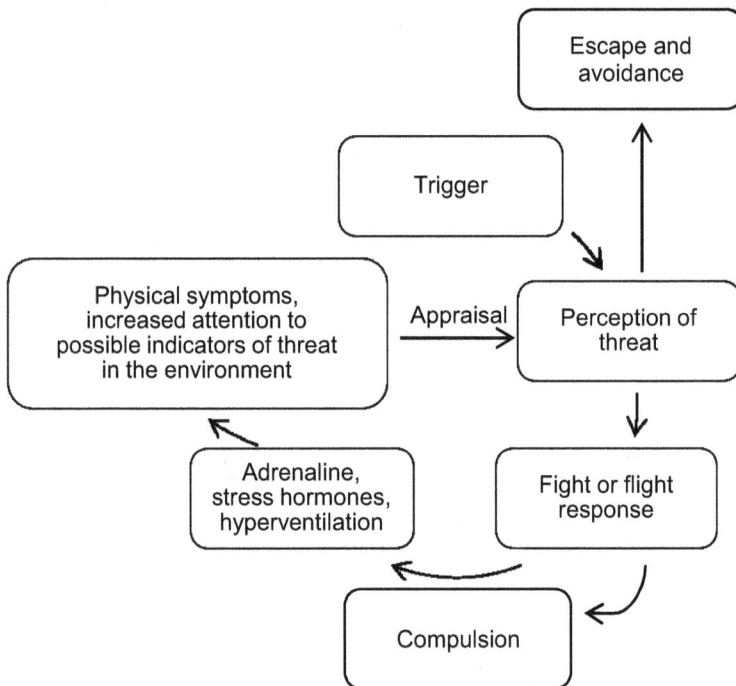

Figure 20.3   Model of OCD

CASE STUDY: ANGELA

Angela is a 25-year-old woman who started having panic attacks after the birth of her baby, Emily. Since then, she tries to avoid being alone in case she panics or develops a critical physical problem. As a result of her avoidance of being alone, she now relies heavily on her husband

Michael. Figure 20.4 is an example of a model that the therapist may have drawn after interviewing Angela. Note that there is no single way to draw a model. This one is somewhat different from the more generic models above. In practice, models often evolve as patient and therapist learn more about the patient's problems.

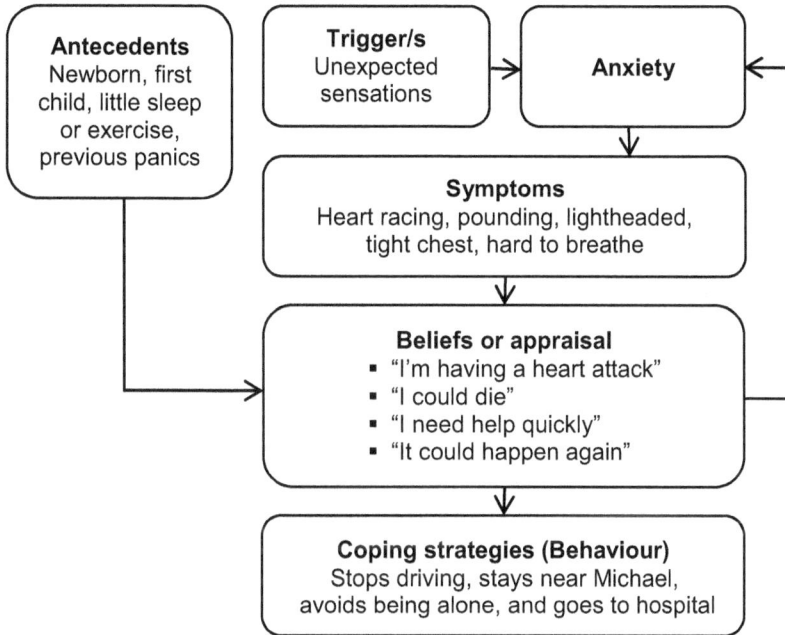

Figure 20.4 Example cognitive model of a patient

VALUE OF THE COGNITIVE MODEL

The case formulation and cognitive model are regarded as important elements of good quality CBT. The cognitive model provides a concise summary of our hypotheses about the patient's problems. It is a useful tool in providing psycho-education. Patients can take it away and discuss it with friends and family, and modify it as appropriate – taking ownership of the model enhances engagement in CBT. The model represents a sound basis on which to begin to plan treatment.

Figure 20.5 illustrates how the cognitive model alerts the therapist to the points at which intervention can disrupt the feedback loops that have been identified. Strategies with an evidence base for efficacy in treating identified problems should be chosen.

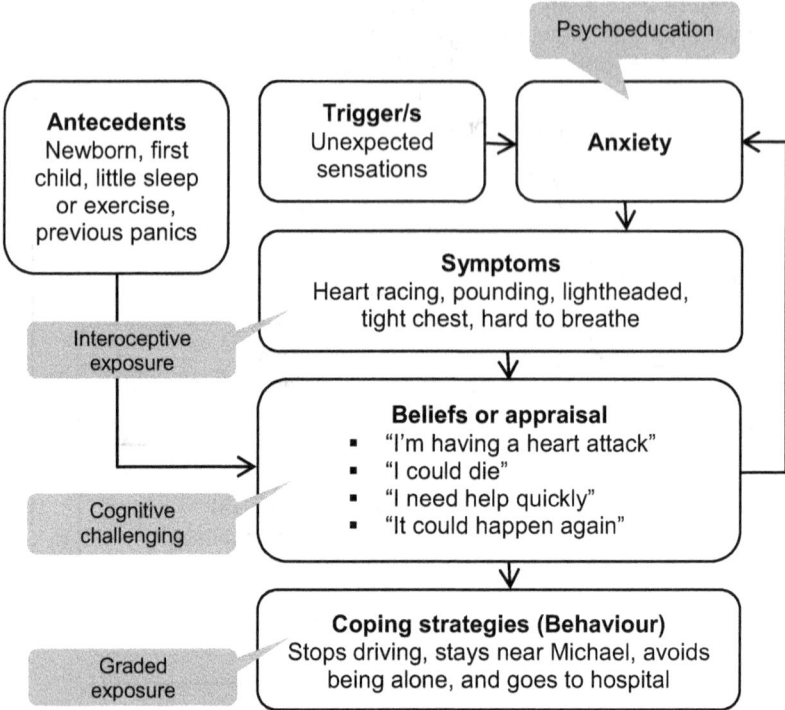

Figure 20.5   Interventions that disrupt the feedback loops of a cognitive model

CHAPTER 21   SCHEMAS

Lisa Lampe

COGNITIVE THEORY OF ANXIETY DISORDERS

The cognitive theory of anxiety disorders is developed out of what is usually referred to as "Beck's cognitive theory of emotional disorder". Cognitive theory represents one of the developments of learning theory.

Jean Piaget (1896–1980) was a Swiss biologist who, in the early twentieth century, described a number of stages of cognitive development. He used the term "schema" in his model of the cognitive development of children, and US psychiatrist Aaron Beck later adopted this term in his new theory of psychopathology.

Aaron Beck (born 1921) was trained as a psychiatrist and psychoanalyst in the United States. He is regarded as the founder of cognitive therapy. Although Beck based his new theory of depression on his clinical observations of patients, he was influenced in the further development of this theory by his readings of Piaget and others.

TIMELINE OF COGNITIVE AND BEHAVIOURAL THERAPIES

There have been three waves of developments that have led to current cognitive-behavioural therapies.

The first wave was the development of behavioural (learning) theories. Ivan Pavlov, who actually received his Nobel Prize for studies into the digestive system, spent many years exploring conditioned reflexes, as in the experiment famously known as "Pavlov's Dog". BF Skinner, the American psychologist, discovered that behaviour is increased because of the consequences that follow, not because of what precedes it.

The second wave of cognitive-behavioural therapy saw the development of cognitive theories of emotion, initially as a protest both against an overly behavioural view and classical psychoanalysis. Although much has been learned about cognitive factors in anxiety disorders, they most commonly act to maintain anxiety by contributing to operant conditioning. This will be explained in more detail later, but to understand cognitive-behavioural formulation and cognitive models, it is essential to have a good grasp of the principles of operant conditioning.

The third wave of development in CBT saw the further development of therapy applications of cognitive and behavioural theories. This has essentially involved modifications and, in some cases, additions to the basic cognitive and behavioural therapy components established over 1960s to 1970s. Additions have included elements of Eastern traditions such as mindfulness, in such therapies as dialectical behaviour therapy (DBT), mindfulness-based therapies and acceptance and commitment therapy (ACT).

HISTORICAL INFLUENCES ON THE DEVELOPMENT OF COGNITIVE THEORY

Piaget linked the stages of cognitive development to development in motor skills. These stages related to various age ranges in childhood. It is now believed that, in reality, the rate and nature of development may vary more from child to child, but Piaget's thinking stimulated further research and was highly influential at the time.

Importantly, it presented a way of understanding cognitive and motor development and the interaction of child and environment, and hence the importance of sensory stimulation for a child.

The term "schema" was used to describe the organisation, or mental representation, of knowledge about a particular subject or object. Schemas may include perceptions, ideas and actions, and will be modified as new information or understanding comes to light.

AARON BECK

In the late 1950s, Beck set out to establish an empirical basis for psychoanalysis, studying the dreams of depressed patients. Beck's thinking was influenced by the work of American psychologist George Kelly (1905–1967) and by that of Jean Piaget, and he eventually chose Piaget's term "schema" to use for his cognitive model of depression.

His cognitive model of depression, along with what is known as "Beck's cognitive triad" of negative outlook on the self, the world and the future, was developed during 1959 and the early 1960s. He published the Beck Depression Inventory in 1961, and this remains a very widely used self-report measure of depression.

Beck's research did not support psychoanalytic theory. Instead, he found that depressed persons had negative self-concepts, which gave them unhappy dreams.

Beck also corresponded with Albert Ellis, who had similarly trained as a psychoanalyst and was pursuing his own ideas about the importance of cognition in psychopathology.

Ellis developed a closely related form of cognitive therapy called Rational Emotive Therapy (or, more recently, Rational Emotive Behaviour Therapy). Beck, Ellis and Donald Meichenbaum (born 1940) are often regarded as the founding fathers of cognitive behaviour therapy.

BECK'S COGNITIVE MODEL OF DEPRESSION

In Beck's cognitive model of depression, negative experiences in childhood, such as excessive criticism or rejection by parents, or loss of a parent, lead to the development of negative beliefs about the self. These beliefs are referred to as schemas, or dysfunctional attitudes and assumptions.

In Beck's theory, these schemas lie dormant until they are activated by a negative event later in life. This negative event would usually be similar in some way, or act as a reminder of, the negative experiences of childhood.

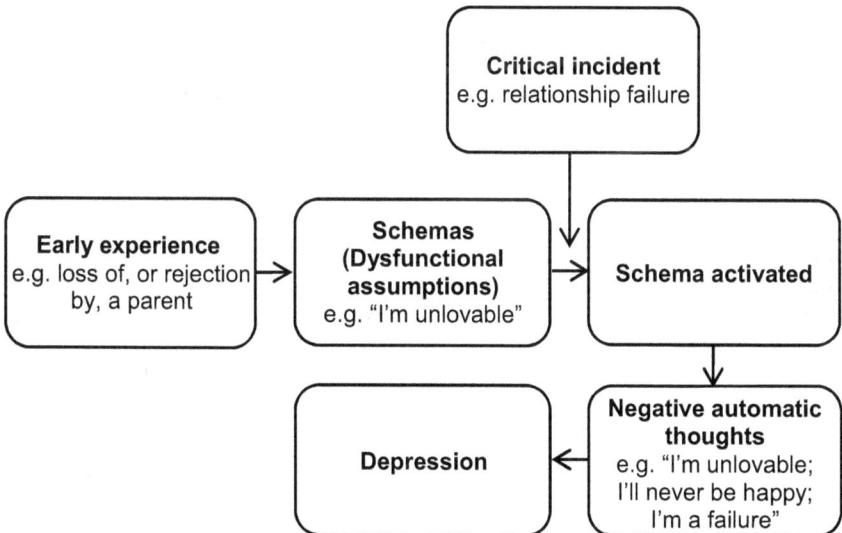

Figure 21.1   Beck's Cognitive Model of Depression

In this model, once the schemas are activated they affect information processing – for example, the person may start to focus on all the negative aspects of things, or start assuming the worst in situations of uncertainty. With all this negative thinking, the person then becomes clinically depressed.

CURRENT STATUS OF BECK'S THEORY OF DEPRESSION

Beck's theory of depression has been highly influential, not least in stimulating research into every aspect of the model. In particular, it has spurred understanding of the cognitive perpetuating factors in mental disorders.

The model of mental disorders based on the concept of environment interacting with a vulnerability is now strongly supported. A number of vulnerabilities in addition to cognitive vulnerabilities have been identified – most importantly, genetic and temperamental. There is good support for cognitive biases in information processing in depression and anxiety.

However, there is less evidence that schemas may be inactive or dormant until activated by an event. Another limitation is that behavioural factors (e.g. social withdrawal, inactivity) that are known to contribute to depression are not included in the model.

SCHEMAS

This chapter deals with one usage of the word "schema". However, this word is also used in many other fields to describe the organisation of knowledge or actions. In the field of psychology and psychiatry, it generally has the meaning as used by Beck's work. Schemas are regarded as deep-seated, long-standing beliefs held by a person, the nature of which contribute to emotional distress and often behavioural problems. A number of commonly problematic themes have been identified. The beliefs underlying schemas are rarely questioned by the individual, who may not even be aware that they hold them. Troublesome schemas are unhelpful, often untrue and usually intensely negative.

> Schemas are deep-seated, long-standing beliefs, the nature of which contribute to emotional distress and behavioural problems.

OTHER TERMINOLOGY

In the field of psychology and psychiatry, other terms may be used which refer to the same concept behind the word "schema". The most common synonyms are "core beliefs" or "dysfunctional assumptions". However, both the words "schema" and "core belief" imply that the beliefs in question are deeply held, central to the sense of self and long-term. "Dysfunctional assumptions" may also be used to describe a more acute experience, akin to "automatic thoughts" that are triggered by a particular situation under the influence of schemas.

ALBERT ELLIS

Albert Ellis (1913–2007) was trained as a clinical psychologist and psychoanalyst in the US. He was influenced by his own experience of overcoming childhood challenges – emotionally unavailable parents, poor health and significant social anxiety – toward a more pragmatic and less abstract view of psychotherapy than psychoanalysis. Ellis read widely in areas of philosophy and cited the influence of the Stoic philosophers of ancient Greece and Rome, especially by Epictetus and Marcus Aurelius. The name Epictetus is often associated with the concept that emotional response has a lot to do with how we think about what happens to us, rather than being solely due to the events themselves.

He was also interested in the ideas of more modern philosophers such as Bertrand Russell, Immanuel Kant and Karl Popper, as well as existential philosophers such as Martin Heidegger and Paul Tillich. Additionally, he found the work of contemporary psychotherapists including Karen Horney and Alfred Adler highly relevant.

Ellis began to believe strongly that, although an individual may hold unhelpful self-beliefs very deeply, these beliefs could be modified by being actively and repeatedly disputed. Ellis emphasised a connection between rational thinking and psychological adjustment. However, using "insight" is not enough; the individual must actively work to change longstanding patterns. Behavioural strategies were also seen as an important part of therapy.

Ellis began to take a less classically analytic approach with his patients. Instead of frequent visits, information and advice giving, he focused more on understanding the links between childhood and present day problems. He felt his patients seemed to do better, faster, with this approach. Based on his research, he published "*Rational Psychotherapy and Individual Psychology*" in 1957.

PRINCIPLES OF COGNITIVE THEORY – BECK AND ELLIS

The following basic principles on which cognitive behavioural therapies are based are widely agreed upon:

- Humans have a biologically based tendency to create and subscribe to deeply held beliefs about themselves, others and the world around them.
- These beliefs can influence emotions and behaviours (and other types of cognitive processes and cognitions) in important ways.
- Certain types of beliefs will contribute to self-enhancing, goal-promoting emotions and behaviours; other sorts of beliefs will contribute to self-defeating emotions and behaviours.
- It is possible to identify and modify the sorts of beliefs that are unhelpful.

FURTHER DEVELOPMENT OF COGNITIVE THEORY – "SECOND AND THIRD WAVE" THERAPIES

Following on from the early developments in cognitive theory and its integration with behaviour therapy, a number of modifications or innovations have been effected.

These may add elements of other philosophies (e.g. mindfulness in mindfulness-based therapies, dialectical behaviour therapy and acceptance and commitment therapy) or focus on particular aspects (e.g. schema-focussed therapy, cognitive behavioural analysis system of psychotherapy), for example.

There are now many therapies loosely or closely based on cognitive behaviour therapy.

DEVELOPMENTS OF THE COGNITIVE MODEL

Additions have been made to Beck's model to take into account research findings about vulnerability factors in contributing to the development of psychological disorders. "Compensatory strategies" include behavioural responses to emotional distress or situational challenges.

The concept of intermediate or conditional assumptions is an attempt to account for mediating factors between core beliefs and the development of longstanding patterns of maladaptive behaviour, especially that seen in personality disorders.

As can be seen from Figure 21.2, the identification of core beliefs or schemas is seen as critical in understanding symptoms, and later in therapy.

Albert Ellis was firmly of the view that the secondary symptoms – the effects of the core beliefs in causing behavioural and emotional disturbance – should be targeted first, followed by the primary problems of troublesome core beliefs.

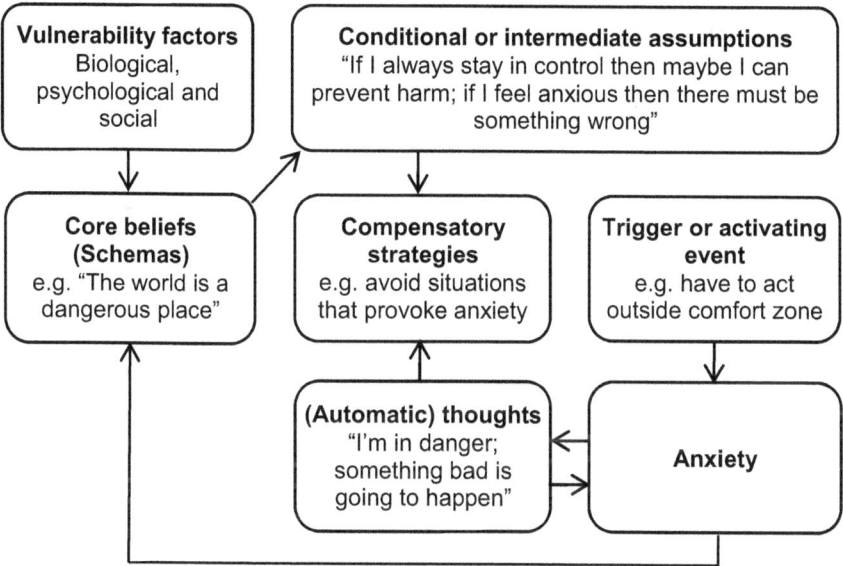

Figure 21.2 Developments of Beck's Cognitive Model

So in this case, the avoidance of anything that causes anxiety would be the initial target of therapy. The underlying schema that "the world is a dangerous place", and assumptions about how this danger should be managed, would be targeted next.

Many therapists, however, might target intermediate beliefs, or would address all these levels simultaneously.

EXAMPLES OF SCHEMAS

As noted before, a number of common themes have been recognised for schemas. Table 21.1 gives each theme an example.

Table 21.1 Common themes and associated cognitions

Theme	Associated cognitions
Shame	"I am a bad person."
Defectiveness	"I am unworthy of love."
Failure	"I don't measure up to others."
Abandonment	"Others will always leave me."
Mistrust	"No-one can be trusted."
Vulnerability to danger	"The world is a dangerous place."
Enmeshment	"I cannot be myself."
Entitlement	"I am better than others."
Subjugation	"My opinions and needs do not count."
Approval-seeking	"I am nothing without the approval of others."

CHAPTER 22   SPECIFIC COGNITIVE DISTORTIONS

Lisa Lampe

ABOUT THIS CHAPTER

The previous chapter looked at some of the philosophical and experiential influences on cognitive theory. This chapter will look at some of the more laboratory-based influences, including those that have arisen from cognitive psychology and neuropsychology.

INFORMATION PROCESSING MODEL

Information processing models inform cognitive theory. Information from the internal and external environment is received and processed by the brain to derive some meaning. This is also referred to as "appraisal".

The stages of information processing include perception of the stimulus information, followed by the initial processing of this information. After this, the information may be discarded (for example, if judged to be irrelevant) or coded for memory. At a later stage it may be retrieved (for example, by deliberate attempts to remember or by the recurrence of the same or similar stimuli). At this time, it may be subject to modification or elaboration, before going back into memory.

Once developed, schemas are further elaborated in the light of ongoing experience. This schema concept of "ongoing elaboration" is quite consistent with an information processing model.

A great deal of research is focused on the ways in which information is stored and retrieved. An information processing model is inherent in cognitive theory. It is the meanings, interpretations or appraisals that are made of events, including internal events such as physical sensations or thoughts, that can give rise both to emotional distress and unhelpful behaviours.

In explaining the information processing model to patients, the concept of "programs" can be helpful. Most patients are now familiar with the concept of computer programs that exist to process many types of data. The program needs to be written by someone, and directs how different pieces of information should be interpreted. Humans do much the same thing, although often they are not aware of it. For example, if an individual was to smell smoke, their prior experience of smoke would have resulted in "programs" that are automatically activated when they smell it, which help them to draw conclusions about its likely origin.

Applying this to an anxiety context, an individual with generalised anxiety disorder and underlying fears that they may make a wrong decision that leads to a catastrophic outcome, may react to a decision-making opportunity with anxiety, because they have appraised such a situation as inherently dangerous.

COGNITIVE BIAS

There are a number of possible influences on the appraisal process, which are usually referred to in the CBT literature as cognitive biases. Cognitive biases can affect information processing in a number of ways and at a number of stages, including attention to stimuli, appraisal or interpretation of the meaning of the stimuli and recall of information. Cognitive biases in anxiety are most likely to be triggered by uncertainty – that is, by situations in which the outcome is not known.

A number of biases in information processing have been described, including probability, cost, attention and attribution.

The particular importance of cognitive biases to the treatment of anxiety disorders is the role that such factors can play in maintaining the anxiety cycle. This is because the appraisal itself may appear to reinforce schemas or negative core beliefs. This will be discussed further after a number of biases are introduced.

PROBABILITY BIAS

A common symptom of anxiety is the overestimation of the likelihood that a particular feared outcome will eventuate. Although in reality there is often a possibility of harm, the anxious person often views even a small possibility as though it is, in fact, very likely. This in turn creates great anxiety. Hence, when faced with the possibility of a feared outcome occurring (e.g. an individual needs to drive across a bridge but fears that they may panic and lose control of the car), an anxious person is likely to appraise the situation as being more likely to result in harm or disaster than it really is. When this overestimation of the likelihood of harm occurring is habitual, it can be referred to as a cognitive bias.

COST BIAS

The degree of anxiety bears a close relationship to the perceived "awfulness" – or cost – of the feared outcome. If an individual is asked to walk across a narrow beam of wood, their anxiety about the task is likely to be much greater if the beam is raised to three metres off the ground than it would be if the beam was only twenty centimetres off the ground. The "cost" of a feared outcome is its perceived seriousness. Individuals with anxiety disorders often overestimate how bad it would be if something they feared (e.g. a panic attack, being disapproved of or disliked by someone) actually happened.

Research in social phobia (social anxiety disorder) indicates that changes in cost appraisals may be associated with a better outcome than changes in probability estimates.

ATTENTIONAL BIAS

The importance of attention focus has been increasingly recognised. Anxious persons become hypervigilant to threat. In other words, they are constantly on the lookout for things they worry about. These perceived threats may be in the external environment, or they may be physical symptoms in the body (the internal environment). For example, individuals with panic disorder or health anxiety commonly focus too much attention on internal sensations; individuals with social phobia may be too focused on external manifestations of anxiety, such as blushing or sweating. This may have the effect of keeping a person focused on these symptoms and may lower the threshold at which they become aware of them, resulting in more anxiety. In this way, someone with generalised anxiety disorder or panic disorder who has excessive anxiety about their health, may spend a lot of time monitoring their own somatic sensations, which might have the effect of increasing awareness and triggering anxiety at a lower threshold.

An excessive focus on internal sensations may also explain nocturnal panic attacks – that is, the person responds in their sleep to some change in physical sensation.

The degree of anxiety bears a close relationship to the perceived "awfulness" – or cost – of the feared outcome.

In the external environment, when an individual is too focused on potential threats, there is a higher possibility of feeling that such cues are extremely common. For example, a person with a severe spider phobia may seem to see spiders everywhere. Similar experiences happen in everyday life. For example, if someone is thinking of buying a new Toyota Camry, they will automatically start noticing these on the road, until it seems that every second car is a Camry. Or someone with OCD who has a fear of contamination by blood may be hypervigilant to red spots or stains in the environment, and seem to see them everywhere. Coupled with this is often a tendency to misinterpret an ambiguous cue. In the previous example, the person with OCD not only seems to see red spots everywhere, but also will tend to misinterpret the nature of these stains as being blood when they are really just paint.

Another consequence of focusing excessive attention resources toward threat is that if attention is taken up by anxiety-related cues, it cannot then be directed effectively to a person's work or interpersonal interactions, thus impairing function.

Self-focused Attention in Social Phobia

The role of attention focus may be especially relevant in social phobia.

Social interaction is a stimulus to increased self-awareness for most people. Two types of self-awareness are recognised, both of which can contribute to increased social anxiety:

- public self-awareness (seeing oneself as others might, or "observer perspective")
- private self-awareness (increased awareness of inner experience).

Increased self-awareness may actually improve performance for people who are naturally low in social anxiety, but it has been shown to impair performance when there is a high degree of fear of negative evaluation. Hence, self-focused attention, if excessive, can be unhelpful in social phobia.

A number of studies have looked at the effect of self-focused attention in social phobia and found that it tends to increase anxiety and reduce performance skill. Individuals with social phobia often devote substantial cognitive resources to generating an image of themselves as they think others see them, as a way to monitor how they are appearing to others. This is referred to as the "observer perspective"; it is as if they were in front of a camera. There are several problems with doing this: it can be distracting and take away from their skill in interacting; it can be inaccurate – individuals with social phobia tend to focus on the negative aspects of their performance and to over-estimate how much their anxiety is obvious to others; and it can be distressing, if they create an image of themselves as doing badly. The opposite perspective is referred to as the "field perspective", in which it is as if the person was behind the camera, and surveying the "field" in front of them.

Treatment Programs

CBT for social phobia now usually includes guidance about keeping attention focused on the task at hand rather than on oneself or on trying to create a picture of how one might look to others. There is some evidence that this instruction itself can be effective in reducing symptoms. Mindfulness approaches may also be helpful, as they encourage the individual to direct their focus mindfully, but also to accept thoughts and feelings as they arise, and avoid reacting with emotional distress or judgments.

There has been some evidence that treatment packages that include such instructions are superior to those without explicit instructions regarding attention focus. Studies have also shown that simply encouraging someone with social phobia to stay task-focused may be effective, even in the absence of cognitive challenging interventions.

ATTRIBUTION BIAS

An attribution bias represents a systematic way in which a person makes a faulty attribution – for example, whenever they confront a particular feared situation.

An everyday example of a misattribution is that of a patient with high blood pressure who, after taking blood pressure pills for a few months, is found to have a normal blood pressure by their doctor, so stops taking the tablets, believing that their high blood pressure is now cured.

With respect to anxiety, examples might include the person with agoraphobia who carries a benzodiazepine tablet with them wherever they go, believing that without that tablet, they would not be able to go out; or the person with any anxiety disorder who leaves a situation as soon as they start to feel anxious and then believes that if they had not left, they would have had a panic attack with the feared consequences (e.g. collapse, embarrassment, serious physical or mental problem). In this example, the avoidance strategy is credited with saving the person from serious harm, and this means they are likely to go on using this strategy to cope with anxiety.

Case Study: Susan

Susan is a 27-year-old woman, who fears that in social situations she will get anxious and vomit, and that others will think that she is weak, odd or incompetent.

"If I become nauseated and my mouth goes dry, I think that this is a sign that I'm about to vomit, so I always leave the situation I'm in and go straight to the bathroom. Then I try to vomit, because I feel that if I do so, I'll 'get it out of my system' so I can go back to what I was doing and be confident that I won't vomit again. Sometimes I don't actually vomit after I've gone to the bathroom, I just dry retch, but even that is enough to reassure me that it's out of my system."

From Susan's perspective, these beliefs do appear to explain her observations: nausea and a dry mouth are signs that vomiting is imminent; vomiting "gets it out of her system", and she is then able to relax. However, she then becomes stuck in a feedback loop where she behaves in a way that produces certain outcomes that seem to prove that her beliefs are correct.

Susan's attributions do not appear to be realistic or helpful. It looks more as though she is making herself vomit, and one wonders what would happen if she simply ignored the nausea and stayed in the situation. The behavioural loop in which she is now stuck is limiting to her life, and she never tests out any alternative hypotheses. Figure 22.1 shows Susan's beliefs and attributions about anxiety and its consequences. Some of them may be unrealistic, or may represent conclusions that are not justified logically, or may simply be unhelpful to her.

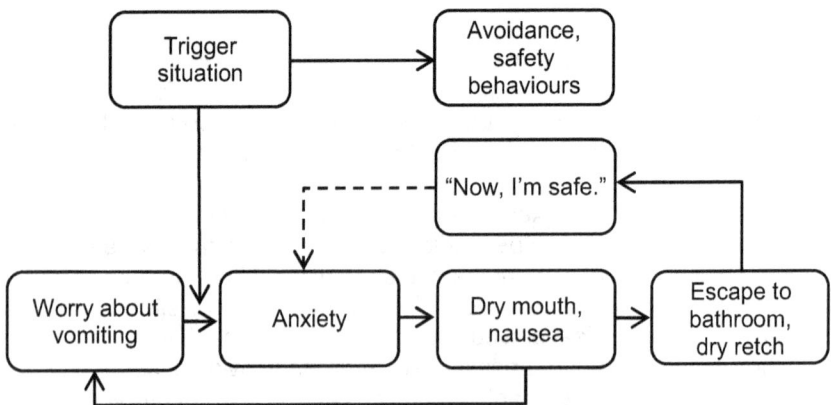

Figure 22.1 A model of Susan's current beliefs and attributions

In this model, her dry mouth and nausea are attributed to her anxiety, rather than evidence that she is about to vomit. It is suggested that she is anxious in social situations because of her fear of vomiting, and the negative consequences it would have. It can also be suggested that vomiting once should have no physiological effect on vomiting again; however, believing that it has this effect will reduce anxiety and therefore reduce the somatic symptoms that are interpreted as signs that she is about to vomit.

Figure 22.2, Susan's attributions are that it is the situation that is causing her dry mouth and nausea and that these are making her anxious because she fears she will vomit.

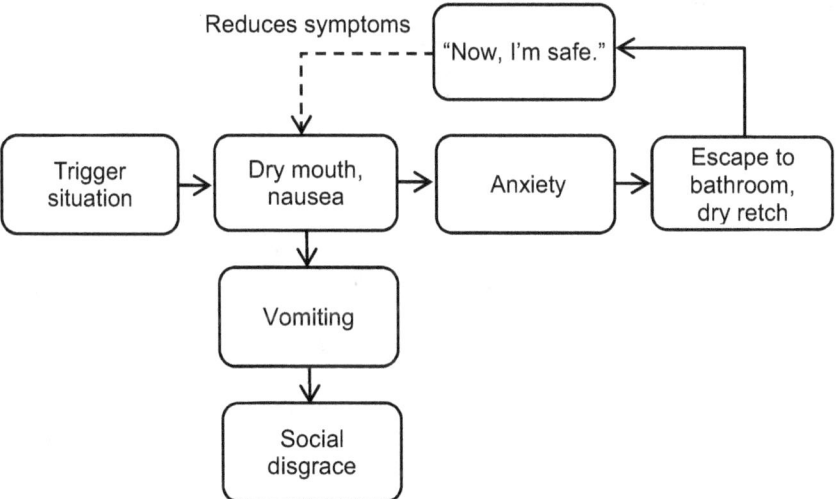

Figure 22.2   Susan's attribution biases

Her escape to the bathroom seems to fix the situation – her dry mouth and nausea improve quickly – but she never tests whether her attributions are really correct, and ends up stuck with a dysfunctional coping style. That is, she will repeatedly escape from anxiety-provoking situations because this makes her feel better quickly, and she believes that the alternative of staying in the situation will make her anxiety worse, lead to vomiting and result in completely unacceptable social disgrace.

COGNITIVE BIASES AS MAINTAINING FACTORS

Cognitive bias plays an important role in perpetuating or maintaining anxiety.

Individuals are usually not aware of cognitive biases. Therefore, the therapist will need to make a careful assessment of the person's responses to anxiety and ask about what is going through their mind, in order to develop hypotheses that can later be tested, regarding probable cognitive biases that act to maintain anxiety.

COGNITIVE "ERRORS" OR DISTORTIONS IN ANXIETY

Another way to discuss the concept of cognitive biases is to use the concept of cognitive errors, or cognitive distortions. Individuals write "programs", just as computers do, to interpret information in various situations. Cognitive errors describe a number of unhelpful patterns of thinking (programs) that have been identified over the years as tending to be associated with emotional distress. Some people find it helpful to look for these patterns in their own thinking when engaging in CBT, and may also find it comforting to know that they are not alone in thinking this way. It should be noted, however, that these do not have the link with cognitive psychology research that the concept of cognitive biases has, but are more of a clinical tool that may or may not be helpful.

Typical cognitive errors that are referred to in clinical practice include catastrophising, mind-reading, fortune-telling, black-and-white thinking, perfectionism, discounting the positive, personalisation and generalising. These are only "errors" in the sense that they tend to be unhelpful and to result in emotional distress: if behaviour (such as avoidance) is based on these beliefs, they can contribute to secondary dysfunction, or impairment in a person's work or relationships. There is no right or wrong way of thinking. The person is encouraged to apply the test of, "Is it helpful?"

Case Study: Rick

Rick was introduced in Part I, when his anxiety was first described. In a further discussion about his anxiety, he admits that he is so afraid of making the wrong decision he even finds it difficult to decide where to go out to dinner with his girlfriend. "I think I'm driving my girlfriend crazy," he says, and worries that he is going to lose her – just as he worries that he could lose his job: "I feel like a loser sometimes. I'm disappointed in myself for not coping better."

When he describes the stress he is under, Rick tends to catastrophise ("I'll lose my job"), mind-read ("I think I'm driving my girlfriend crazy"), and use fortune-telling ("She'll get fed up and leave me"). These are all examples of cognitive errors.

Rick admits that he sometimes misattributes the cause of tension in his head to being a sign of stroke rather than anxiety, although he is aware of this. If he made this assumption habitually, it could be an example of an attribution bias.

Rick has beliefs that maybe his worry will actually prevent harm somehow: "I worry that if I'm not worrying I will miss something, and that's when things will go terribly wrong." This is referred to as a positive metabelief (or metacognition), and will be covered in Chapter 24.

CHAPTER 23   RUMINATION AND WORRY

Michelle Moulds

CASE STUDY: JUN

"I wish I'd never gone to my cousin's engagement party. I hardly knew anyone. He has so many friends. Seeing them all there made me feel so nervous and inadequate. I bet people could tell I didn't have any friends. I should have talked more. I just stood there like a statue. I looked like an idiot, a mute idiot. I was the only one not saying anything.

"Why didn't I talk more? I bet I made people feel really uncomfortable. Everyone must have thought how quiet and boring I was. I'm so pathetic. Why am I so scared to say anything? Why am I so socially inept? Is it because of my family? Mum and Dad are both quiet people. Did I inherit it off them?

"Great, now I'm doomed for life. I'll never have a girlfriend. I'll never get married and have kids. People will always wonder what's wrong with me. They'll think I'm some kind of a weirdo. How will I cope going to the wedding? I can't face those people again. Next time I'll know better. I'll just make an excuse that I'm sick and I won't go."

WHAT IS RUMINATION

Rumination refers to a recurrent, persistent and passive style of thinking.

In terms of content, when patients ruminate they tend to focus on themselves and on their current mood and anxiety symptoms. They also replay events from the past, and think over and over about their current concerns and stressors.

Patients often describe feeling "stuck" in their ruminative thought. That is, once they start to ruminate, patients report that is extremely difficult to stop their stream of thought.

Qualitatively, rumination tends to be abstract, non-specific and evaluative in nature. For example, a patient may repetitively pose questions such as "Why me? Why can't I get over this? Why do I feel this way?" These questions are often unanswerable.

RUMINATION IN DEPRESSION

Susan Nolen-Hoeksema, the US psychologist who investigated why women are twice as prone to depression as men, coined the term "depressive rumination", and developed a highly influential model of rumination known as the response style theory. This theory states that, while everyone experiences low moods at times, individuals who respond to their sadness by thinking about the causes, meanings and implications of their symptoms are more likely to go on to develop clinical depression, and to stay depressed for longer. A large number of studies have provided support for this account.

While this theory was developed and tested in the context of depression, rumination has also been identified as an important feature of the cognitive profile of patients with anxiety disorders.

RUMINATION IN SOCIAL PHOBIA

One such example is social phobia. Theoretical models of this disorder emphasise the role of anticipatory rumination. That is, prior to social events, socially anxious individuals think over and over about what could go wrong, how they might behave in an embarrassing way or how others will respond to them.

Similarly, following social events, socially anxious patients frequently engage in a "post-mortem" of the event, in which they replay the social encounter and ruminate about their (presumed) poor performance. Post-event rumination is also referred to as "post-event processing".

Both of these processes increase anxiety and encourage individuals to avoid social situations. In this way, rumination contributes to the persistence of social anxiety.

RUMINATION IN POSTTRAUMATIC STRESS DISORDER

Patients with posttraumatic stress disorder also ruminate, following their traumatic experience. In many cases, the content of rumination focuses on the individual's appraisal of their actions leading up to or during the trauma. They ruminate about their responsibility for the event (e.g., "It's my fault that my friend was stabbed – I should have seen that the guy had a knife and tackled him").

The content also focuses on the individual's thoughts about their PTSD symptoms (e.g., "I can't stop thinking about the accident – I'm losing my mind"; or "These nightmares are a sign that I'm going crazy").

Rumination can also fuel patients' anger if they perceive that another person was responsible for the trauma (e.g., "It's not fair - the other driver was speeding and she is fine. Why am I the one who is lying in a hospital bed?").

Persistent rumination on these types of themes contributes to the maintenance of PTSD by reinforcing unhelpful beliefs.

In addition, rumination results in affected individuals thinking about the trauma and its sequelae in a very abstract and vague way, rather than helping them to process the trauma memory and their associated emotions.

WHAT IS WORRY

Tom Borkovec, one of the pioneers of research on worry as a disorder, and his colleagues defined worry as a chain of thoughts and images that elicits negative affect (mood or emotions), and that is experienced by an individual as uncontrollable.

In terms of content, anxious individuals worry about a broad range of themes – health, finances, relationships, the safety of their family members, to name just a few. Worry is focused on negative situations and events that could happen in the future.

Qualitatively, worry, like rumination, tends to be vague, non-specific and lacking in concrete detail. That is, worry tends to focus on "big picture" themes, such as, "What will become of me in the future? What if I lose my job? Then everything will be ruined."

WORRY IN GENERALISED ANXIETY DISORDER

Persistent anxiety and worry are the primary DSM-5 symptoms of generalised anxiety disorder. As previously described, individuals with GAD worry about a broad range of themes and topics.

Their worry tends to be catastrophic; individuals with GAD worry endlessly about a multitude of possible negative situations that could feasibly occur in the future. They usually ask "what if" questions.

Worry and rumination both tend to be vague, non-specific and lacking in concrete detail.

RUMINATION AND WORRY: COMMONALITIES

Rumination and worry share a number of features. Both are repetitive, worsen psychological symptoms (mood, anxiety), and are vague and abstract. While rumination has primarily been studied in the domain of depression, worry has been examined in the context of anxiety. The primary distinction between these two types of thought is their temporal focus; that is, while rumination tends to focus on events that have happened in the past, worry is typically about events that could happen in the future. However, this distinction may over-simplify things, as the different temporal focus is not always clear-cut. For example, a patient with PTSD might ruminate about a previous assault and, as a result, worry over and over about the chance of being assaulted again in the future.

REPETITIVE THINKING

The shared features of rumination and worry have led a number of researchers to suggest that a more useful way to conceptualise rumination and worry might be, instead, to conceptualise both under a more general umbrella of "repetitive thinking"; that is, irrespective of whether an individual repeatedly dwells on something negative that happened to them in the past, or thinks over and over about something negative that could happen in the future. This is an important step because, rather than focusing solely on theoretical definitions, it encourages therapists to focus on the important issue of developing more effective treatments for repetitive thinking – regardless of the disorders in which these types of thinking occur.

WHY DO ANXIOUS INDIVIDUALS ENGAGE IN REPETITIVE THINKING

If rumination and worry cause distress, why do patients persist in thinking this way?

Research on individuals with anxiety and mood disorders has shown that there are a number of factors that contribute to the likelihood that patients will continue to think in these ways. For example, individuals often report that they think repeatedly about the past and how they currently feel in order to determine why they feel badly, so they can understand themselves and their behaviour. In these instances, patients start out ruminating or worrying with good intentions, but these styles of thinking ultimately prevent them from reaching their goals.

Individuals also often believe that rumination will help them to solve their problems. Other patients endorse beliefs such as the idea that replaying past events helps them to avoid making the same mistakes again.

All these examples have in common that they reinforce the idea that repetitive thinking is a useful process. It is, therefore, not surprising that individuals who hold such beliefs persist in ruminating and worrying, despite their aversive outcomes.

CONSEQUENCES OF REPETITIVE THINKING

Rumination and worry are associated with a range of negative consequences. For example, repeatedly dwelling on negative themes, such as one's worthlessness, as well as all of the bad things that could happen in the future, can strengthen such maladaptive cognitions and make them seem more realistic and believable.

Avoidance is another consequence of repetitive thinking. If a person recurrently thinks about all of the bad things that could happen, they will be driven to avoid situations in which their fears might be realised (e.g., going to a party or giving a presentation at work).

Repetitive thinking can also result in inaction. The more an individual thinks about and mulls over the past and possible negative events in the future, the more they delay engaging in active problem solving that could, in fact, help them to take steps to improve how they feel now.

Another consequence of ruminating or worrying is that these streams of thought can have a snowball effect; once rumination starts, it triggers other negative thoughts and memories. In response, individuals may employ additional maladaptive habits (e.g., thought suppression), that further fuel the repetitive thinking and keep them locked in a vicious cycle.

CAN REPETITIVE THINKING BE ADAPTIVE?

A recent line of thought that has been developed by Ed Watkins of Exeter University, is that not all repetitive thinking is necessarily bad. That is, there are times in which thinking about how we feel, replaying the past and thinking about the future can actually be helpful and adaptive.

Watkins suggests that it is not the process of repetitive thinking itself that is problematic. Instead, it is the manner in which one reflects on this content that is important. Specifically, he proposes that the mode of processing that is adopted during repetitive thinking determines its consequences. While an analytical mode of processing results in negative outcomes, an experiential mode of processing has adaptive consequences.

Note that the content of the repetitive thoughts in these modes of processing is the same. However, while the analytical example is vague, abstract and is made up of "why" questions, in comparison, the experiential example is specific, concrete and focused on the direct experience of the symptoms rather than posing questions about why the symptoms are occurring, and what they mean (Table 23.1).

Table 23.1 Analytical and experiential examples

Analytical mode	Experiential mode
"Why do I feel anxious?"	"I feel anxious."
"Why am I the only one who feels anxious about asking a question in class?"	"I need to focus on how I can best ask the question, given how I'm feeling."
"Why is my heart beating madly, and why is my mouth so dry?"	"My heart is beating madly and my mouth is dry."
"Why can't I just get over it?"	"What do I need to say?"

These two modes of processing repetitive thought are clearly qualitatively different. They also have very distinct consequences.

An analytical mode of thinking encourages avoidance and procrastination (rather than a direct plan of action) and prompts more "why" questions. As such, this mode maintains rumination and increases anxiety symptoms.

By contrast, the experiential mode encourages direct reflection on the problem at hand, without pondering about "why" the problem arose or what it might mean. In this way, an experiential mode of processing encourages problem-solving, prompts specific action and limits generalising to other thoughts and situations.

CHAPTER 24   OTHER IMPORTANT COGNITIVE PERPETUATING FACTORS

Lisa Lampe

POST-EVENT PROCESSING

Sometimes, an individual might think about events a lot, especially if those events have been particularly challenging, exciting or enjoyable. It is also common to mull over events or experiences that have an element of ambiguity. The concept of post-event processing was introduced in the previous chapter. The intensity and frequency of post-event processing can be high.

EMOTIONAL TONE OF POST-EVENT PROCESSING

Individuals can have positive or negative reactions to things; the emotional tone of a person's experiences is often referred to as a "valence", either positive or negative in tone. So post-event processing can be described as having a positive or negative valence, or emotional tone.

NEGATIVE POST-EVENT PROCESSING AND SOCIAL ANXIETY

In the case history of Jun in the Chapter 23, Jun wishes he had never gone to his cousin's engagement party because he did not know anyone and did not say anything. He ruminates intensely about his recent experience.

People who engage in negative post-event processing are more likely to be highly anxious when they enter situations, and are also more likely to make negative appraisals of their performance in social situations.

Post-event processing can thus act to reinforce both the fear and the expectation of negative evaluation.

MODEL OF POST-EVENT PROCESSING

Figure 24.1 shows a number of reinforcing factors for fear of negative evaluation.

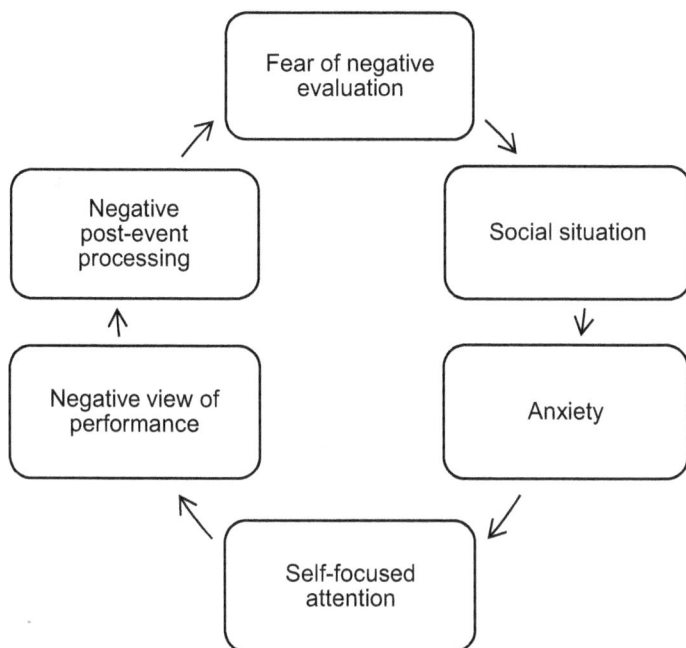

Figure 24.1   Model of Post-Event Processing

Some people focus their mind on what they perceive to have been a bad performance and on negative evaluation from others. This will only reinforce their beliefs that they are socially inept and their expectations of future bad performances. By contributing to emotional distress, this way of thinking also reinforces the "cost" of how bad a negative evaluation is; it feels bad, so it must be. Hence, a number of feedback loops are maintained. This diagram also shows how post-event processing (PEP) interacts with some other cognitive factors, such as self-focused attention and cognitive attribution biases.

Other factors have also been identified, including a possible memory bias. A memory bias may result when post-event processing (that is, focusing on what is perceived to be a negative performance, and on highly aversive consequences of negative evaluation) is so intense or frequent that it leads to the negative view being remembered in preference to anything positive that might have happened. These memories may then be triggered easily by the individual thinking about a future social event, and this in turn contributes to anticipatory anxiety about the event.

IMPLICATIONS OF POST-EVENT PROCESSING

Unlike many other types of phobia, which often improve significantly if a person, often without any formal treatment, decides to make themselves confront the situation, clinicians often hear from people with social phobia that although they frequently made themselves go to social events, the situation did not get any easier.

Sometimes, patients even report that the frequent exposure to social events made their phobia worse. Understanding about post-event processing can contribute to an understanding of how exposure could be counterproductive, or even unhelpful, in social phobia if cognitive factors are not addressed. That is, if a person's experience of social situations is of having performed badly, then all their memories of attempts to confront the problem will be negative. This will suggest to them that such attempts are doomed to failure, and will reinforce their beliefs about themselves as being socially inept.

It is, therefore, important for people to recognise any cognitive biases they may have, such as only focusing on the negative, and biased attributions, but also to refrain from unhelpful post-event processing. Instead, one session of balanced review to ask themselves what they can learn from the experience to apply in the future, and then refraining from further post-event processing, is likely to be most helpful therapeutically. It is also likely to be helpful to take a more experiential approach to accepting the anxiety rather than ruminating in an overly analytic, repetitive way.

METABELIEFS

A recent development in CBT is the concept of "metabeliefs". Adrian Wells from the University of Manchester, has written extensively on this topic and its application, particularly to the anxiety disorders. Wells refers to worry about a particular bad thing happening as "Type 1 worry", and worry about worry itself as "Type 2 worry". Metabeliefs are thoughts or beliefs about your own mental events. This may include beliefs about the helpfulness of thoughts, harmfulness of thoughts and cause or meaning of thoughts.

INFLATED RESPONSIBILITY

A sense of inflated responsibility has been identified as a common cognitive bias in OCD.

Examples of thoughts and beliefs in OCD around inflated responsibility include:

- "Failing to prevent (or failing to try preventing) harm occurring to others is the same as having caused the harm in the first place."
- "I should be able to control my thoughts."
- "If I have the chance to prevent it and I don't, it will be my fault if it happens."
- "Just because it's unlikely to occur wouldn't absolve me from responsibility if it did happen."

This sense of inflated responsibility contributes to the urge to complete compulsions, which are designed to remove or reduce the likelihood of harm, since the sense of responsibility creates additional anxiety about a negative or catastrophic outcome, e.g., "It would be bad enough that it happened, but even worse, it would be all my fault." Some overlap with "cognitive errors" is also evident in this instance: catastrophising, personalising and some black-and-white thinking can be identified.

THOUGHT-ACTION FUSION

Some people talk about "magical thinking" such as children experience, where thoughts, fantasies, dreams and reality often are mixed together and the child has trouble telling them apart.

Thought-action fusion is a type of magical thinking, in that it affords some type of almost supernatural power to thoughts themselves. If someone thinks hard enough that they are going to win the lottery, would that make it happen? It is certainly true that thoughts can influence behaviour, in what is sometimes referred to as a self-fulfilling prophecy. For example, if someone spends all their time worrying that their relationship is going to fail, and this makes them grumpy, preoccupied or overly clingy, then it may have the result they are trying to avoid. However, thought-action fusion is the sense that merely having a thought about acting in a certain way makes an action more likely.

There are two types of thought-action fusion: probability, where there is a belief that having a thought about an action or behaviour increases the probability of the action occurring; and morality, where the belief is that having the thought is morally equivalent to having carried out the action.

THOUGHT-EVENT FUSION

A related concept is thought-event fusion, where there is a belief that having a thought about an event makes that event more likely to happen.

For example, a woman has an image of her daughter getting run over by a car, and she worries that this means it is going to happen. This can be very distressing and often leads to futile attempts to suppress such thoughts, or to take actions to "undo" or prevent them – for example, compulsions like saying prayers or repeating the opposite thought over and over.

METACOGNITIONS AND OCD

Metacognitions can be activated by several mechanisms: for example, by some other thought occurring, such as reassurance seeking, hypervigilance or avoidance, or by another type of trigger – for example, for someone worried about contamination, hearing about someone who is Human Immunodeficiency Virus (HIV) positive or has cancer.

Case Study: Carlos

Carlos is a young man who is worried that he will come into contact with the Human Immunodeficiency Virus (HIV) and become infected. He overestimates the probability of this occurring from contact with a blood spot or casual contact with an ill person. He feels anxious when using public transport.

Carlos's obsessive belief is that he will come into contact with something contaminated with HIV and catch it himself. He further worries that something must have made him worry about HIV, perhaps that he actually has HIV – this is a metabelief.

Carlos is hypervigilant for situations in which he might come into contact with any HIV contaminant, and he tends to misinterpret any type of brown or red spot as being blood. He reminds himself to look out for potential blood spots or individuals who look sick, and to avoid using public facilities. There is also often doubt about his own experiences, for example, asking himself, "Did I touch that spot or not? Was it infectious?"

There may be metacognitions about even thinking of HIV infections. This provokes more anxiety and leads to compensatory strategies such as attempts to reduce the risk by washing his hands repeatedly with bleach, or seeking certainty about the presence or absence of danger by, for example, repeated HIV tests (since there are repeated opportunities to be infected again). This in turn only reinforces beliefs about the danger posed by HIV and contributes to a feedback loop where all the same strategies are repeated.

Carlos also has thought-action fusion in that he thinks something must have made him worry. The role of this thought-action fusion here is to exacerbate anxiety about the situation.

PERCEIVED BENEFITS AND COSTS OF WORRY

Beliefs about worry (i.e., metacognitions about worry) can be positive, as in the perceived benefits of worry.

Most people are not aware that they have any good feelings at all about worry. However, some researchers, such as the Canadian psychologists Michel Dugas and Robert Ladouceur, have identified the central role of uncertainty in contributing to anxiety. That is, that anxious people find it very hard to tolerate the uncertainty around a possibility that something bad could happen. Worry represents a strategy for dealing with uncertainty, since it can create a sense of preparedness or problem-solving, which relieves anxiety in the short term. For example, worry can give a sense of "covering all the bases". If we worry about something, it may not happen. Some people say that if they don't worry and something bad does happen, they would feel guilty. Worry can give a sense of preparing for the worst, and may feel like a search for the "right" answer. However, most people are more aware of their negative metacognitions about worry ("It will give me a heart attack or cause cancer", "It makes me too anxious to sleep") and it can take deeper exploration to uncover the positive metabeliefs that keep people using worry as a strategy to try to reduce anxiety.

In cognitive behaviour therapy, individuals will be asked to let go of worry as a strategy. Therefore it is important that beliefs about the helpfulness of worry are identified, or the individual might find themselves seemingly inexplicably anxious about *not* worrying. It is also important to identify better strategies to cope with the problems, such as uncertainty or feeling out of control, that worry was intended to solve.

Beliefs about worry can also be negative. Most people find it much easier to identify their negative metabeliefs about worry; after all, this is often one of the reasons they come for help.

Examples of negative metacognitions include:

- "All this worry might send me crazy."
- "This worry could give me cancer or make me sick."
- "I worry so much; I'm not good company."
- "I can't control my worry."

PART VI SUMMARY

Cognitive neuroscience research into cognitive processing in anxiety has greatly increased understanding of the nature of both normal and pathological anxiety, and has informed advances in treatment. An information processing model assists in understanding the reactions of an individual to their internal and external experiences, and how the way in which they process this information can contribute to the development and maintenance of anxiety disorders.

Biases may be identified in information processing that result in the individual paying too much attention to certain stimuli at the expense of others, and lead to appraisals that overestimate the likelihood of danger or a negative outcome, as well as the magnitude of any adverse outcome.

Information processing occurs following an internal or external sensory stimulus, and has a number of stages. In the first stage, an individual attends to the stimulus. They then appraise the nature and meaning of the stimulus – this process is influenced by memories of previous experiences (which have been stored and then retrieved when a similar situation arises in the future) and heuristics – "rules" that the individual has developed to guide them in such situations, analogous to programs that are written to enable computer analysis. Behavioural, emotional and cognitive responses will be based on these appraisals. Both the appraisals and the behavioural responses can become habitual.

Rumination and worry are two types of cognitive processes that feature prominently in anxiety, and may contribute to the persistence of anxiety symptoms. Negative post-event processing may be particularly relevant in social phobia.

Other cognitive factors that may contribute to the persistence of anxiety disorders include an unhelpful focusing of attention on threat-related cues, "magical thinking", and "thinking about thinking" or metacognitions.

Identification of cognitive factors that contribute to the persistence of anxiety disorders is important so that effective treatment strategies may be developed to target and reduce these factors.

PART VII   ASSESSMENT OF ANXIETY DISORDERS

Anxiety is associated with a number of medical conditions. An important component of the assessment of patients with anxiety disorders is to rule out whether the anxiety is due to these medical conditions, or whether it is due to a primary anxiety disorder.

Part VII will explain the medical presentation of anxiety disorders and how anxiety might be related to a variety of medical conditions. It will also discuss "what anxiety as a symptom" means, and what it means in the medical setting.

The structured instruments that are used to assess for anxiety disorders in a formalised manner will also be outlined. While these instruments are most commonly used in research settings, e.g., for clinical trials and epidemiological studies, they can also be used in clinical practice.

A broad range of substances are implicated in the aetiology and maintenance of anxiety disorder. It will be explained in the following chapters why it is necessary to screen broadly for possible substance abuse when assessing a person with anxiety disorders.

CHAPTER 25   ASSESSMENT INTERVIEW

Philip Boyce

GOALS OF THE ASSESSMENT INTERVIEW

The cornerstone of assessing a patient with an anxiety disorder is a clinical interview.

There are a number of specific goals for the assessment interview.

First, it is important to find out whether the patient is experiencing normal or pathological anxiety. For example, it is common to experience anxiety in stressful circumstances, such as sitting an exam or giving a presentation. This normal anxiety can be helpful, as is shown by the Yerkes-Dobson curve in Part I.

Second, the type of anxiety disorder from which the patient suffers must be confirmed, but it is also important to find out about the context of the disorder, what triggered it, what maintains it and why this particular patient has developed an anxiety disorder.

To achieve these goals, it is necessary to develop a good working relationship with the patient. Not only will this help in eliciting the patient's history, but will lay the foundation for therapeutic work with them.

The essence of establishing the therapeutic relationship is in good communication skills.

BENEFITS OF GOOD COMMUNICATION

Clinicians who have good communication skills are able to identify a patient's problems better, as the patient is more able to talk openly and comfortably about their problems.

If the patient feels confident in the clinician, then the patient's anxiety will come down again, improving the quality of communication.

A consequence of the improved communication is that the patient is more likely to adhere to any treatment that is being offered to them, which in turn leads to a better outcome for them.

GOOD COMMUNICATION SKILLS

The right setting is important; that is, an environment where the clinician will not be interrupted while interviewing the patient, and the patient can feel comfortable. Rather than sitting directly opposite the patient over a desk – a setting that may feel like an interrogation – it is better to sit at a slight angle from the patient, so they can be observed comfortably, without feeling confronted.

A key element of good communication skills is to maintain eye contact with the patient. This does not mean staring at the patient throughout the interview, but maintaining a comfortable eye contact with them so they know that they are being listened to. It also allows the clinician comfortably to observe any changes to their facial expression.

The interview should start with open-ended questions, so the patient can feel free to give out the information that the clinician needs. This is followed by closed questions, to confirm symptoms.

The crucial element of good communication skills is letting the patient know that they are being listened to. This can be done by both verbal and non-verbal means.

Non-verbal ways of showing that one is paying attention include maintaining appropriate eye contact with the patient, having an attentive posture – perhaps leaning forward to show interest at appropriate times – and nodding (or sometimes shaking the head) as appropriate whilst the patient is telling their story. All these actions convey to them that their words are being paid attention to.

Verbal ways of demonstrating this include utilising techniques such as summarising what the patient has said. This has two purposes. First, it is a way for the clinician to sort out what the patient has been saying and to make sure that they have heard it correctly, and second, it demonstrates to the patient that they are being attended to. It is also possible to demonstrate attentiveness by paraphrasing what the patient said.

> The crucial element of good communication skills is letting the patient know that they are being listened to.

GOALS OF THE ASSESSMENT INTERVIEW

The first goal for the clinician is to get some understanding about the patient's anxiety, particularly to understand whether it is normal or pathological anxiety.

The type of anxiety disorder from which the patient is suffering then needs to be identified.

OPEN-ENDED QUESTIONS

After finding out some basic demographic details about the patient, the clinician can use open-ended questions to elicit the symptoms of the patient's anxiety.

For example:

Interviewer: "Please could you tell me about the problem that you want help for, how it started and what happens to you?"

Patient: "I get very anxious when I'm around people."

IDENTIFYING SPECIFIC SYMPTOMS OF ANXIETY

Once it has been established that the patient is experiencing anxiety, the clinician can then move on to identifying specific symptoms of anxiety.

For example, the patient can be asked, in straightforward language, whether they have been experiencing palpitations. The patient may then endorse the symptom and go on to elaborate some more about the fear that they might be having a heart attack.

For example:

Interviewer: "You've told me about these anxiety attacks you have around people. When you experience the anxiety attacks, do you feel your heart pounding?"

Patient: "Oh yes, sometimes it feels as if I might be having a heart attack."

In this example, the patient endorses the symptom, and then elaborates some more about her fear that she might be having a heart attack.

CONFIRMING COMMON SYMPTOMS OF ANXIETY

The clinician can then go on through the common symptoms of anxiety such as shaking, and ask whether the patient experiences them or not.

For example:

Interviewer: "Do you feel shaky?"

Patient: "Yes, that can be very embarrassing."

Interviewer: "Do you have trouble getting your breath?"

Again, the patient endorses the symptom, but goes on to collaborate more, highlighting her fear of negative appraisal.

UNDERSTANDING THE CONTEXT OF ANXIETY

Once the symptoms have been established, their context needs to be understood.

First, it is necessary to find out what happened when the symptoms first came on; what was the precipitant to the patient developing his or her anxiety. Anxiety disorders are often triggered by life events, so it is important to understand what was happening in the patient's life at the time the symptoms arose; what stressors the patient was under when they started to develop anxiety. Knowledge of the patient's general physical health at the time is also important, as is knowing whether they were taking any medications that could have contributed to the onset of the anxiety.

An understanding of the course of the illness should also be developed; that is, when the anxiety comes on and when it eases.

Anxiety is not present all the time, so the triggers for the patient's particular anxiety need to be understood in order to develop a treatment plan.

Finding out the triggers of the anxiety is also important in clarifying the diagnosis.

For example, in distinguishing between social anxiety disorder and agoraphobia, it is important to identify the triggers for the patient's anxiety; that is, whether it is a fear of not being able to escape from the situation, or a fear of negative evaluation.

It is also important to identify what maintains the anxiety disorder; what the patient gets from having the disorder. The impact of the anxiety on the person and their key relationships needs to be examined here, as the anxiety might be a way of dealing with interpersonal difficulties.

Other lifestyle-only factors that seem to maintain anxiety disorder include excessive caffeine intake and substance or alcohol misuse.

The most important issue is to find out what the anxiety disorder is preventing the person from being able to do. Sometimes this is an important clue to what is happening with the patient.

OBSERVATION – SIGNS OF ANXIETY

While eliciting the symptoms and the context of the symptoms of the patient's anxiety, the clinician should also be observing the patient, looking for signs of anxiety.

Observation of the patient starts at the moment of contact and sometimes even before then. For example, if a patient needs to check the time of their appointment a number of times, this would suggest significant anxiety.

Patients who are very anxious will often arrive early for an appointment, again demonstrating their fear of negative appraisal. Even when waiting to come in for an appointment, they may show signs of their anxiety, such as being restless in a waiting room, or paying repeated visits to the toilet.

Again, the observation of the patient may suggest some signs of anxiety; for example, it may be possible to see chewed fingernails from their anxiety, or constant fiddling with objects to help give reassurance. In some cases the patient may bring along a companion to help reduce anxiety during the course of an assessment.

While interviewing the patient and paying attention to what they are saying, the clinician needs to observe them throughout, to note any tell-tale signs of anxiety coming through, particularly signs of autonomic arousal.

Common symptoms of anxiety include: sweating, shakiness, fidgeting, having blotches appear on the skin, etc. It is important to observe, not only that the patient is anxious, but what leads to increases in their anxiety level. For example, when they are talking about a particularly difficult situation, blotches may appear on their skin, which demonstrates increased anxiety associated with the issue.

PREDISPOSING FACTORS

The factors that may have predisposed the patient to developing an anxiety disorder then need to be identified. This is done by using open-ended questions, with follow-up direct questions. These need to encompass any genetic predisposition.

For example: "Does anyone else in your family suffer from anxiety... or depression... or any other mental health problem?"

PREDISPOSING FACTORS: TEMPERAMENT AND CHILDHOOD TRAUMA

Childhood experiences that may have predisposed the patient to developing an anxiety disorder should be identified. The patient may have been an anxious or timid child, or may have experienced anxiety very early on as a child, in the form of separation anxiety. The clinician can enquire about this by using open-ended questions to get some understanding about the patient's childhood.

For example:

- "Could you tell me about what your childhood was like?"
- "Did you ever experience anxiety as a child, for example, going to school or staying over with a friend?"
- "How did you get on with the other kids; did you have lots of friends or just a few close friends?"
- "What sort of a child would you say you were?"

After finding out about the patient's childhood and early life experiences, the question of whether they may have experienced any specific traumas can be explored. Such questions have to be asked very sensitively, and it is important to observe whether the questions increase discomfort for the patient (this could be an indication of possible early trauma).

For example: "Did you have any unpleasant or traumatic experiences as a child?"

After being asked general questions, the patient can be asked whether they had experienced any abuse. The questions should start with physical abuse, before moving on to the most sensitive area, sexual abuse.

For example: "Did you ever experience any abuse as a child... such as being hit... or being criticised... or being interfered with?"

Finally, the clinician needs to explore with the patient the issues that might be contributing to their mental health problems and maintaining their anxiety disorder. This includes asking about their current relationship, and whether they are experiencing any difficulties.

They should also be asked whether they are experiencing any difficulties in the workplace. Sometimes the anxiety disorder is a means of avoiding going to work, because the person may be having difficulty coping, or there may be interpersonal difficulties.

The patient's social network also needs to be discussed. A supportive social network will, to some degree, protect against anxiety and depression. A sparse social network may contribute to the maintenance of anxiety.

CHAPTER 26   MEDICAL ASSESSMENT ISSUES

Christopher Ryan

ALL THAT QUIVERS IS NOT ANXIOUS

When diagnosing a person as suffering an anxiety disorder, one of the most important tasks is to ensure, as far as possible, that their apparent anxiety is not due to a medical illness such as diseases of the thyroid, heart, lung or adrenal, which can look like a primary anxiety order because it causes the same symptoms as a subjective sense of panic (such as sweating or palpitations).

Symptoms that are due to general medical illnesses are unlikely to get better unless the underlying condition is treated. It is important to be aware of the possibility of these illnesses, because apparent anxiety may be an early symptom of a serious underlying medical condition that should be treated in its own right. Some of the medications used to treat a variety of general medical illnesses may themselves cause anxiety symptoms as a side effect. Missing the true cause of the symptoms will probably mean that even the best therapeutic efforts won't work.

This chapter provides an introduction to this fascinating, important but confusing aspect of anxiety.

WHAT IS HAPPENING HERE

Many of the somatic, or bodily, symptoms of the anxiety disorders are also commonly encountered in a range of general medical illnesses. This is particularly true for panic disorder and generalised anxiety disorder. Not only that, but, if an individual does happen to suffer intermittent palpitations, difficulty breathing, sweating or any other such symptoms, they will become anxious about them. They are then likely to pick up some of the psychological symptoms of the anxiety disorders and with both types of symptoms on board, their physical illness will begin to look a lot like an anxiety disorder.

> Apparent anxiety may be an early symptom of a serious underlying medical condition.

Even without a person worrying about their physical symptoms, some medical conditions directly cause the psychological symptoms of anxiety, such as feeling of dread, irritability, panic, anticipation, inner tension, decreased concentration, initial insomnia and inability to relax. People with thyroid disease, for example, may often feel anxious if they have not got a single other symptom.

There are a number of physical diseases that can cause somatic symptoms of anxiety such as palpitations, difficulty breathing, dry mouth, nausea, urinary frequency, dizziness, muscular tension, seating, abdominal churning, tremor and cold skin.

There is a wide range of medical conditions that can look like anxiety disorders. Table 26.1 shows a number of symptoms of anxiety and the physical diseases that can cause these symptoms. As the table reveals, a number of conditions appear on more than one row. Hyperthyroidism and pheochromocytoma are the archetypal physical illnesses that can look like anxiety disorders.

Table 26.1   Symptoms of anxiety and physical diseases that can cause these symptoms

Symptom of anxiety	Physical diseases
Difficulty breathing	Angina, congestive cardiac failure, pulmonary embolism, hypoglycaemia or hypoxia
Palpitations	Arrhythmias, hyperthyroidism, carcinoid or pheochromocytoma
Abdominal churning	Carcinoid, hyperparathyroidism, irritable bowel syndrome or pheochromocytoma
Dizziness	Hypoglycemia, hypoxia or Parkinson's disease
Tremor	Hypoglycemia, hyperthyroidism, pheochromocytoma or Parkinson's disease
Sweating	Hyperthyroidism, pulmonary embolism, severe pain, thyrotoxicosis or carcinoid

MEDICATIONS CAUSING ANXIETY SYMPTOMS

There are also a number of drugs and medications that cause anxiety symptoms, so it is essential to consider other causes when a patient presents with an apparent anxiety disorder.

It is possible that they only became anxious after starting to take a new antidepressant, and unless this is recognised, there is little hope of helping them with their anxiety.

TAKING A CAREFUL HISTORY

The obvious next question is: "How does one pick out the people whose anxiety symptoms are due to medical illness or medication, from the majority of people who have an anxiety disorder?"

The answer is two-fold.

- The clinician should always be alert to the possibility that symptoms are not due to an anxiety disorder.
- They should always take a careful history and spend some time putting the pieces of the history together.

Sometimes these cases will be obvious. If the patient only began getting panic attacks when they first started their steroid medication, the panic attacks are probably related to the steroids. However, without taking a history it would be impossible to know when the panic attacks started, that the patient is taking steroids, or that the timing of the two coincided. One of the old sayings of medicine is that "many more mistakes are made by not asking than by not knowing", and that is certainly true here.

WHAT TO LOOK OUT FOR

Sometimes, even with a good history, the answers will not be easily apparent, but a bit of knowledge, and a curious and sceptical attitude certainly help.

Timing is important; it is significant if a person's anxiety symptoms have developed for the first time late in life. People aged over 40 can develop anxiety disorders, but the older people get, the more likely it is that they will develop a medical illness or two. Anxiety symptoms present for the first time in someone over 60 strongly suggest either a depressive illness or a new physical illness.

It is important to know exactly when the physical symptoms arose and what their relationship is to the psychological symptoms. People with pheochromocytoma, a tumour of the adrenal gland that can mimic panic, often describe a full-blown panic attack – sweating, palpitations, abdominal churning, but their internal state and level of anxiety can sometimes seem lacking. They can be quite anxious, but are not as anxious as people usually are when experiencing such a bad panic attack.

There may also be extra symptoms that do not usually go with anxiety disorders, and which the patient may not mention if they are not asked about them. People with anxiety disorders can get some concurrent weight loss, but when they do, it is usually mild and associated with their not eating as much as usual. People with hyperthyroidism can lose a lot of weight, even though they report eating more than usual.

The patient may also have symptoms that might usually suggest anxiety, but which seem slightly unusual, or much more severe than the other anxiety symptoms. Chest discomfort is a common complaint in panic disorder, and is probably due to the muscles that move in the rib cage becoming tired as the person hyperventilates. Crushing central chest pain, as if someone were sitting on the chest, is not a part of panic disorder and is more suggestive of angina. This is particularly true if the pain is also felt down one of the arms or into the jaw.

It is important to look carefully at the patient. A number of conditions have specific characteristics, but if the clinician does not look carefully at the patient, these can be missed. Examples include people with early Parkinson's disease, who tend not to swing their arms as they walk; and people with acromegaly, who have extremely large hands, big heads and prominent jaws.

Finally, it is important to remain sceptical about the patient's diagnosis. Even if an anxiety disorder has been diagnosed, the clinician should be prepared to re-think the diagnosis, particularly if the patient does not improve as they might be expected to.

TESTING A HYPOTHESIS

If it is possible that a patient's symptoms might be due to a medical illness or medication, the clinician has a number of options.

If it is possible that a medication is the cause, the easiest option is to stop or decrease the medication, in conjunction with the doctor who prescribed it, and see if that improves things.

If a medical illness may be the cause, the patient should be referred back to their general practitioner or to a specialist who can have another look at their history, and consider some tests. Some of these illnesses, for example hyperthyroidism, can be identified with a simple, cheap blood test. These thyroid function tests are so simple and cheap, and hyperthyroidism is so common, that many authors suggest that anyone suspected of having an anxiety disorder should get a thyroid blood test. Other tests are not so easy or so cheap, but they are worth pursuing if it is possible that the patient's anxiety symptoms are really a medical illness in disguise.

CHAPTER 27   DIAGNOSIS AND DIFFERENTIAL DIAGNOSIS

Philip Boyce

BACKGROUND

The cornerstone for the treatment of anxiety disorders lies in an accurate diagnosis. The specific treatment, whether behavioural, cognitive or pharmacological, depends on the specific anxiety disorder from which the patient is suffering. On the surface, this appears to be a straightforward task. But there are pitfalls along the way.

It is most important for the clinician to work out whether they are dealing with a primary anxiety disorder, whether the anxiety is the consequence of medications or medical illnesses that can cause anxiety, or whether the anxiety arises from another psychiatric disorder.

NEUROTIC, STRESS-RELATED AND SOMATOFORM DISORDERS

The 10th revision of *The International Classification of Diseases* (ICD-10), the diagnostic system used by the World Health Organisation, classifies the anxiety disorders in the chapter on "neurotic, stress-related and somatoform disorders". The anxiety disorders are grouped under a number of headings. The first of the anxiety disorders is labelled phobic anxiety disorders. Under this group are categorised agoraphobia with and without panic disorder, social phobia, specific phobias and other phobic anxiety disorders. Under the ICD-10 system, panic disorder is classified under the other anxiety disorders, along with: generalised anxiety disorder, mixed anxiety and depressive disorder, other mixed anxiety disorders, and anxiety disorder, unspecified.

Obsessive-compulsive disorder is a separate anxiety disorder within the ICD-10 system and is subdivided into:

- predominately obsessional thoughts
- predominantly compulsive acts
- mixed obsessional thoughts and acts
- other obsessive-compulsive disorders.

Posttraumatic stress disorder is one of the disorders of the "reaction to severe stress, and adjustment disorders". Acute stress reaction was also classified here, along with adjustment disorders.

ICD-10 also includes dissociative disorders, somatoform disorders and a catch-all term of "other neurotic disorders".

PRIMARY OR SECONDARY

Anxiety is a normal human emotion that can be triggered by a number of different things, including both illicit and prescription drugs, alcohol and medical illness. A key feature in assessing patients with anxiety is to determine whether the patient has a primary anxiety disorder, or whether it is associated with, or arises from, a medical illness or a medication. The association between anxiety and medical illnesses is complex.

COMMON CULPRITS

Anxiety symptoms can be triggered by a range of both prescribed and non-prescribed drugs, the most common of which is probably caffeine. An overdose of caffeine can lead to the full range of anxiety symptoms and can trigger a panic attack in someone who is prone to panic disorder.

In assessing patients for an anxiety disorder, it is important to check whether they are using excess caffeine, either in multiple cups of coffee or in energy drinks. If they are, this could be a contributing factor to panic.

Other non-prescription drugs can also lead to anxiety symptoms, particularly alcohol and some of the recreational drugs such as amphetamines, ecstasy, cannabis and other hallucinogenic drugs, but we need to be aware that anxiety symptoms will also accompany withdrawal from drugs and alcohol, especially from alcohol.

PRESCRIPTION MEDICATIONS

Anxiety can also be a side effect of a number of prescription medications, so the clinician needs to ask patients, as a matter of routine, if they take any prescription medication or any other substances.

Many drugs can cause palpitations, but these can be easily distinguished from anxiety in a clinical examination. The most common medications that cause anxiety include some of the anticonvulsants, such as carbamazepine. Bronchodilators, namely drugs used in the treatment of asthma, can lead to jitteriness and anxiety. Antidepressants, especially the SSRIs, can cause an initial increase in anxiety, before having an anxiolytic effect. It is important to be aware of this, when initiating treatment with such medication. The antihistamines that are often used for problems such as travel sickness, or for treating allergies, can cause anxiety. Medications that contain adrenaline noradrenaline can also cause anxiety.

Patients being treated for thyroid disease, who are on replacement thyroxine, can also report anxiety symptoms, particularly when the thyroid levels are too high.

MEDICAL ILLNESS AND ANXIETY

Anxiety can accompany a number of medical illnesses. In some instances, anxiety may be the initial problem of which the patient is aware, and the reason why they are seeking treatment. A typical example of this would be anxiety associated with disturbances in the endocrine system.

The relationship between anxiety and medical illness is complex. Anxiety may be a major symptom of a medical illness such as in thyroid disease. It may also be a person's response to the illness that they have. A typical example would be a patient diagnosed with cancer, who would be anxious both about the cancer itself, and its effects on them.

Anxiety disorders commonly co-occur with a number of medical conditions, which is known as comorbidity. Such an association may most commonly be seen when patients present with "medically unexplained disorders" or "functional disorders" – high rates of anxiety disorder existing with a functional bowel disorder, such as irritable bowel syndrome or functional dyspepsia.

MEDICAL COMORBIDITY

The Anxiety Disorders Association of America convened a multidisciplinary conference to review current data on the relationship between anxiety disorders and specific mental illness.

Anxiety may be a major symptom of a medical illness such as thyroid disease, or a person's response to the illness that they have.

In their review, they examined the association between the various anxiety disorders and hypertension, arthritis, asthma and ulcers. These disorders are of particular importance as these associations occur more commonly than expected by chance, and may have some common underlying mechanisms.

It is important to remember that anyone with an anxiety disorder can have any medical disorder, with the association occurring purely by chance.

As Figure 27.2 shows, the anxiety disorders have strong associations, as measured by the odds ratios, with all these chronic physical conditions.

This chapter will go through each of the body systems, and discuss their associations with the anxiety disorders.

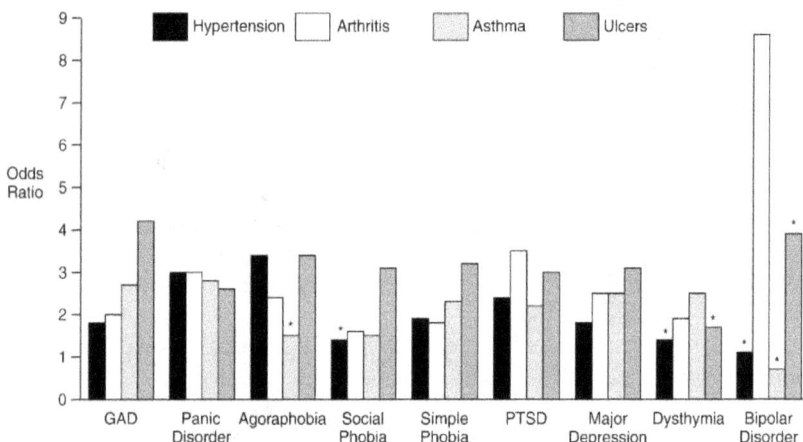

Figure 27.2 Associations of *DSM-III-R* mental disorders among NCS-R respondents with chronic physical disorders. * indicates not statistically significant at p ≥ 0.05. From Roy-Byrne et al. (2008). Reproduced with permission of Elsevier.

CARDIOVASCULAR SYSTEM

The most common associations in this system are the symptoms of a panic attack and that of a heart attack, or myocardial infarction.

The chest pain, difficulty in breathing, palpitations and sweatiness of a panic attack may, when they occur for the first time, lead some individuals to think they are having a heart attack. In such a situation, they may present at an emergency department complaining of a suspected heart attack. Sometimes, patients presenting in this way will undergo extensive investigations before the diagnosis of panic disorder is made.

Panic attacks are more likely in younger patients below thirty years of age, females and those with a history of anxiety. In addition, panic attacks are usually triggered by a stressful event, although this can also happen with heart attacks.

This emphasises the importance of taking a careful history from the patient. Patients with acute myocardial infarction will generally be older than those experiencing a first-time panic attack and, generally, will not have a history of anxiety.

It is important to remember that common things commonly occur, so a young person presenting with these symptoms in the emergency department will be more likely to be having a panic attack than an acute myocardial infarction.

Another association between disorders of the central cardiovascular system and panic disorder is in regard to mitral valve prolapse. Mitral valve prolapse is found in about 3% to 5% of adults. The incidence of mitral valve prolapse in panic disorder is reported to be much greater - in the order of 20% to 50% in some studies.

Anxiety disorders may contribute to a poorer outcome, following a myocardial infarction.

ENDOCRINE SYSTEM

Illnesses emerging from disturbances to the endocrine system can contribute to anxiety symptoms. This is partly because the adrenal glands are part of the endocrine system, and they produce adrenaline and noradrenaline, which leads to arousal and anxiety symptoms.

There are rare conditions of the adrenal such as pheochromocytoma that can contribute to panic disorder. However, as they are very uncommon they are not necessarily worth investigating for in every anxious person.

Perhaps the most commonly recognised association between disorders of the endocrine system and anxiety disorders is in relationship to the thyroid gland.

Overactivity of the thyroid, or thyrotoxicosis, is perhaps the most widely known thyroid abnormality that presents as an anxiety disorder.

When assessing patients for this, it is worth asking about associated symptoms of thyroid disease, such as: changes to the skin, hair and eyes – in thyrotoxicosis, the hair skin becomes greasier, the person more heat intolerance and the eyes develop exophthalmos.

Hypothyroidism can also present with anxiety symptoms.

GASTROINTESTINAL SYSTEM

The functional gastrointestinal disorders are all very closely associated with the anxiety disorders. This has raised an important question as to whether these disorders share some common aetiological factor (such as neuroticism).

The two most common such disorders are irritable bowel syndrome (IBS) and functional dyspepsia. There are very high rates of anxiety disorder found among patients suffering from IBS or functional dyspepsia, with high rates of social anxiety disorder associated with IBS.

The treatment of IBS and functional dyspepsia are essentially the same as the treatment for anxiety disorders, with CBT and the SSRIs and other antidepressants commonly being used.

RESPIRATORY SYSTEM

There are a number of associations between disorders of the respiratory system and anxiety disorders.

Hyperventilation syndrome can be part of a panic attack; patients who are prone to developing panic disorder will have a panic attack if they hyperventilate.

When patients or individuals are struggling to get their breath, or have a build-up of carbon dioxide in the blood (i.e., hypercapnia), they can, as a result, have a panic attack.

One of the more common diseases of the respiratory system is asthma. There are close associations between asthma and the anxiety disorders. It is important to remember that this is a bidirectional relationship, with increased anxiety contributing to asthma attacks, and an attack of asthma increasing the level of anxiety.

It is also important to remember that some of the medications used to treat asthma can also contribute to anxiety symptoms.

CANCER

Cancer patients commonly experience anxiety alongside the disease. In most cases, the anxiety is related to the diagnosis of cancer and its prognosis. In some cases, where there is pre-existing anxiety, a cancer diagnosis will unmask the anxiety disorder and make it become more prominent.

Many of the treatments used for cancer will increase anxiety, and may lead to the onset of an anxiety disorder.

COMORBIDITY WITH OTHER PSYCHIATRIC DISORDERS

Anxiety disorders frequently occur in conjunction with other psychiatric disorders. When they do, the patient requires appropriate treatment in addition to the major Axis I disorder from which they may be suffering.

Many patients suffering from schizophrenia have a comorbid anxiety disorder that often goes unrecognised and untreated.

Panic disorder commonly accompanies bipolar disorder, and may be an early sign of bipolar relapse. This needs to be recognised and treated in its own right, as well as the bipolar disorder being appropriately managed.

Anxiety symptoms frequently co-occur with major depression. Here, it is important to tease out whether the anxiety is a part of a depressive illness (when the depression is treated, the anxiety disorder goes), or whether it is genuinely comorbid with a depressive illness, where both need to be treated separately.

Anxiety disorders are frequently comorbid with cluster B and cluster C personality disorders.

The cluster C personality disorders, also known as the "anxious–fearful" personality disorders, have anxiety at their basis. With some, such as the avoidant personality disorder, it is hard to disentangle whether the anxiety is part of the personality or whether it is a disorder in its own right.

When there is a comorbid Axis 2 personality disorder in conjunction with an anxiety disorder, it will have a profound effect on the prognosis and outcome. Those with a borderline personality disorder will have a poor outcome.

PURE AND COMORBID ANXIETY DISORDERS

For the majority of anxiety disorders, having a pure anxiety disorder is not that common. Specific phobias are the disorders most likely to occur in a pure form. In contrast, panic disorder occurs in a pure form in only around 30% of patients, with many patients having one other comorbid condition, and 20% having three or more comorbid conditions.

COMORBIDITY IN AUSTRALIA

There are also high rates of comorbidity between the anxiety disorders, affective disorders and substance use disorders, as demonstrated in Table 27.1.

Table 27.1   Comorbidity between the anxiety disorders, affective disorders and substance use disorders in Australia

Comorbid 12 month mental disorder class	Any affective disorder	Any anxiety disorder	Any substance use disorder
Any affective disorder	-	25.4%	21.4%
Any anxiety disorder	58.5%	-	33.5%
Any substance use disorder	17.6%	11.9%	-

Note. From Teesson, Slade, & Mills (2009). Reproduced with permission of the Royal Australian and New Zealand College of Psychiatrists.

Over half of the people with an affective disorder such as depression, dysthymia or bipolar disorder, also had an anxiety disorder. About a quarter of the people with an anxiety disorder also had an affective disorder, and one in ten had a substance use disorder.

ANXIETY DISORDERS: ONE OR MANY

It is unusual to have a "pure" anxiety disorder. When assessing patients with an anxiety disorder, it is common to find that they will have more than one anxiety disorder present. This has raised an important question as to whether there is one anxiety disorder or whether there are many different anxiety disorders. It is difficult to find clear data about the likelihood of having another anxiety disorder, once one has been diagnosed. The *National Comorbidity Survey Replication* was a large epidemiological study conducted in the USA. The prevalence rates for the anxiety disorders were calculated. The correlations were high between the various anxiety disorders, with the exception of obsessive-compulsive disorder (Kessler et al., 2005).

CHAPTER 28   SUBSTANCE ABUSE AND ANXIETY

Anthony Harris

INTERACTION BETWEEN SUBSTANCE ABUSE AND ANXIETY DISORDERS

A broad range of substances, both legal and illicit, are implicated in the aetiology and maintenance of anxiety disorders. When one is considering the interaction of substances of abuse and anxiety disorders, a number of general points need to be kept in mind. Firstly, the nature of the substance abused: is it sedating like an opiate, or stimulating like methamphetamine? Secondly, the stage of use; for example, whether the person is intoxicated or experiencing withdrawal symptoms. Thirdly, the presence or absence of symptoms of dependence and, finally, the nature of the anxiety disorder. When considering the interaction between the substance abuse and anxiety disorders, it is important to keep in mind that both are common, and the co-occurrence may be by chance rather than causal.

TOBACCO

Tobacco abuse is still the leading cause of preventable illness and mortality in the world, killing nearly six million people a year.

Tobacco use is increased in people with a past or present history of psychiatric illness generally, and anxiety disorders in particular.

Of the anxiety disorders, panic disorder and social phobia have increased rates of smoking. The relationship of panic disorder with smoking is complex. Smoking may precede the onset of panic, and it is thought that the hyperventilation that accompanies smoking may be a trigger for panic disorders. In social phobia, social fears predict the development of nicotine dependence.

Tobacco use is increased in people with a past or present history of psychiatric illness generally, and anxiety disorders in particular.

SMOKING

Smoking has a biphasic effect on anxiety, determined by the time since it was last administered and by the dose of nicotine.

Initially, when the smoker first ingests or inhales nicotine, it has an anxiolytic effect, probably due to the action of nicotine on pre-synaptic $5HT_{1A}$ and $\alpha 4\beta 2$ nicotinic receptors. However, with chronic use, tolerance develops to this effect.

The late response is anxiogenic, due to withdrawal, so for many people, the cigarette smoked to "help them calm down" is, in all probability, one to satiate their symptoms of withdrawal. Very high doses of nicotine are also anxiogenic.

CAFFEINE

Caffeine is typically ingested by drinking tea, coffee or caffeinated soft drinks, but is also found in a wide variety of processed foods and over the counter medications.

Caffeine in moderate to high doses – that is, greater than 500 mg a day (equivalent to four strong coffees) – can trigger panic attacks in people who are susceptible to them. People with panic disorder frequently moderate their caffeine intake because of the anxiogenic effect of caffeine. Caffeine use may be associated with increased rates of generalised anxiety disorder and, of course, sleep disorders. However, there does not appear to be any association with social anxiety or OCD.

An older term, caffeinism, refers to a syndrome of chronic intoxication which is manifested by anxiety, tremulousness, insomnia, headache, palpitations and nausea or vomiting. If used, this term should be reserved for very heavy use – i.e., exceeding 1000 mg of caffeine a day.

ALCOHOL

Alcohol is legal in most countries, and it remains the world's most widely abused substance, other than tobacco. The *2007 National Survey of Mental Health and Wellbeing* found that, over a 12-month period, approximately 2.9% of Australians had a pattern of harmful use and 1.4% were dependent upon alcohol (Australian Bureau of Statistics, 2007).

Increased rates of anxiety disorders are seen in those who are alcohol dependent. It is important to note that alcohol abuse by itself does not cause increased rates of anxiety disorders.

A point that has caused some debate is the J curve pattern associated with alcohol use in mood and anxiety disturbance (Figure 28.1). Drinkers who report using a small dose of alcohol (defined as one to two standard drinks a day), have lower levels of anxiety and depression than those who either abstain or who drink heavily.

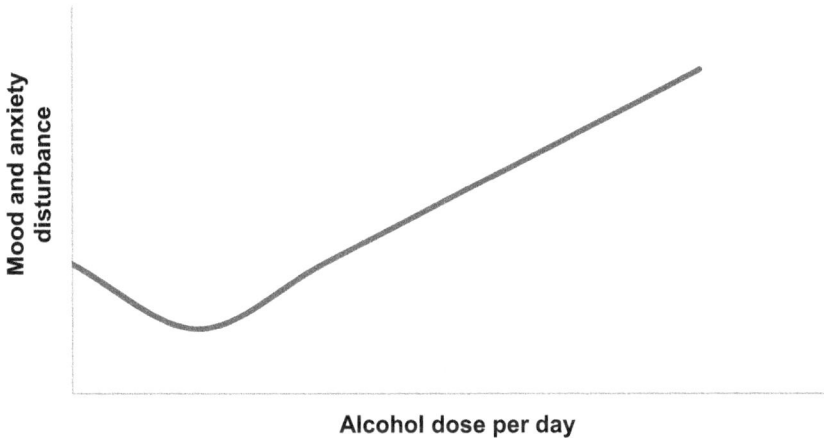

Figure 28.1 The J curve pattern

A hangover experienced by many people the day following a period of alcohol abuse may also include anxiety as part of the range of symptoms that include nausea, headache, sensitivity to noise, dysphoria and thirst.

There is a possible specific increase in alcohol abuse and dependence in people with social phobia, panic disorder and posttraumatic stress disorder. However, no consistent relationship has been described between social anxiety and alcohol use.

A prominent symptom of alcohol withdrawal is anxiety. Anxiety tends to be an early sign of withdrawal, accompanying the physiological signs such as, increased heart rate, increased blood pressure and sweating, and the psychological symptoms of increased salience of drinking and alcohol seeking behaviour. These signs and symptoms form part of the clinical spectrum experienced in alcohol withdrawal syndrome that includes nausea, vomiting, palpitations, tremors and agitation, and extends to hallucinations, delusions, seizures, coma and death. The more severe end of this spectrum is sometimes known as delirium tremens.

Recovering from alcohol dependence will lead to improved anxiety and mood-related symptoms, which suggests that at least part of the problem of anxiety and mood symptoms in alcohol abuse disorders is artifact.

There are not a large number of studies examining the treatment of comorbid alcohol-anxiety disorders. Those that have been performed suggest that cognitive-behavioural or behavioural approaches can successfully reduce both alcohol dependence and anxiety symptoms.

CANNABIS

Cannabis is one of the most widely abused substances, with a 12-month prevalence of harmful use being 0.6% and of dependence being 0.4% of the population. Rates of occasional use are much higher.

However, its relationship to anxiety is complex. Chronic users sometimes nominate the self-treatment of anxiety and depression as the reason for its use.

Increased rates of anxiety observed in people who use cannabis do not appear to be significant when factors such as age, the presence of other substances and other disorders, such as mood disorders, are taken into account.

Nonetheless, the initial use of cannabis is associated with panic-like symptoms, as is high dose consumption and polysubstance abuse.

First time users of cannabis frequently report anxiety symptoms or even panic. However, longer term users cite the reduction of anxiety and mood symptoms as one of the primary reasons why they continue using the drug. High dose, dependence and other substance abuse have all been associated with higher rates of anxiety disorder.

This confusion may be at least partly due to the complexity of the pharmacological effects of the many psychoactive compounds in cannabis. Some component compounds, e.g., cannabidiol are anxiolytic, whilst others, e.g., tetrahydrocannabinol (or THC), are anxiogenic. The common practice of combining tobacco with cannabis when smoking the drug has further obscured the relationship of cannabis with anxiety.

In summary, it seems likely that high dose use of THC rich cannabis is likely to contribute to anxiety, while the withdrawal state from cannabis dependence is marked by raised anxiety symptoms.

PSYCHO-STIMULANTS

Psycho-stimulants such as amphetamines and MDMA, or ecstasy, are important substances of abuse that can cause anxiety disorders.

In particular, amphetamine abuse, or dependence, is associated with very high rates of anxiety symptoms and disorders. Up to 39% of people who abuse methamphetamine report a lifetime history of anxiety disorders.

On the other hand, MDMA, or ecstasy, has a more complex association with anxiety. Use at low doses may be anxiolytic, however at high doses it is also associated with substance related anxiety disorders.

The effects of these drugs are mediated through dopaminergic, serotoninergic and noradrenergic agonist effects.

The onset of symptoms and their severity are influenced by the mode of administration, which can be oral, intravenous, intranasal or via inhalation. Those who inhale have the most rapid onset of the effects and thus most prominent anxiety related symptoms.

The effects of stimulant use most commonly experienced are arousal, tachycardia, hypertension and feelings of anxiety and panic. Panic is experienced by up to 58% of people using methamphetamines.

During withdrawal from methamphetamine use, the symptoms are characterised by sleepiness, hunger, dysphoria and, again, anxiety.

BENZODIAZEPINES

Benzodiazepines are widely used hypnotics and anxiolytic medications that are commonly abused.

High rates of prescription continue to be seen, especially in elderly people, despite the risks of confusion, falls and other serious consequences. It is thought that up to 10%-30% of people who are prescribed therapeutic doses of benzodiazepines become dependent over the long term.

In cross-sectional studies, it is difficult to differentiate between continued symptoms of anxiety and those of withdrawal.

However, withdrawal phenomena have all the hallmarks of acute anxiety, in which can be included a range of more severe symptoms, such as perceptual abnormalities and seizures. The time of onset of withdrawal phenomena reflect pharmacokinetic properties of the benzodiazepine in question. Those with a short half-life, (e.g., alprazolam), or those used at higher doses, will have a more severe and more rapid onset of withdrawal phenomena including symptoms of anxiety.

OPIOID-RELATED DISORDERS

People who abuse opiates also have an increased lifetime prevalence of anxiety disorders, which ranges from 26% to 35%.

There is a suggestion that in at least some people, anxiety disorders, and especially phobias, may have preceded the onset of opiate use.

Anxiety is commonly seen as part of the withdrawal syndrome from opiates, accompanying the other symptoms of tachycardia, arousal, chills, cramps, rhinitis, nausea, vomiting, diarrhoea and an intense craving, among other symptoms and signs.

Partly because of this, benzodiazepines can be used to help treat some of the symptoms of opiate withdrawal, and are commonly abused by addicts to help cover withdrawal symptoms.

CHAPTER 29   ASSESSMENT TOOLS

Caroline Hunt

STRUCTURED DIAGNOSTIC INTERVIEWS

When making a diagnosis based on unstructured clinical interviews, clinicians often find it difficult to reach an agreement.

Structured and semi-structured interviews are an important assessment tool. They were first developed in response to the recognition of poor agreement between clinicians in making diagnoses based on unstructured clinical interviews.

Structured interviews are designed to minimise the sources of variability that cause diagnostic disagreement between clinicians. These sources include the questions that are asked, and the decision-making rules around whether or not a disorder is present.

In other words, structured interviews aim to maximise the reliability and validity of diagnostic interviews. Structured interviews standardise the content, format and order of questions, and provide clear algorithms for making a diagnostic decision. Interviews will vary in the degree to which they are structured and meet with these specifications.

The use of structured interviews for making diagnoses is essential in research, especially if findings are to be published in a peer-reviewed journal and are to be used in empirically-driven clinical practice.

The use of structured diagnostic interviews is effective in the teaching of trainees and interns about diagnostic criteria and how questions about these criteria might be phrased. They also add weight to medico-legal reporting, help in obtaining a second opinion if, for example, a web-based computerised version is being used which the patient can complete independently, and are advantageous in keeping up to date with changed diagnostic systems.

> Structured interviews aim to maximise the reliability and validity of diagnostic interviews.

RELIABILITY

Reliability is an important concept in understanding the usefulness of structured interviews. It refers to how stable or consistent the diagnostic outcome from a given interview will be, across different contexts.

There are different types of reliability.

- *Inter-rater reliability* is the agreement of two or more independent assessors considering the same material by, for example, live observation or via videotape.
- *Test-retest reliability* assesses the stability of the interviews (using the same informant) on two separate occasions, usually a week apart. The closer the result, the greater the test-retest reliability of the measure.

Reliability is most commonly assessed with the use of Cohen's Kappa statistic, which is an index of change-corrected agreement.

Kappa can range from -1, indicating perfect disagreement, or where two interviews result in complete disagreement of diagnoses, to 0, which is no better than chance agreement, through to 1, meaning perfect agreement.

Table 29.1 Cohen's kappa

Kappa	Reliability
-1	Perfect disagreement
0	No better than chance
> 0.40	Acceptable
> 0.75	Good or excellent
1	Perfect agreement

By convention, a kappa of 0.40 is thought to be at the lower bounds of acceptable reliability, while a kappa of 0.75 is thought to represent good or excellent reliability.

Kappa is, however, sensitive to base rates, resulting in lower kappas for less prevalent disorders.

VALIDITY

Validity is a second important concept for assessing the usefulness of a structured interview.

Validity is the degree to which the interview accurately assesses the diagnosis, or diagnostic system that it is proposed to assess. In simple terms, validity concerns what the interview assesses, and how well it does so. Therefore, the validity of a diagnostic interview will be linked to the validity of the diagnostic system.

There are also different types of validity.

- *Criterion validity* is the agreement between the diagnostic outcome and an independent criterion, often an accepted standard such as another well-established assessment, an expert clinical interview or a consensus of information from multiple sources.
- *Convergent validity* is the amount of agreement between an interview's diagnostic outcome and other variables with which, in theory, it should agree.
- *Discriminant validity* is the amount of disagreement between the interview outcome and factors that should not be associated with the diagnosis.
- *Predictive validity* is the degree to which the outcome is associated with another expected outcome, which is measured over time.

HOW TO CHOOSE A SUITABLE INTERVIEW

If a clinician wants to use a structured diagnostic interview, they would choose on the basis of the sample they want to assess, and why they want to make a diagnosis. Interviews can be assessed on a range of variables, including sound psychometric properties; that is, the interview needs to have evidence that it is reliable and valid.

The degree of structure can be an important difference. Some interviews are semi-structured and allow some flexibility in how questions can be asked and how the information can be followed up. These interviews usually require clinical experience and significant training to be administered reliably and validly. Other interviews are fully structured and allow no flexibility, and can be administered by non-clinicians; some have been computerised. Fully structured interviews have often been developed for epidemiological research. They tend to make more diagnoses than semi-structured interviews conducted by expert clinicians.

Other considerations include the range of disorders assessed, the time taken to administer, information provided in addition to diagnosis (such as severity ratings or the course of illness), the expertise or training required for administration, the available support and guidelines for use and, finally, the cost.

KEY BROAD-BASED DIAGNOSTIC INTERVIEWS FOR ADULTS

A number of diagnostic interviews cover a broad range of disorders, but have modules for the diagnosis of anxiety disorders that can be administered separately. Those listed have been updated to provide DSM-5 diagnoses and, on the whole, have sound reliability and validity.

However, these differ in a number of ways. For example, the following interviews are semi-structured:

- *Anxiety Disorders Interview Schedule for DSM-5* (ADIS)
- *Structured Clinical Interview for DSM-IV* (SCID) – soon to be replaced by a DSM-5 update
- *Schedule for Affective Disorders and Schizophrenia* (SADS).

In contrast, the *Composite International Diagnostic Interview* (CIDI) and *Diagnostic Interview Schedule* (DIS) are fully structured and the CIDI has been computerised as the CIDI-Auto.

The CIDI and DIS tend to be used in epidemiological surveys, and their agreement with the semi-structured interviews has often been found to be poor.

ADIS is considered by many to be the most comprehensive diagnostic assessment of adult anxiety disorders, so deserves to be looked at in more detail.

ANXIETY DISORDERS INTERVIEW SCHEDULE

The ADIS covers the full range of DSM-5 anxiety disorders, as well as mood disorders and commonly comorbid conditions. It also screens for substance use and psychotic disorders. The interview provides comprehensive data on onset and course of illness, and a dimensional severity rating of essential features.

The interview requires clinical experience and training in administration. The inter-rater reliability for the ADIS-IV ranges from 0.67 to 0.86. The ADIS is an excellent choice when a clinician needs to assess a range of disorders and, if differential diagnosis is needed, it provides clinically useful information. The length of administration may restrict its use to research settings.

STRUCTURED CLINICAL INTERVIEW FOR DSM-IV AXIS 1 DISORDERS (SCID-I)

The SCID is one of the most widely used diagnostic instruments. The coverage of the SCID is broader than the ADIS, but the interview lacks some of the more detailed questions and severity ratings; only dichotomous data is recorded at the item level. Questions tend to be limited to the information needed to make a DSM diagnosis. An updated DSM-5 version is being developed.

Two versions of the SCID have been developed to meet different needs:

- the SCID-CV (the clinician version)
- the SCID-I (the research version).

The SCID requires clinical experience and training, and good support materials are available. Inter-rater reliability has been found to range from 0.40 to 0.86.

Overall, the SCID is user-friendly and efficient, with a potentially broad coverage of diagnoses.

KEY BROAD-BASED DIAGNOSTIC INTERVIEWS FOR CHILDREN AND ADOLESCENTS

A number of diagnostic interviews for children and adolescents cover a broad range of disorders, but also have modules for the diagnosis of anxiety disorders that can be administered on their own. Those listed provide DSM-5 diagnoses and on the whole have sound reliability and validity.

However, they differ in a number of ways. For example, the following interviews are semi-structured:

- *Anxiety Disorders Interview Schedule for Children - Child and Parent version* (ADIS-C)
- *Schedule for Affective Disorders and Schizophrenia for School-Age Children* (K-SADS)
- *Diagnostic Interview for Children and Adolescents* (DICA)
- *Diagnostic Interview Schedule for Children, Adolescents and Parents* (DISCAP).

In contrast, the *National Institute for Mental Health Diagnostic Interview Schedule for Children* (DISC) is highly structured, can be scored with a computer program, and the administration has been computerised.

ISSUES WITH THE USE OF STRUCTURED DIAGNOSTIC INTERVIEWS WITH CHILDREN AND ADOLESCENTS

There are a number of issues that are specific to the use of structured diagnostic interviews with children and adolescents. Most interviews for childhood disorders have both child and parent versions.

One important issue is the degree of agreement between the diagnostic outcome, when child responses are compared to parent responses; this is referred to as parent-child reliability. It is accepted that parent-child reliability is poor across most assessments, particularly for disorders that require ratings of internal emotional states such as anxiety or affective disorders.

However, it may be best to see child-parent discrepancies as informative rather than problematic. The current view is that diagnostic assessments need to include multiple informants - children are valuable informants regarding their subjective thoughts, behaviours and emotions.

One source of variability in poor child-parent reliability is the issue of whether younger children have the capacity to understand questions posed in structured diagnostic interviews. Some studies have suggested that younger children are less reliable, especially with regard to the reporting of complex detail such as the duration or onset of symptoms, so the lower age cut-off point should be ten years.

Some assessment has tried to increase comprehension; for example, the ADIS-C includes descriptions and visual representation of the scale for rating behaviour – the "feelings thermometer". There is probably a need for further work to be done on child diagnostic interviews in this regard.

The ADIS-C and K-SADS are probably the most widely used diagnostic interviews and will be reviewed now in more detail.

ADIS-C/P

The ADIS-C covers anxiety disorders and other related childhood disorders, such as ADHD. The child and parent versions are similar, but the parent version contains additional disorders, such as conduct disorder, oppositional defiant disorder and enuresis, and requests more detail regarding history and consequences. The interview requires clinical experience and training.

The psychometric properties are strong, with test-retest reliability kappas of 0.61 to 0.80 for child interviews, 0.65 to 1 for parent interviews, and 0.62 to 1 when the information from children and parents is combined.

Inter-rater reliability is sound, with kappas of 0.59 to 0.82 using videotaped interviews, and 0.35 to 1 using live observation. There is also good agreement between face-to-face and telephone delivery, with reported kappas of 0.69 to 0.91.

The ADIS-C is an excellent choice when clinically useful information is needed, although the length of administration may restrict its use to research settings.

K-SADS-PL

The primary focus of the K-SADS is affective disorders and schizophrenia, but the interview also contains modules on anxiety disorders. The PL (Present and Lifetime) version provides both current and lifetime diagnoses.

The format of the K-SADS includes a screening interview with five diagnostic supplements - affective, anxiety, behavioural, psychotic and substance use/other. An introductory interview collects background information and includes questions about school, peer relations, family relations and other activities such as hobbies and sports. Many structured interviews have this section, which aims to build rapport before the structured questions commence.

The test-retest reliability of the K-SADS using live observation is good to excellent, with kappas of 0.63 to 0.90. The K-SADS takes one and a half hours to administer per child and parent, or 3 hours in total. The interview requires clinical experience and training, but the length of the interview perhaps limits its use to research settings.

KEY DIAGNOSTIC INTERVIEWS THAT FOCUS ON SPECIFIC ADULT ANXIETY DISORDERS

Lastly, a number of diagnostic interviews have been developed specifically to diagnose PTSD. The *Clinician Administered PTSD Scale* (CAPS) is a widely used and psychometrically strong diagnostic interview, and is often used as the standard against which other, newer, measures are assessed. It provides a comprehensive assessment of, and provides severity ratings for, the 20 DSM-5 symptoms of PTSD as well as some other areas of functioning. It takes one hour to administer and may not be suitable for routine clinical use. On the other hand, the *PTSD Symptom Scale – Interview Version* (PSS-I) is similar in coverage and psychometric strength to the CAPS, but can be completed in less than 15 minutes.

PART VII SUMMARY

Part VII explained the medical presentation of anxiety disorders, how anxiety might be related to a variety of medical conditions and how it can be confused with some medical illnesses.

In assessing patients, it is important to confirm the type of anxiety disorder from which the patient is suffering, to find out about the context of the disorder, what triggered it, what maintains it and why it has developed.

In order to do this, it is necessary to develop a good working relationship with the patient and the key to this is in good communication skills. The crucial element of good communication skills is letting the patient know that they are being listened to.

To elicit the symptoms of a person's anxiety, the clinician can use open-ended questions, but should also be observing the patient for signs of anxiety. Common symptoms of anxiety include: sweating, shakiness, fidgeting and having blotches appear on the skin. It is also important to observe, not only that the patient is anxious, but what leads to increases in their anxiety level.

When diagnosing a person as suffering an anxiety disorder, one of the most important tasks is to ensure, as far as possible, that their apparent anxiety is not due to a medical illness. Apparent anxiety may be an early symptom of a serious underlying medical condition that should be treated in its own right. Some of the medications used to treat a variety of general medical illnesses may also cause anxiety symptoms as a side effect.

There are a number of diseases that can look like a primary anxiety disorder because they cause the same symptoms. For instance, diseases of the thyroid, heart, lung or adrenal cause the same symptoms as a subjective sense of panic.

Anxiety disorders also have strong associations with chronic physical conditions such hypertension, arthritis, asthma and ulcers. The most common associations in this system are the symptoms of a panic attack and that of a heart attack, or myocardial infarction. The chest pain, difficulty in breathing, palpitations and sweatiness of a panic attack may, when they occur for the first time, lead some individuals to think they are having a heart attack

Part VII went through each of the body systems, and discussed their associations with the anxiety disorders.

For the reasons outlined above, it is crucial to take a careful history of the patient. It is also important to take their age into account; anxiety symptoms present for the first time in someone over 60 suggest either a depressive illness or a new physical illness

The clinician needs to ask patients as a matter of routine if they take any prescription medication or any other substances.

The most common medications that cause anxiety include some of the anticonvulsants, such as carbamazepine. Bronchodilators can lead to jitteriness and anxiety, while some antidepressants can cause an initial increase in anxiety, before having an anxiolytic effect.

Anxiety symptoms can also be triggered by non-prescribed drugs such as caffeine and alcohol. An overdose of caffeine can lead to the full range of anxiety symptoms.

A broad range of substances are implicated in the aetiology and maintenance of anxiety disorder. Commonly abused substances include tobacco, alcohol, cannabis and opioid. It is important to screen broadly for possible substance abuse when assessing any person with anxiety disorders.

Finally, Part VII explained that structured and semi-structured interviews are an important assessment tool because they help minimise the sources of variability that cause diagnostic disagreement between clinicians.

There are sound structured interviews available to diagnose anxiety reliably, and the choice of instrument will depend on the needs of the assessment.

However, while most interviews have good to excellent reliability, more work is needed to confirm the validity of the diagnostic outcomes, although these can only be as valid as the diagnostic system they are developed to assess.

PART VIII   BEHAVIOUR THERAPY

Angela is a 25-year-old woman who started having panic attacks after the birth of her baby, Emily. Since then, she tries to avoid being alone in case something happens and now relies heavily on her husband Michael.

"I felt I needed him there because if something happened, then who would look after our daughter? He arranged for me to work with him in the office so we could drive in together every day…

"I don't do the shopping on my own any more. He likes driving and he's not a very good passenger so it suits us both… But I think it's starting to annoy Michael. He doesn't get to do what he used to do."

Avoidance is a key behavioural feature of all patients with anxiety disorders. On the surface, it makes sense for people to avoid things that make them feel anxious; not only does avoidance reduce anxiety in the short-term, but the anxious individual believes it also prevents the bad thing from happening.

Avoidance comes in many forms, from overt avoidance of entering feared situations, such as shopping centres and trains in people with panic disorder and agoraphobia, to avoidance of snakes or spiders in specific phobias.

However, avoidance can be more subtle or covert, where people use safety-seeking behaviours to protect themselves against their feared outcomes, such as avoiding eye contact in social phobia.

Sometimes avoidance can just be cognitive, where people avoid thinking of things that make them anxious; for example, people with PTSD will avoid traumatic memories. In OCD, the avoidance behaviours often take the form of rituals or compulsions, which are designed to avoid the consequences associated with the obsession; for example, compulsive hand-washing is designed to avoid being contaminated.

> Avoidance is a key behavioural feature of all patients with anxiety disorders.

Behaviour therapy for anxiety disorders involves combating these avoidance behaviours through exposure to feared situations, sensations or memories. This type of treatment is called exposure therapy. A primary goal of exposure therapy is to decrease the person's anxiety, while they remain in the feared situation, without avoiding in any way. In lay terms, exposure therapy is all about "facing your fears".

Part VIII will introduce the principles underlying exposure-based treatments.

Different methods of exposure therapy will be described, in particular imaginal and in vivo exposure, and these will be linked to clinical examples across different anxiety disorders.

The evidence base for behaviour therapy for the anxiety disorders will also be explored.

CHAPTER 30   PRINCIPLES OF BEHAVIOUR THERAPY

Rocco Crino and Juliette Drobny

CLASSICAL CONDITIONING

Part V described the work of Ivan Pavlov and the phenomenon of classical conditioning, a type of associative learning that has been useful in understanding the acquisition of fear. As the meaning of terms such as unconditioned stimulus and conditioned response can be confusing or difficult to remember, they are revisited here.

PAVLOV'S DOGS

As illustrated in Figure 30.1, in the original classical conditioning paradigm with Pavlov's dogs, food acts as the unconditioned stimulus, which triggers a natural or unconditioned response, namely salivation.

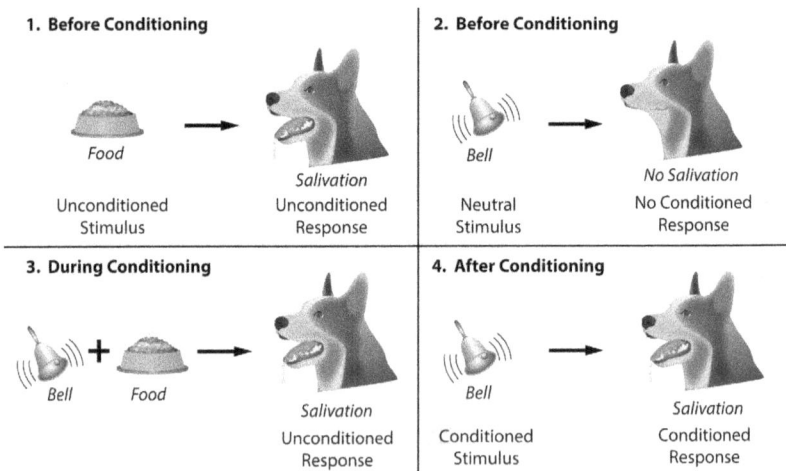

1. Before Conditioning

Food
Unconditioned Stimulus

Salivation
Unconditioned Response

2. Before Conditioning

Bell
Neutral Stimulus

No Salivation
No Conditioned Response

3. During Conditioning

Bell   Food

Salivation
Unconditioned Response

4. After Conditioning

Bell
Conditioned Stimulus

Salivation
Conditioned Response

Figure 30.1   Pavlov's dogs

Before conditioning occurs, a neutral stimulus such as a bell or a light is presented, which initially leads to no conditioned response (i.e., no salivation).

During conditioning, the bell is paired with food, and the dog naturally salivates to the food.

However, after repeated pairings of the bell with the food, the dog learns that the bell signals the delivery of food, so begins to salivate to the bell alone. The bell has become a conditioned stimulus, and the dog displays a conditioned response of salivation to the bell.

In summary, in classical conditioning a neutral stimulus can take on a new meaning if paired with an unconditioned stimulus, which then provokes a conditioned response.

CLASSICAL CONDITIONING OF HUMAN FEAR

As discussed in Part V, the birth of modern behaviour therapy can be traced back to the 1920s with the work of Watson and Rayner who demonstrated, with the case of Little Albert, that human fears could be conditioned by the use of Pavlovian learning principles.

Albert, an 11-month old boy with no known fears or anxiety, was conditioned to fear a white rat. The production of a loud noise alone (the unconditioned stimulus), resulted in a startle response and crying (the unconditioned response) by Albert. The white rat was then presented to Albert accompanied by the loud noise, resulting in a startle reaction and crying. After repeated exposure, the presentation of the white rat alone (the conditioned stimulus) without the loud noise resulted in the fear response (conditioned response). Interestingly, the fear generalised to include other furry animals and toys. Thus it is evident that classical conditioning is involved in fear acquisition and, as discussed in Part V, is often involved in the development of anxiety disorders.

OPERANT CONDITIONING

The highly influential American behavioural psychologist, B. F. Skinner, introduced the concept of operant conditioning, another type of associative learning. Here, learning occurs through rewards and punishments for behaviour. In operant conditioning, the learner makes an association between a behaviour and its consequence.

The components of operant conditioning involve reinforcers and punishments. A reinforcer is any event that strengthens or increases the behaviour, while a punishment is any adverse event, or outcome, that causes a decrease in the behaviour. Reinforcers and punishments can be either positive or negative. For the purpose of this chapter, only reinforcement will be discussed.

POSITIVE AND NEGATIVE REINFORCEMENT

The terms *positive* and *negative* are not the same as those used in everyday language. Here, positive refers to the addition of something and negative refers to the withdrawal of something.

Positive reinforcement occurs when a behaviour is followed by the addition of something pleasant, which then increases or strengthens the behaviour. Examples of positive reinforcers include the use of praise for doing a good job, or receiving a financial reward or bonus for achieving a goal at work. In animal training, food rewards are often used to reinforce the desired behaviour – for example, a dog sitting when told to sit. All of these rewards increase the chances that the desired behaviour will be repeated.

Negative reinforcement, however, occurs when a behaviour is followed by the removal of something unpleasant. This, too, strengthens the behaviour. An example of negative reinforcement is taking a painkiller for a headache. The decrease in pain is reinforcing, and will increase the likelihood of taking a painkiller the next time a headache occurs. Negative reinforcement is very relevant to the maintenance of anxiety disorders.

NEGATIVE REINFORCEMENT AND AVOIDANCE

In anxiety provoking situations, avoidance or escape is a common behaviour. In the case of a dog phobic, for example, the person's anxiety rapidly increases on seeing a dog. This anxiety feels terrible and triggers the urge to avoid or escape the dog. By avoiding, the anxiety rapidly decreases, which feels good and is therefore very reinforcing.

Therefore, in the short-term, avoidance is an effective method in reducing anxiety (Figure 30.2).

In positive reinforcement, a behaviour is followed by the addition of something pleasant, which strengthens the behaviour, whereas in negative reinforcement, a behaviour is followed by removal of something unpleasant which also strengthens the behaviour.

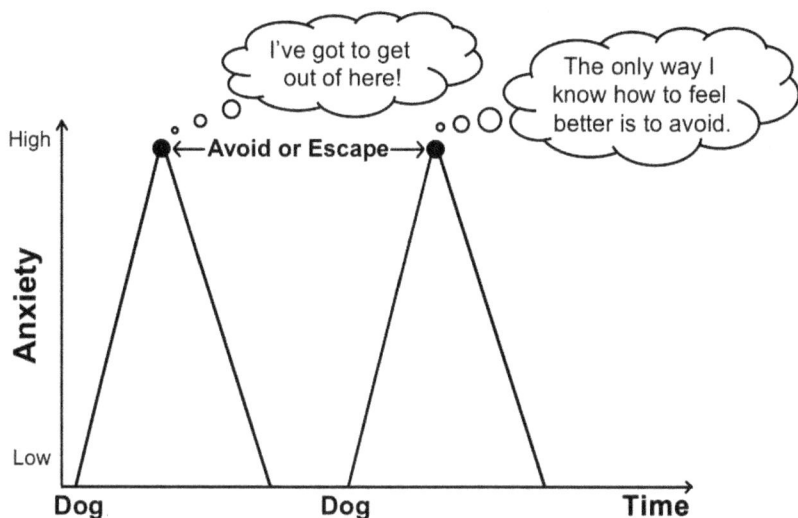

Figure 30.2 Effect of avoidance on anxiety over time

However, the next time the person sees a dog, their anxiety will continue to rise. By previously avoiding the dog, they learned their anxiety decreased, so they continue to use avoidance to manage their anxiety. Thus, in the long-term, avoidance actually serves to maintain anxiety.

Perhaps most importantly, by avoiding, the person never finds out what would actually happen if they remained in the situation with the dog. Does the bad thing they fear actually happen? As most dogs are not dangerous, by avoiding, the person does not have the opportunity to disconfirm their fear. Hence, through negative reinforcement avoidance behaviours are strengthened, which in turn maintains the person's fear of dogs.

The negatively reinforcing properties of avoidance are relevant to the maintenance of all anxiety disorders. Although it is not always labelled as avoidance, different behaviours used to decrease anxiety, such as safety behaviours and compulsions, all operate in the same way.

The following scenarios describe the triggers in different anxiety disorders:

- a person with agoraphobia who experiences panic symptoms in a shopping centre
- a person with social phobia at a party
- a person with OCD who has touched something they think is contaminated.

When people with these three anxiety disorders are confronted with the triggers described in the scenario, their anxiety increases, which makes them feel distressed. At this point, the person with agoraphobia wants to avoid or escape the situation, the person with social phobia uses a safety behaviour (e.g., avoids eye contact) and the person with OCD performs a compulsion (e.g., hand-washing). As a consequence, their anxiety decreases, which makes them feel good. The next time these people are faced with a similar trigger, anxiety once again rises and they have learned that if they want to feel better, they should use their avoidance behaviour.

Hence, the reduction in anxiety reinforces the avoidance behaviour, which in turn prevents them from learning that nothing bad will happen, thus perpetuating their anxiety. In summary, avoidance is reinforcing, and prevents new learning.

LEARNING THEORY

The role of different types of associative learning, namely classical and operant conditioning, has contributed to the understanding of the acquisition and maintenance of fear and anxiety disorders. Learning theory also provides insights into how learned associations can be unlearned, an approach that has guided the development of behavioural treatments for anxiety disorders. Concepts involved in the weakening of learned associations, namely extinction, counterconditioning and habituation will now be discussed.

EXTINCTION

The concept of extinction learning was previously discussed in Part V. Extinction refers to a reduction in a conditioned response (e.g., salivation), when a conditioned stimulus (e.g., a bell) is repeatedly presented *without* the unconditioned stimulus (e.g., food).

Returning to Pavlov's dogs, during the first trial of an extinction phase, the dog will continue to salivate to the bell. However, after repeated trials where the bell is rung and no food is delivered, the dog comes to learn that the bell no longer signals food, and therefore stops salivating to the bell.

COUNTERCONDITIONING

Counterconditioning is another procedure that can reduce or extinguish a learned fear response. In counterconditioning, a conditioned stimulus (e.g., snake) is paired with a *positive* or non-aversive unconditioned stimulus (e.g., enjoyable food). Here, the new unconditioned response (e.g., pleasure or relaxation) to the positive unconditioned stimulus is substituted for the fear response, which results in the modification of the conditioned fear response.

HABITUATION

Another type of learning is habituation. Habituation is a simpler type of learning that leads to decreased behavioural responses to repeated stimuli. It is a basic biological process that does not require conscious motivation or awareness, which has been shown in every animal species. Habituation is learning to ignore irrelevant stimuli that are neither harmful nor helpful.

Habituation can be easily demonstrated in a snail. If a snail's tentacles are touched gently, they will sharply retract. After some time the tentacles will re-emerge. If the process is repeated, over time the snail will learn that no harm occurs, and will stop retracting its tentacles.

ORIGINS OF EXPOSURE THERAPY

An American psychologist by the name of Mary Cover Jones, who was aware of the work of Pavlov and Watson, was amongst the first to report the treatment of human fears. She treated Little Peter, a 3-year-old child with a fear of rabbits. The aetiology of his fear was unknown. The logic behind the approach used by Mary Cover Jones was based on learning principles – specifically, counterconditioning (Figure 30.3).

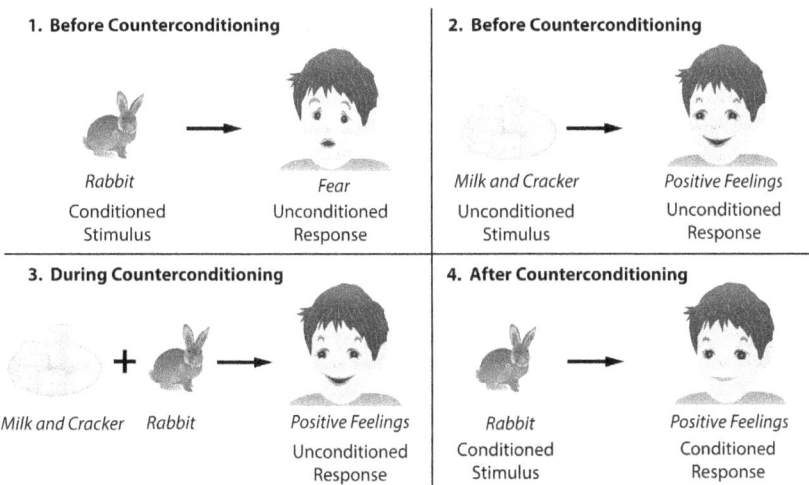

1. Before Counterconditioning

Rabbit
Conditioned
Stimulus

Fear
Unconditioned
Response

2. Before Counterconditioning

Milk and Cracker
Unconditioned
Stimulus

Positive Feelings
Unconditioned
Response

3. During Counterconditioning

Milk and Cracker   *Rabbit*

Positive Feelings
Unconditioned
Response

4. After Counterconditioning

Rabbit
Conditioned
Stimulus

Positive Feelings
Conditioned
Response

Figure 30.3   Little Peter

Little Peter was provided with a snack of milk and crackers (alternative positive unconditioned stimulus), food he enjoyed and associated with positive feelings (unconditioned response). As he ate the snack he was presented with the feared rabbit, firstly at a comfortable distance. Subsequent sessions involved moving the rabbit closer and closer to Peter while he enjoyed the milk and crackers. By doing this, Jones was able to establish a relationship between the rabbit and a positive stimulus, so that Peter eventually played comfortably with the rabbit.

Jones' work was somewhat revolutionary for its time in the application of learning principles to the treatment of human fears and, eventually, other behavioural problems.

SYSTEMATIC DESENSITISATION

The work of South African psychiatrist Joseph Wolpe is also paramount in the early development of behavioural interventions. Wolpe's original work with cats, in which he used a counterconditioning paradigm, led to the development of systematic desensitisation. He used food as the non-aversive, unconditioned stimulus to overcome the cats' fear of their original cages. However, he settled on relaxation, assertion and a sexual response as possible positive unconditioned stimuli in humans.

Wolpe's systematic desensitisation process was described in terms of counterconditioning. Typically, when using systematic desensitisation, the attempt is made to substitute a relaxation response in place of the maladaptive anxiety response. The procedure involves developing a hierarchy of feared situations, ranging from mildly to extremely anxiety provoking. The anxious patient is gradually exposed to the feared stimulus, while practicing previously learnt relaxation. It can be conducted in imagery or in vivo.

Work by other researchers around this time led to the further development of exposure-based treatments. They called into question the notion of counterconditioning and the need for an inhibitory response to anxiety. Experimental psychologist Richard Solomon, for example, examined the persistence of the avoidance response in conditioned animals, and reported that exposure alone, in the absence of the aversive event, resulted in the extinction of avoidance.

Similarly, Joan Malleson used a hierarchy not unlike that used in a desensitisation program, but instructed patients to feel more and more frightened as they progressed through the hierarchy. Although anxiety increased initially, it gradually faded, so the stimulus no longer elicited the fear response. Such research raised questions about the necessity of relaxation as an inhibitory response.

MECHANISMS OF CHANGE

Treatment outcome studies suggest that relaxation is not a necessary component for successful anxiety reduction. As a result, the counterconditioning model was subsequently superseded by the *habituation model*. The habituation model suggests that prolonged exposure in imagery or in vivo, without an incompatible response, is sufficient to result in a decrease in the associated anxiety. It is now generally acknowledged that repeated, and prolonged exposure in the absence of dangerous consequences results in a decrease in the intensity of the emotional response and, eventually, results in the feared stimulus no longer eliciting the emotional response. Relaxation may therefore be of little utility as the same results were achieved through exposure alone.

It would appear, then, that the common and most important element to systematic desensitisation, imaginal, or in vivo exposure and flooding, is the *exposure* to the feared stimulus. Exposure is considered, at least in part, to be based on Pavlovian extinction; that is, repeated and continuous presentation of the conditioned stimulus in the absence of the unconditioned stimulus.

However, the notion that exposure is based solely on the extinction paradigm has been questioned by Mark Bouton and colleagues whose work suggests that exposure may be efficacious through the learning of new information, so that the conditioned stimulus is no longer associated with one unconditioned stimulus, but may be associated with a number of unconditioned stimuli. Thus, a stimulus that was associated with danger may become associated with outcomes other than danger. In other words, the original association is not unlearned as such, but new associations, for example safety, co-exist with the old learning, and the resultant response is dependent on contextual retrieval.

The mechanism of change during exposure is still not clearly understood. The reduction in anxiety may occur through extinction, habituation, new learning or a combination of these processes.

ESSENTIAL ELEMENTS OF EXPOSURE

Irrespective of the mechanism of action, the essential elements of effective exposure, whether in imagery or in vivo, are that:

- The exposure to the feared stimulus is prolonged, so that it allows the anxiety to dissipate.
- The emotion consistent response, such as avoidance or escape, is prevented.
- Exposure is repeated to allow new learning to take place.

As a therapeutic intervention, exposure remains one of the most powerful treatments in overcoming situational fears and avoidance. Exposure has been successfully applied to a variety of clinical problems, especially where fear and anxiety are central features.

CHAPTER 31   IMAGINAL EXPOSURE

Rocco Crino

IMAGINAL EXPOSURE

Imaginal exposure involves exposing the individual to emotionally provocative cues in imagination. Although in vivo exposure is the most efficacious form of exposure, imaginal techniques are used when it is difficult, or impractical, to expose the individual to real life cues, for example, a storm phobia. In some circumstances, it is difficult to access the phobic situation or stimulus. This may be because it is too expensive, for example, having repeatedly to take flights for a person with a fear of flying, or having repeated visits to the dentist for someone with a dental phobia. In some cases, it is simply difficult to obtain a specimen of the phobic stimulus, for example, fears of certain animals such as snakes, spiders or dogs, for the purposes of in vivo exposure. Imaginal exposure is also used when the anxiety provoking cues are internal, for example, traumatic memories in PTSD, or catastrophic future-oriented fears such as a death of a loved one. It is also used when the anxiety provoked by the real life cue is of such intensity that in vivo exposure is difficult to implement in the first case.

FOUR STEPS TO IMAGINAL EXPOSURE

Four steps are required when conducting imaginal exposure:

Step 1: Rationale

When using imaginal exposure, as with any other treatment, a thorough rationale and explanation of the procedure is the first step in developing a collaborative approach. Every day examples of the desensitisation process will assist the individual to understand the process – for example, the effects of repeatedly watching a horror movie.

> Imaginal techniques are used when it is difficult, or impractical, to expose the individual to real life cues.

Step 2: Relaxation Training

If the traditional systematic desensitisation is going to be used, some form of relaxation training is taught – for example, Jacobson's progressive muscle relaxation or another relaxation procedure. As was discussed previously, this step is optional, as relaxation training does not enhance the outcome of exposure alone.

Step 3: Hierarchy Construction

The hierarchy is collaboratively constructed with the patient, who lists the feared scenes or situations, which are then rated in terms of the degree of anxiety that each situation provokes. The situations are then ranked from least to most anxiety provoking.

Step 4: Graded Imaginal Exposure

The fourth step is actually conducting the imaginal exposure, starting with less anxiety provoking situations, then gradually progressing to more anxiety provoking ones.

HIERARCHY CONSTRUCTION

When constructing a hierarchy for imaginal exposure, typically eight to ten scenes or situations are described in detail. The patient provides ratings of the level of discomfort or anxiety associated with each scene on a SUDS (i.e., Subjective Units of Discomfort) scale ranging from 0 to 10, where 0 reflects no anxiety, 5 reflects moderate levels of anxiety and 10 reflects severe anxiety.

When constructing the steps of the hierarchy, an attempt should be made to include the key stimulus elements that illicit fear or anxiety in the individual. Generally, imaginal exposure commences with items reflecting low to moderate levels of anxiety – for example, a SUDS rating of 2 to 4.

EXAMPLE IMAGINAL EXPOSURE HIERARCHY

Table 31.1 is an imaginal exposure hierarchy used in the treatment of a person with a lift phobia. The key elements that influence the level of anxiety experienced include:

- position of the lift doors
- number of levels

- proximity to the lift doors and console
- visibility of the lift doors
- crowdedness of the lift.

Table 31.1 Example imaginal exposure hierarchy

Step	Scene
1	Stand outside the lift with the doors open
2	Stand inside the lift with the doors open, press the "doors open" button
3	Stand inside the lift, press the "doors closed" button and remain stationary in the lift with the doors closed
4	Stand inside the lift facing the console, move up one level and exit
5	Stand inside the lift, facing the console, move up three levels and exit
6	Stand away from the console, move up three levels and exit
7	Facing the back wall, move up three levels and exit
8	Stand at the front of a crowded lift, move up three levels
9	Stand at the back of a crowded lift, move up one level
10	Stand at the back of a crowded lift, move up three levels

GRADED IMAGINAL EXPOSURE

When commencing imaginal exposure, the patient is instructed to sit comfortably in their chair with their eyes closed. If anxiety is too great, they can start with their eyes open and later go on to repeating the scene with their eyes closed. Each scene is then described in considerable detail, with the patient being prompted to imagine and describe their sensory experiences. For example:

- "What do you see?"
- "What can you hear?"
- "How does it feel?"

SUDS ratings are taken at various points. The scene is repeated until the SUDS ratings decrease to low levels. Recordings of the exposure session may be used for between session exposure homework. As the individual becomes desensitised or habituated to the scenario, that is, their SUDS ratings are quite low reflecting little or no anxiety, the next step in the hierarchy is introduced. Similar procedures are followed until the hierarchy is completed.

TYPES OF IMAGINAL EXPOSURE

The previous example of the exposure hierarchy to lifts was one of graded imaginal exposure. However, there are other imaginal exposure techniques that can be considered on a continuum, in terms of the amount of anxiety provocation associated with each.

Systematic desensitisation with the use of relaxation is perhaps the least distressing intervention. Graded imaginal exposure without relaxation, or any other competing response, results in a slightly higher level of discomfort. Imaginal flooding is prolonged presentation of the most anxiety provoking scene until anxiety subsides, and this results in the greatest level of discomfort.

Interestingly, the outcome for each procedure is similar, and the utilisation of each is on the basis of the tolerance the patient has to the degree of discomfort, and a collaborative approach when dealing with the anxiety.

CHAPTER 32   IN VIVO EXPOSURE

Rocco Crino

PRINCIPLES OF IN VIVO EXPOSURE

As suggested by the name, in vivo exposure is carried out in real life. Essentially, the procedure is very similar to that used in imaginal exposure, except that the fear provoking stimulus or situation is encountered in real life. There is some suggestion that in vivo exposure results in better transfer to actual situations than imaginal exposure and the results are achieved in a shorter period of time.

As with imaginal exposure, in vivo exposure procedures can be considered on a continuum, with graded exposure at one end and flooding procedures at the other. Flooding involves exposure to the major fear-evoking stimulus until the anxiety subsides. Graded exposure, on the other hand, is conducted in a structured, hierarchical and systematic manner and is considerably more palatable for the patient than flooding procedures.

RATIONALE OF IN VIVO EXPOSURE

When utilising in vivo exposure, as with all cognitive-behavioural procedures, a clear and understandable rationale is critical. Exposure will involve some level of discomfort for the patient, so a clear rationale will assist the individual to engage in what may appear to be an uncomfortable procedure.

Education about in vivo exposure should involve real life examples of exposure occurring in daily life.

For example, when the individual first learned to swim, their first day of school, or when they learned to drive a car. Each of these situations provoked some level of anxiety. However, repeated exposure resulted in those behaviours no longer eliciting any anxiety whatsoever.

It is also important to reinforce the idea that repeated exposure results in habituation and/or new learning. Thus, the individual will be required to engage in tasks repeatedly until the anxiety is minimised.

ESSENTIAL ELEMENTS OF IN VIVO EXPOSURE

There are three essential elements to in vivo exposure.

- The exposure needs to be prolonged, continuing until the anxiety ratings reduce by some 50%. If not 50%, some reduction is essential before termination.
- Avoidance, escape or safety-seeking behaviours are prevented, or if initially incorporated in earlier steps of the hierarchy, are faded out before completion of the hierarchy.
- The exposure needs to be repeated. Repetitive exposure is essential in promoting habituation and/or new learning, and providing disconfirmation of the feared outcome.

EXPOSURE GOALS

As with imaginal exposure, construction of the in vivo exposure hierarchy requires a collaborative approach. The goal of exposure needs to be clearly defined, and there also needs to be clear, definitive descriptions of each step required to achieve the goal.

Vague goals such as "I want to travel on the train", or, "I want to get over my anxiety in shops", are not suitable for the construction of the hierarchy. Specific goals however, such as, "I want to be able to travel to the city from home by train", or, "I want to do the grocery shopping at the local shopping centre", are clear and definitive goals that are suitable for the construction of the hierarchy.

EXPOSURE STEPS

As with imaginal exposure, the in vivo exposure hierarchy should have multiple steps of varying degrees of difficulty. Usually 8 to 12 steps are used to achieve the goal.

Steps should at all times be chosen collaboratively, with the patient encouraged to adopt a co-therapist approach.

HIERARCHY CONSTRUCTION

Each step is rated in terms of expected degree of difficulty or expected level of anxiety or discomfort, using the SUDS rating scale where 0 is no anxiety or discomfort, 5 is moderate levels of anxiety or discomfort and 10 is severe anxiety or discomfort.

The steps are arranged from least anxiety provoking through to most. The initial anxiety ratings will be used to determine the actual steps of the hierarchy. However, a flexible approach is certainly warranted as patients may have underestimated the actual level of anxiety elicited.

In vivo exposure aims to expose the patient to the feared stimulus in the absence of avoidance, safety behaviours or compulsions. However, if the anxiety experienced is too severe, safety behaviours and compulsions can be built into the exposure hierarchy and gradually reduced.

For example, take a patient with OCD who normally checks the stove is switched off ten times before leaving the house. If, as part of therapy, they are unable not to check the stove at all, then the first step in their hierarchy might involve checking the stove five times instead of ten, then reducing it to only two checks in the next step, then one check, followed by no checking behaviour. Again, a collaborative approach is required when developing exposure goals and steps.

EXAMPLE IN VIVO EXPOSURE HIERARCHY

Table 32.1 is an example of an exposure hierarchy for a person with agoraphobia who has a fear of travelling on a train.

As you can see, the goal is very specific: to travel to the city by express train. There are ten steps required to achieve this goal, and the degree of difficulty is manipulated by incorporating factors that increase or decrease the person's anxiety. Note that the presence of safety behaviours is incorporated into the exposure hierarchy to decrease the level of difficulty. However, these are gradually faded out towards the end of the hierarchy.

> In vivo exposure aims to expose the patient to the feared stimulus in the absence of avoidance, safety behaviours or compulsions.

Table 32.1 Example in vivo exposure hierarchy

Step	Goal: Travel to the city by express train
10	Travel to city on an express train in peak hour alone, without mobile phone or water bottle
9	Travel to city on an express train in peak hour alone, with mobile phone and water bottle
8	Travel to city on an all-stops train (six stations) alone, on a weekday, in peak hour, without mobile phone or water bottle
7	Travel to the city on an all-stops train (six stations) on the weekend, alone, without mobile phone or water bottle
6	Travel on a train to work in peak hour (four stations) alone, without mobile phone or water bottle
5	Travel on a train to work in peak hour (four stations) alone, with mobile phone and water bottle
4	Travel on a train to work in peak hour (four stations) with friend, without mobile phone or water bottle
3	Travel on a train (two stations) on a weekday but not in peak hour with friend, without mobile phone or water bottle
2	Travel on a train (two stations) on weekend with friend, mobile phone and water bottle
1	Sit at the train station alone and read the time table

As can be seen, factors that influence the level of anxiety experienced include:

- number of stations
- presence of friend
- use of safety behaviours (mobile phone, water)
- crowdedness of the train
- express versus all-stops train.

CONDUCTING IN VIVO EXPOSURE

In the initial stages of implementing the exposure hierarchy, a step with a lower anxiety rating may be chosen to demonstrate the procedure, or demonstrate the mechanism of change. It is also useful to choose an easier situation to ensure early successful experiences, which will serve to enhance patients' confidence in the procedure and in themselves. Commencing exposure with an item that is too difficult is likely to lead to a failure experience that may demotivate the patient and, potentially, reinforce their fear.

Implementation of the actual exposure hierarchy usually commences with moderate anxiety provoking situations, defined as having a SUDS rating of about 4–5. In order to maximise the effectiveness of exposure, it needs to be repeated and prolonged, and conducted in a variety of contexts and situations, in order for habituation and/or new learning to occur. As each step is mastered, the individual moves on to the next step. Mastery of the step is defined as at least a 50% decrease in their SUDS rating.

In vivo exposure is conducted in a similar manner across the different anxiety disorders. However, in OCD, in vivo exposure is typically referred to as "Exposure plus Response Prevention", or ERP for short. This simply means that the patient is exposed to a situation that triggers their anxiety (e.g., a surface they perceive to be contaminated), and are then prevented from performing their neutralising response (e.g., hand-washing). Despite the difference in name, ERP operates in exactly the same way as graded in vivo exposure.

EXPOSURE THERAPY AND ANXIETY OVER TIME

Figure 32.1 displays the typical pattern of anxiety experienced during exposure therapy. As can be seen, in the first trial anxiety rises sharply to high levels. At this point, the patient often has a strong urge to avoid, use a safety behaviour or perform a compulsion. However, if they are prevented from doing so, their anxiety will remain high for some time and then gradually start to decrease on its own.

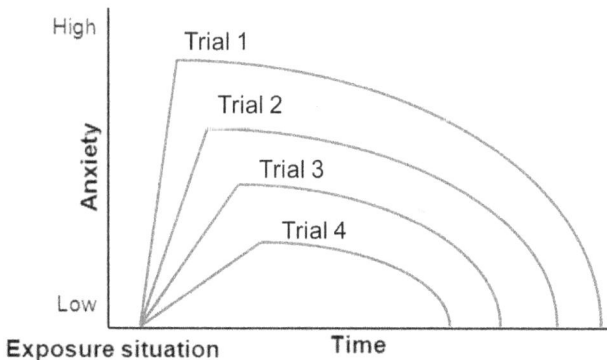

Figure 32.1   Effect of exposure therapy on anxiety over time

The next time they expose themselves to the situation (Trial 2), their anxiety will still rise, but not as high as the first exposure trial. The anxiety will continue to remain high but will gradually decrease, often taking less time than the time before. As exposure to the situation continues, the initial anxiety experienced becomes lower and lower, and takes less and less time to decrease.

SAFETY BEHAVIOURS IN THE FINAL STEP

It is important to note that conducting exposure therapy with safety behaviours artificially reduces the person's level of anxiety, and habituation is unable to be achieved. Moreover, the person is less likely to acquire new learning from the situation, as the lack of the feared outcome may be attributed to the use of the safety behaviour. Therefore, they are likely to remain fearful in the situation without the continued aid of the safety behaviour. Hence, safety behaviours need to be eliminated before completing the exposure hierarchy.

As a final note, it also important to ask about the presence of any new safety behaviours or compulsions that may have emerged throughout treatment as these will also need to be removed.

CHAPTER 33   THE EVIDENCE BASE FOR EXPOSURE THERAPY

Juliette Drobny

ABOUT THE EVIDENCE

To examine the effectiveness of behaviour therapy for anxiety disorders, the Cochrane Library was searched to obtain the highest quality independent evidence. Where Cochrane reviews were not available, meta-analyses from the Centre of Reviews and Dissemination, or other meta-analyses, were examined. Where there were no meta-analyses, individual reports were identified that evaluated the effectiveness of behaviour therapy.

In this chapter, reference will be made to effect sizes (ES) of treatment. To interpret effect sizes, a common guideline is where 0.2 reflects a small effect, 0.5 reflects a medium effect and 0.8 and above represents a large effect. In short, the larger the number, the greater the effect size.

Reference will also be made to:

- odds ratio (OR), the odds that an outcome will occur given a particular event, compared to the odds of the outcome occurring in the absence of that event
- confidence interval (CI), a measure of the reliability of an estimate
- standardised mean difference (SMD), a summary statistic in meta-analysis when the studies all assess the same outcome but measure it in a variety of ways
- weighted mean difference (WMD), a standard statistic that measures the absolute difference between the mean value in two groups in a clinical trial
- *p*-value, the probability of obtaining a test statistic result at least as extreme or as close to the one that was actually observed, assuming that the null hypothesis is true.

In the literature, an active treatment is often compared to a control group, such as a waitlist, a placebo or treatment as usual. A large between-group effect size indicates that the active treatment is more effective than the control group, while a small between-group effect size indicates little difference between the two groups.

PANIC DISORDER WITH AND WITHOUT AGORAPHOBIA

Sanchez-Meca et al. (2010) conducted a meta-analysis reviewing the effect of exposure therapies compared to a waitlist or placebo control group.

In vivo exposure comprised either interoceptive exposure or exposure to feared situations, while imaginal exposure consisted of exposure to feared situations or sensations in imagination.

Interoceptive exposure is a form of behavioural therapy in which *internal* physical sensations (e.g., feelings of choking, dizziness) are reproduced, and the patient is exposed to them in a controlled setting. This is in contrast to exposure to *external* stimuli, as in in vivo exposure. Interoceptive exposure therapy is often used in panic disorder. However, it has also been studied in claustrophobia.

As shown in Figure 33.1, large effect sizes were found for in vivo exposure for panic (ES = 1.25, 95% CI = 1.05 to 1.44) and agoraphobic (ES = 0.89, 95% CI = 0.68 to 1.11) measures. Imaginal exposure was also effective, but yielded smaller, yet moderate, effect sizes (Panic measures: ES = 0.65, 95% CI = 0.13 to 1.17, Agoraphobic measures: ES = 0.61, 95% CI = -0.20 to 1.42).

An active treatment is often compared to a control group, such as a waitlist, a placebo or treatment as usual. A large between-group effect size indicates that the active treatment is more effective than the control group, while a small between-group effect size indicates little difference between the two groups.

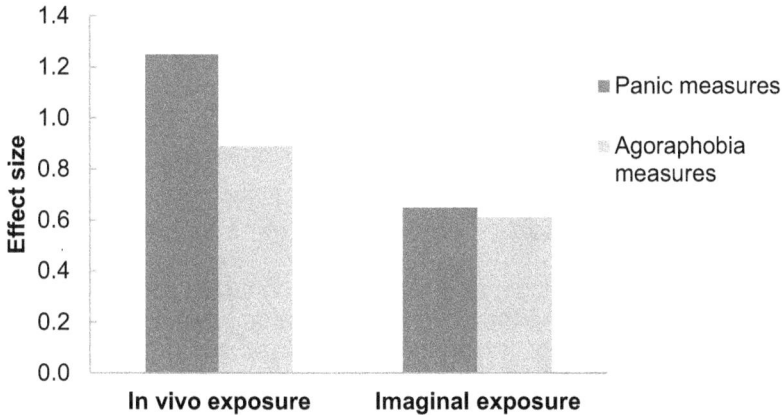

Figure 33.1 Post-treatment effect sizes for exposure versus waitlist/placebo in panic disorder and agoraphobia. Data adapted from Sanchez-Meca et al. (2010).

A randomised controlled trial conducted by Ito et al. (2001) compared interoceptive exposure and in vivo exposure to external situations, against a waitlist control for patients with panic disorder.

As shown in Figure 33.2, both groups yielded large effect sizes on phobic avoidance at post-treatment (Interoceptive: ES = 2.5, External in vivo: ES = 3.0). There were no significant differences between these exposure treatments at post-treatment or at 12-month follow-up.

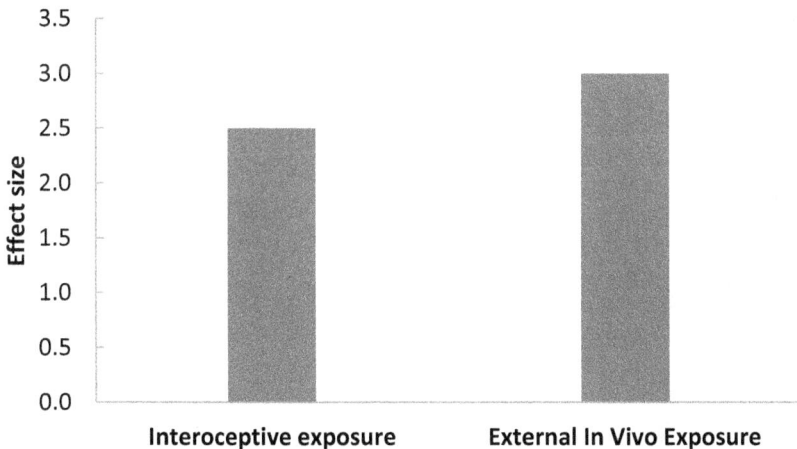

Figure 33.2 Post-treatment effect sizes for phobic avoidance across exposure treatments versus waitlist control. Data adapted from Ito et al. (2001).

SOCIAL PHOBIA

A meta-analysis by Acarturk et al. (2009) reviewed eight studies of exposure therapy for social phobia, compared with a control group. Exposure therapy was more effective than control conditions, producing a large effect size of 0.79 (ES = 0.79, 95% CI = 0.50 to 1.09).

GENERALISED ANXIETY DISORDER

In a study from 2009, Hoyer and colleagues conducted a randomised controlled trial examining the effectiveness of worry exposure and the empirically supported treatment of applied relaxation for GAD when compared to a waitlist control.

For worry exposure, no reference was made to the role of thought challenging. Instead, patients were instructed to expose themselves to their worry following a habituation-based rationale.

As shown in Figure 33.3, at post-treatment, worry exposure resulted in significant reductions in anxiety (SMD = -1.15, $p < .01$), worry (SMD = -0.65, $p < .01$), metacognitive beliefs (SMD = -0.64, $p < .01$) and depression (SMD = -1.15, p < .01), with moderate to large between group effect sizes. Interestingly, as can be seen in Figure 33.4, there were no differences on any measures (Applied Relaxation v. WL: anxiety SMD = -1.23, $p < .01$; worry SMD = -0.82, $p < .01$; metacognitions SMD = -0.70, $p < .01$; depression SMD = -1.15, $p < .01$) when worry exposure was compared to applied relaxation. Although operating via two different mechanisms, both treatments appear equally effective.

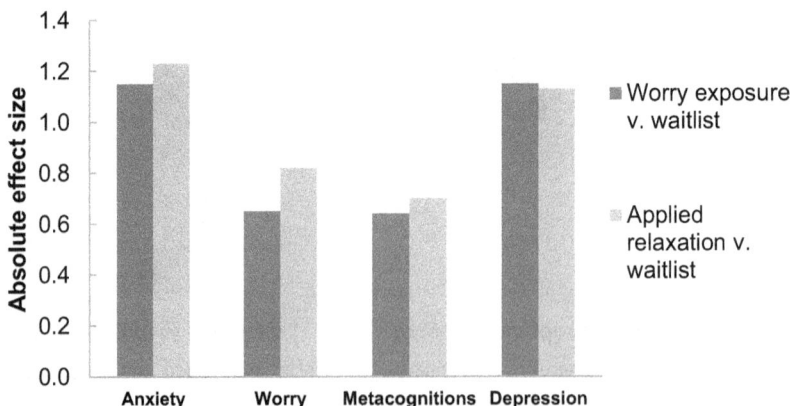

Figure 33.3 Post-treatment effect sizes for worry exposure and applied relaxation versus waitlist (Hoyer et al., 2009)

OBSESSIVE-COMPULSIVE DISORDER

A Cochrane review by Gava et al. (2007) reviewed three studies with a total of 72 participants, comparing exposure and response prevention (ERP) with treatment as usual. ERP was found to be more effective than treatment as usual for reducing obsessive-compulsive symptoms (WMD = -11.73, 95% CI = -14.52 to -8.95). They also found that drop-out rates were higher for ERP than treatment as usual (OR = 1.66, 95% CI = 0.57 to 4.86).

Research and clinical experience indicates that patients find ERP very challenging. Some of the more severe patients are unwilling, or unable, to engage in treatment due to their fear. This is not overly surprising, as some patients believe they or their loved ones will die if they do not perform their rituals. This has implications for the effectiveness of ERP.

No differences were reported for general anxiety (SMD = -0.78, 95% CI = -1.97 to 0.40) or depression (WMD = -4.14, 95% CI = -9.30 to 1.02). Therefore, it seems that ERP specifically targets obsessions and compulsions.

POSTTRAUMATIC STRESS DISORDER

A randomised controlled trial conducted by Bryant et al. (2008) compared two behavioural treatments, both with each other and combined. Sixty-six patients with PTSD received either imaginal exposure alone, in vivo exposure alone, or imaginal and in vivo exposure combined.

All three treatments significantly reduced symptoms of PTSD at post-treatment and 6-month follow-up. However, as can be seen in Figure 33.6, there were no differences between the three exposure treatments, as evidenced by the very small between-group effect sizes (post-treatment: imaginal v. in vivo ES = 0.03, 95% CI = -0.48 to 0.54; imaginal v. imaginal + in vivo ES = 0.01, 95% CI = -0.48 to 0.51; 6-month follow-up: imaginal v. in vivo ES = 0.02, 95% CI = -0.49 to 0.53; imaginal v. imaginal + in vivo ES = 0.10, 95% CI = -0.40 to 0.60).

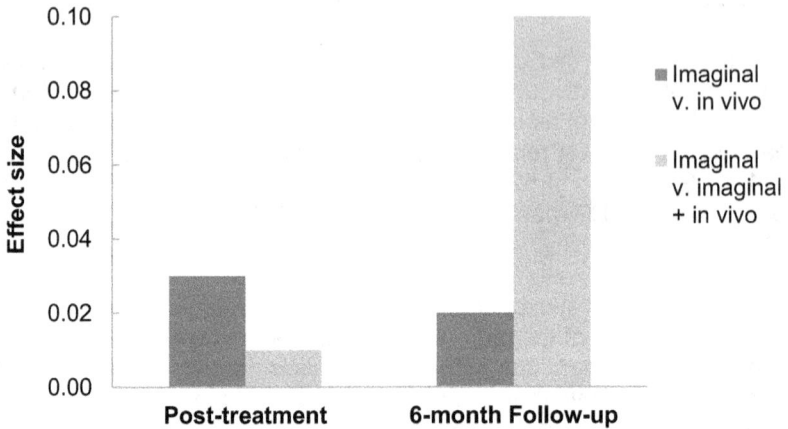

Figure 33.4 Effect sizes for imaginal exposure v. in vivo exposure v. imaginal + in vivo exposure on PTSD symptoms. Data adapted from Bryant et al. (2008).

Furthermore, no differences existed between the groups in the percentage of participants achieving high end-state functioning (imaginal = 10%, in vivo = 18%, imaginal + in vivo = 16%) or clinically significant change (imaginal = 42%, in vivo = 29%, imaginal + in vivo = 42%, see Figure 33.5).

This suggests that these behavioural treatments are equally effective, and combining them does not enhance treatment outcome.

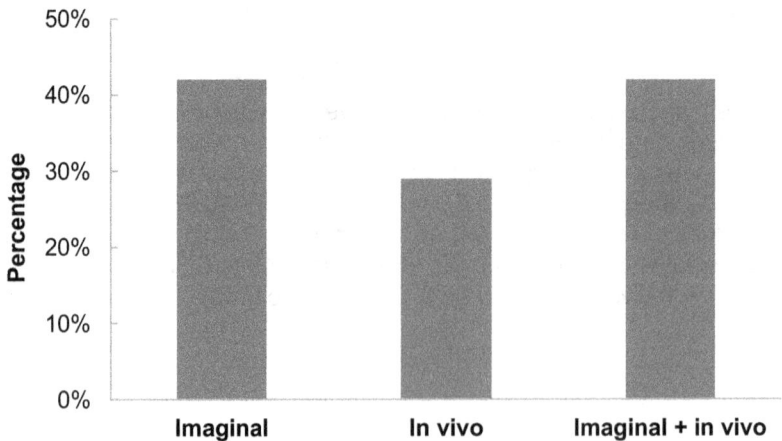

Figure 33.5 Percentage of participants achieving clinically significant change. Data adapted from Bryant et al. (2008).

SPECIFIC PHOBIA

There are five different behavioural treatments targeted toward the treatment of specific phobias. They are:

- systematic desensitisation
- in vivo exposure
- interoceptive exposure
- imaginal exposure
- applied muscle tension.

Systematic Desensitisation

In a review of specific phobias conducted by Choy, Fyer, & Lipsitz (2007), five studies compared systematic desensitisation (SD) against a placebo or waitlist control. These studies included two animal phobias, two height phobias and one flight phobia. Across all five studies, self-reported anxiety was lower for the systematic desensitisation group than controls. However, for measures of avoidance, one animal study found no effect on avoidance, while the other found that eleven of twelve subjects in the systematic desensitisation group were able to touch, or hold a live snake at post-treatment, in comparison with one of the twelve control subjects (Figure 33.6). In the flight phobia study, most patients in both the treatment and control group were able to complete a test flight. Other studies did not assess avoidance.

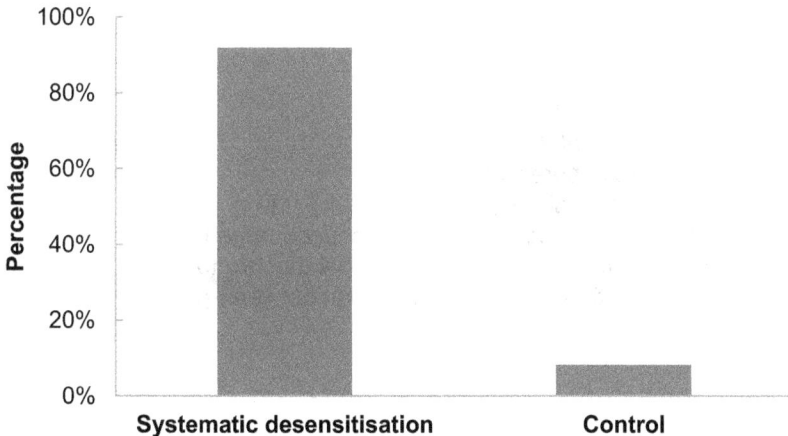

Figure 33.6   Percentage of snake phobics able to handle a snake at post-treatment across systematic desensitisation (SD) and control groups. Data adapted from Choy et al. (2007).

Four long-term follow-up studies found that initial treatment gains were maintained at 6-months to 3.5 years.

In Vivo Exposure

Of eight studies comparing in vivo exposure with a placebo or waitlist control group for phobias involving animals, height, driving, flying or claustrophobia, in vivo exposure consistently resulted in reduced subjective anxiety and avoidance. One animal phobia study found that 92% of patients treated with in vivo exposure were able to handle their feared animal after treatment, compared with 0% in the control group.

Of sixteen studies that examined long-term treatment effects, most reported that treatment gains from in vivo exposure were maintained or improved further over time. However, less favourable outcomes were reported for flight and blood phobics. Relative to post-treatment improvement rates, fewer patients were considered clinically significantly improved at 1-year follow-up.

Interoceptive Exposure

Among patients with claustrophobia, the interoceptive exposure group resulted in greater improvement in physiological and cognitive symptoms of anxiety compared with the control group. It also performed equally well as in vivo exposure on reducing subjective, physiological and cognitive symptoms of anxiety.

Imaginal Exposure

A study by Rentz et al. (2003) on exposure treatments for dog phobia found imaginal exposure treatments were associated with large pre- to post-treatment effect sizes (ES = 0.76 to 1.41, M = 1.09). As can be seen in Figure 33.7, in vivo exposure also produced large treatment effects (ES = 1.55). There was a trend for in vivo exposure to produce stronger effects. However, there were no significant between-group differences.

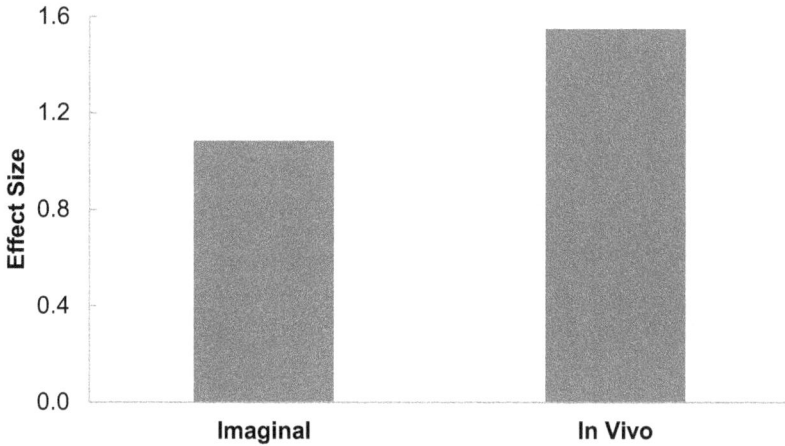

Figure 33.7 Pre- to post-treatment effect sizes across imaginal and in vivo exposure treatment for dog phobia. Data adapted from Rentz et al. (2003).

APPLIED MUSCLE TENSION

Perhaps the main exception to the superiority of in vivo exposure is for blood-injury phobia. As previously discussed, blood-injury phobia is a special case of phobia, as it has a unique two-phase physiological response comprising an initial sympathetic reaction with increased blood pressure and heart rate, followed rapidly by a parasympathetic response with a sudden drop in blood pressure and heart rate. This explains why people with a blood-injury phobia often faint at the sight of blood.

To treat this special kind of phobia, applied muscle tension is incorporated into the in vivo exposure to reverse the drop in blood pressure and prevent fainting. Rentz et al. (2003) reported 90% of patients with a blood-injury phobia improved with applied muscle tension, compared to only 40% receiving in vivo exposure alone (Figure 33.8).

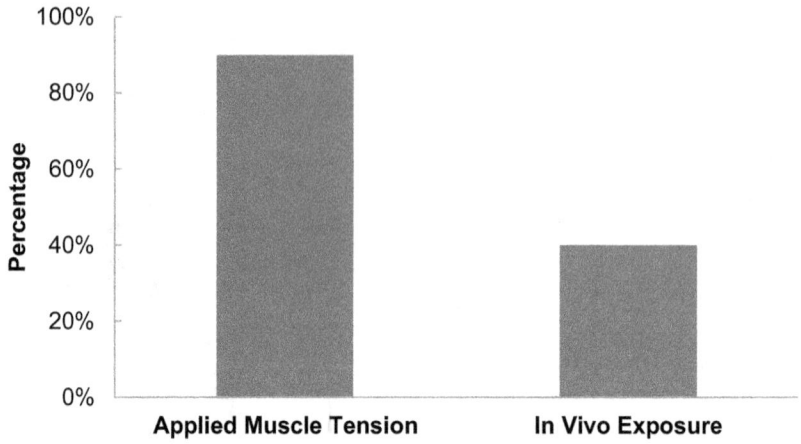

Figure 33.8 Percentage of improved patients with blood-injury phobia. Data adapted from Rentz et al. (2003).

PART VIII SUMMARY

Behaviour therapy and, more specifically, exposure-based strategies, have been found to be effective treatments across all the anxiety disorders.

The effectiveness of these treatment strategies relies heavily on the principles of learning theories, such as classical conditioning and operant conditioning.

Part VIII demonstrated how these well-known paradigms relate to the acquisition and maintenance of fear in a clinical setting. It also addressed the specific mechanisms involved in exposure therapy, namely, extinction, habituation and new learning.

Specific forms of exposure therapy, namely, imaginal and in vivo exposure, were discussed in relation to their use in various clinical presentations. The steps involved in designing and implementing imaginal and in vivo exposure were outlined.

Lastly, Part VIII addressed the empirical basis for behaviour therapy, demonstrating that all forms of exposure are superior to waitlist or placebo control groups, and typically yield moderate to large effect sizes for all anxiety disorders.

More specifically, research has found in vivo exposure to be more effective than imaginal exposure in disorders such as panic and agoraphobia. However, particularly with exposure and response prevention for OCD, attrition rates are often elevated due to the confronting and challenging nature of exposure therapy. Methodological limitation of this research will be discussed in Chapter 40.

PART IX   COGNITIVE THERAPY

Glen is a 50-year-old man presenting with social anxiety.

"The last time I went out socially was about a month ago. It was awful. I went out to a bar with a friend and a couple of his friends, but it was terrible. I had a few drinks before we went to calm me down a little bit, but when we got there I was worried about what I was going to say, so I stuck pretty close to my friend. I thought that would be a little bit easier. A few times I pulled out my mobile phone and made out that I was making a call or answering the phone, so I could leave the situation."

Glen hints at the reason he is anxious in social situations, saying that: "I was worried about what I was going to say."

However, this thought is vague; he has not identified a clear, threat-based thought. He might be concerned that he would say something boring, leading others to think he was a boring person and, therefore, reject him. He might worry about saying something incorrect, leading others to think he was stupid. He might have nothing to say at all, leading others to think he was weird or that there was something wrong with him. He might worry about unknowingly saying something insensitive and, therefore, offending one of the people there. Or he might even suffer from Tourette's disorder and be concerned about suddenly swearing and embarrassing himself. Identifying the specific threat that Glen perceives in social situations is essential in cognitive therapy.

Cognitive therapy is based on the premise that our thoughts about situations affect our emotions. In cognitive therapy, the clinician aims to change a person's emotions by changing their thoughts. But before thoughts can be changed, they must first be identified.

Some people are more cognitively minded than others. It is not uncommon in therapy for people to say they simply do not have any thoughts, they just feel anxious, or that the anxiety comes on so quickly that there is no time for thoughts. However, according to the cognitive model, there is *always* a thought driving a person's emotion.

In cognitive therapy, the clinician aims to change a person's emotions by changing their thoughts.

One of the fundamental skills in cognitive therapy is helping patients *identify* their underlying thoughts. It is only then that the process of thought challenging (or cognitive restructuring) as a means of reducing anxiety, can begin.

Part IX will introduce the principles underlying cognitive therapy. Methods of identifying thoughts will be described, followed by a discussion of different thought challenging methods. The evidence base for cognitive therapy for the anxiety disorders will also be examined.

CHAPTER 34 COGNITIVE MODEL OF EMOTION

Ross Menzies

COGNITIVE MODEL OF EMOTION

It is important to understand the cognitive model of emotion, also known as the ABC model of emotion (Figure 34.1), in order to understand cognitive therapy or more broadly, cognitive-behavioural therapy (CBT), for anxiety disorders.

In the ABC model, A refers to the *Activating Event* (or situation), B refers to *Beliefs* (or thoughts) and C refers to the *Consequence* (or emotion).

When individuals present with anxiety states, they tend to believe that situations or events (A) are the driver of emotions. What has to be brought home to the individual with the anxiety disorder is that it is not the event itself but their thoughts or beliefs (B) about the event that are the real driver of emotion (C).

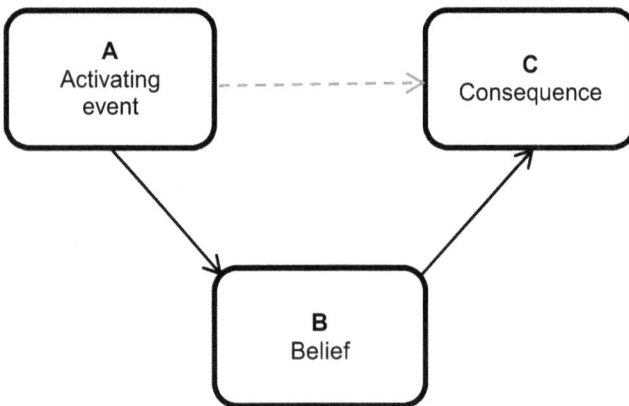

Figure 34.1 ABC model of emotion

EVENTS AND EMOTION: A SPURIOUS LINK

Classic events triggering anxiety for people with anxiety disorders include:

- You see a hair in your coffee.

- Your wrist inadvertently touches the toilet seat.
- You see a spider on the wall.
- Your friend fails to reply to your email.
- You read a report on rising interest rates.
- You notice a tightening in your chest.
- Your boss yells at you.

A person with a spider phobia might be having a very nice morning until they see a spider on a wall. Somebody with social evaluative anxiety, or social anxiety disorder, might be doing fine until they notice their friend hasn't replied to their email. Or perhaps their boss has yelled at them. The patient with panic disorder notices a tightening in the chest and gets anxious. The person with generalised anxiety disorder reads a report in the paper on rising interest rates and gets anxious.

In each of these cases, the individual might point to the activating event as the cause of their emotion, often saying, "I was fine until that happened". The first task in cognitive therapy is to undermine this spurious link between events and emotion.

COGNITION AS THE REAL DRIVER OF EMOTION

The following is an example of how to get the anxious person into the frame of mind to identify thoughts as the real driver of emotion.

A socially anxious woman reported that she became anxious after her boss yelled at her over some typing errors. She claimed, "It was the boss yelling that made me anxious. I was fine until the boss began to yell."

But it is fairly easy to demonstrate to her that it cannot possibly be the boss yelling that drove her anxiety because she admits that, on some other occasions when he yells at her, she is more angry or sad than anxious, and she certainly admits that many other people would be more angry or sad than anxious in such a situation.

So if the boss yelling could be followed by anxiety or anger or sadness, it cannot be the cause of these emotions; it cannot simultaneously cause three very different emotional responses. Something else must be mediating the relationship between the boss yelling and the emotional consequence. And that is where cognition, or thinking, comes in.

When asked, "What thoughts did you have about your boss yelling at you?", she answered, "He might sack me." Hence, this threat-based thought was driving the anxious emotion.

Different emotions will be driven by different thoughts. One might get angry in this situation because of a thought like, "He shouldn't yell at me", and individuals with a tendency toward sadness might have thoughts like, "I'm hopeless at everything I do."

In summary, these activating events, such as the boss yelling, the hair in the coffee, touching the toilet seat or a feeling of tightening in the chest, lead to the activation of thoughts or beliefs. It is the individual's thoughts that drive the emotional consequence, not the event per se. The patient needs to be on board with the cognitive model of emotion in order to engage with cognitive therapy.

NEGATIVE THOUGHTS THAT DRIVE ANXIETY

There have been nearly 100 years of laboratory research into the drivers of anxiety, beginning with the early work of Ivan Pavlov, who first identified classical conditioning, the early work in the 1920s of John Watson and Rosalie Rayner with Little Albert and very important work by Joseph Wolpe, Stanley Rachman and others in the 1950s and 1960s. A hundred years of research has made it very clear that the sorts of cognitions that drive anxiety disorders are *threat* or *danger* thoughts.

In the last 20 years, it has become increasingly clear that, in human fear conditioning in the laboratory, fear arises when humans perceive threat or danger. So, it is threat thoughts, or danger thoughts, that drive anxiety states.

Below are some of the threat thoughts regularly seen in anxiety disorders:

- "I'll get sick if I touch that door handle."
- "I'm having a heart attack."
- "No one will like me at the party."
- "I'm too high up… I might fall."
- "The house will burn down if I've left the iron on."
- "I might fail this exam."

These different thoughts are characteristic of different anxiety disorders. The individual who fears having a heart attack might have panic disorder. The person who does not want to touch the door handle might have obsessive-compulsive disorder, the person who worries about not being liked at the party might have social anxiety disorder and so on. Although the nature of the thought varies across anxiety disorders, they share a common theme: thoughts about threat or danger. Threat or danger thoughts are at the heart of anxiety disorders.

HOW DO WE IDENTIFY DANGER THOUGHTS

To identify danger thoughts, one could simply ask the anxious patient, "Why were you anxious? What threat were you perceiving?", but this method has a number of problems. Many individuals, particularly children and adolescents, say they are unaware of the danger thoughts. Even some adults will say they don't know why they were anxious. Many will also incorrectly attribute their anxiety to the wrong thought. That is, they will claim they are anxious for one reason, yet closer analysis of their behaviour suggests they were anxious for an entirely different one.

It should also be remembered that much of the relevant brain activity involved in threat appraisal occurs below consciousness, that is, out of awareness. To this respect, Freud was right in saying that many of the drivers of anxiety will be unconscious. So identifying danger thoughts is not as simple as just asking people, "Why were you anxious?" They may get it very wrong when asked that question.

There are a number of rules and procedures used in cognitive therapy to help clinicians identify unhelpful, danger thoughts.

Rule 1 – Thought Monitoring

Firstly, the individual may be asked to record the thoughts that arise in consciousness when they are anxious. Thought records or thought monitoring forms are commonly used in cognitive therapy (Table 34.1).

The individual is encouraged to write down the thoughts that occurred in situations that triggered anxiety. Thought monitoring in this way enhances the person's awareness of the thoughts that might be driving their anxiety.

Table 34.1 Thought record form

Date	Situation	Thought	Feeling
2/12	Waiting in line at the supermarket	"Oh no, my heart's racing!" "I'm feeling dizzy and lightheaded." "My legs feel weak and wobbly." "I feel like I'm going to faint!" "This will be so embarrassing!" "No one will help me!" "Who will look after my children?"	Anxious Panicky Worried

Rule 2 – Generate Hypotheses Based on Behaviour

Secondly, clinicians can generate hypotheses about what is driving anxiety based on the individual's behaviour, not just on the thinking that is arising in their mind.

Case study: Viktor

Viktor has an obsessive-compulsive disorder of the washer subtype. He bathes in disinfectant, uses antibacterial wipes, scrubs surfaces with antibacterial cleaning agents, but interestingly, if asked why he does these things, he claims he is not afraid of germs. He says he cleans because "People won't visit me if my house isn't perfect."

Viktor's behaviour suggests something about the cause of his anxiety other than the thoughts he offered. Viktor says it is just about having a clean house, because people won't visit him if the house is not clean. But, of course, no-one would be able to tell whether it was an antibacterial product or a non-antibacterial product that he used on the kitchen bench. So his behaviour suggests there is more going on than just wanting clean surfaces and a clean looking house. If Viktor only wanted a clean looking house, he would not need to pay for the expensive antibacterial products he is using. His behaviour suggests he is concerned about bacteria even if he does not hear these thoughts about germs and illness in his conscious mind. It suggests that beliefs about illness underlie his behaviours and his anxiety.

There is a lot of laboratory research into OCD, conducted by the team at the University of Sydney, which suggests that in OCD contamination cases (that is, in washers), fear of germs and illness is the driver of their anxiety. Viktor's case is one where the clinician should pursue danger thoughts about germs even when the individual says that is not what they are thinking.

Rule 3 – Downward Arrowing

A third technique to identify danger thoughts is to use *Downward Arrowing*. This is a technique that is used to peel away the layers of thinking, to find the deeper thinking that might be driving anxiety in the individual.

Case study: Mary

Mary, a 21-year-old university student was very anxious about her examinations. She said she felt anxious in the lead up to the exam because she was afraid that she would fail it.

In downward arrowing the clinician asks the question, "What would be so bad about that?" and then repeats this question again and again until the underlying thought driving the anxiety is uncovered. An example with Mary illustrates the technique, as shown in Figure 34.1.

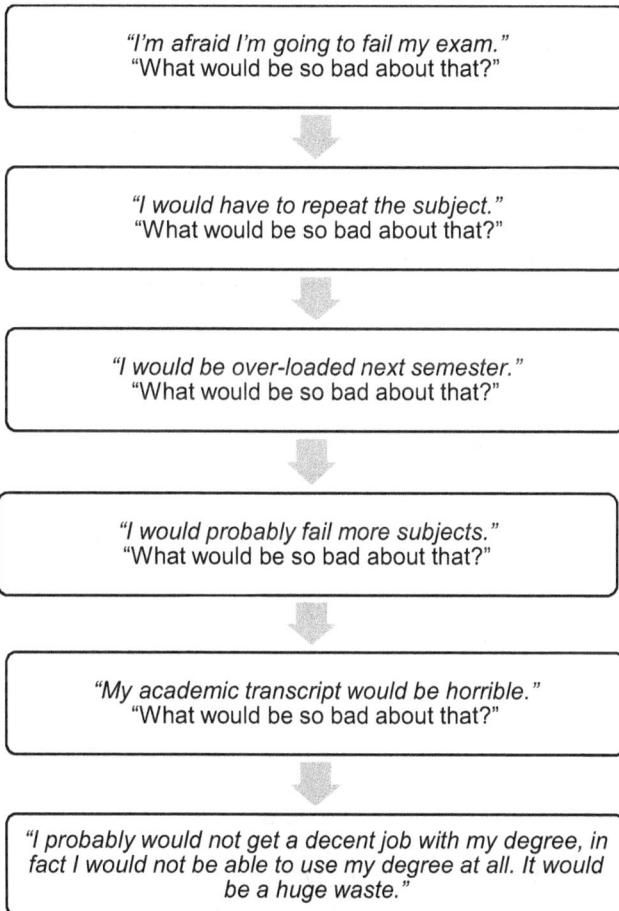

> *"I'm afraid I'm going to fail my exam."*
> "What would be so bad about that?"

> *"I would have to repeat the subject."*
> "What would be so bad about that?"

> *"I would be over-loaded next semester."*
> "What would be so bad about that?"

> *"I would probably fail more subjects."*
> "What would be so bad about that?"

> *"My academic transcript would be horrible."*
> "What would be so bad about that?"

> *"I probably would not get a decent job with my degree, in fact I would not be able to use my degree at all. It would be a huge waste."*

Figure 34.1 Example downward arrowing

By using downward arrowing, the clinician has been able to drill down to Mary's core fear. This is not a small fear about failing one exam but a much broader threat about never being able to use her degree.

CHAPTER 35   COGNITIVE RESTRUCTURING

Ross Menzies

COGNITIVE RESTRUCTURING

As discussed in Chapter 34, it is a person's threat or danger thoughts that lead to anxious feelings. It follows, therefore, that if you want to change the way you feel, you need to change the way you think. Cognitive restructuring uses a set of questions designed to undermine the person's belief in their negative, threat-based thought. It is useful to conceptualise these questions into a series of five tests, as shown in Table 35.1.

Table 35.1   Questions for cognitive restructuring

Test	Questions
Evidence Test	What is the evidence for and against the negative thought?
Utility Test	What is the thought doing for you? Is it helpful in any way?
Externalising Test	What would you tell a friend (to help them) if they had the same thought? What would your most relaxed, rational and supportive friend or family member say?
Control Test	Are you worrying about an outcome beyond your control? Is there any point to this type of worry?
Badness Test	If the thought is true, is it as bad as you think? What is the worst outcome?

EVIDENCE TEST

Individuals with anxiety disorders tend to get anxious about thoughts or beliefs for which, often, they have little or no evidence at all. One of the first questions a patient with an anxiety disorder will be asked is, "What is the evidence for or against the anxious thought?" This is known as the Evidence Test.

The patient with panic disorder believes they are having a heart attack, despite hundreds of previous panic attacks and no heart attacks, despite numerous investigations that have shown their heart function to be normal, despite numerous trips to Emergency only to be discharged as all clear shortly after. Often, the anxious individual has tremendous evidence that their thoughts are not accurate, but they are not using that evidence to undermine their thinking. The evidence test is a fundamental part of cognitive restructuring. Cognitive therapy essentially aims to produce evidence-based thinkers. If the person has strong evidence to support their thought, then their anxiety is justified and a problem solving approach to their situation is warranted. However, if they do not have evidence to support the thought, their thought needs to be challenged and replaced with an alternative, more realistic thought.

UTILITY TEST

The second test, the Utility Test, involves questioning the client about what the thought is doing for them, whether it is useful or helpful in any way. These are very important questions. Sometimes, an individual will have evidence for a thought, but the thought may lack utility such that it's simply not useful to think it. For example, a socially anxious individual might think, "I might feel awkward at the party tonight." Perhaps they do not know anyone going to the party, and they have felt awkward on previous occasions like this. So they might say they have some evidence that they may feel awkward. However, does this thought have utility? Does it help them? What is the consequence of ruminating about this, and going over and over the various scenarios in which they could feel awkward? It will drive anxiety and increase avoidance. The thought may prevent them from going to the party, thus reducing opportunities to broaden their social network. The thought will confine them, stop them from enjoying their life, and keep them imprisoned in their anxiety. So anxious thoughts often lack utility, even when there is a sprinkling of truth in them. They are not helpful.

EXTERNALISING TEST

The third test, the Externalising Test, involves asking, "What would you tell a friend if they had the same thought?" This is a very useful question as anxious people are often very good at knowing how they would advise someone else. They know what other individuals should be thinking, but they are not applying that thinking to themselves. So the socially anxious individual might very quickly respond, "Well, who cares if you feel awkward, you've got to get out there, you've got to confront life, you've got to be open to new experiences. How else are you going to meet people? How else are you going to move your life forward?" They might be very good at generating these sorts of sentences if it is for someone else. So, externalising the fear to think about other people can be very useful.

> Anxious people are often very good at knowing how they would advise someone else.

An interesting probe question frequently used in cognitive restructuring is, "What would your most relaxed, rational and supportive friend or family member say?" If thoughts drive emotion and threat thoughts drive anxiety, it follows that the very relaxed, rational friend must have very rational, evidence-based thinking. They do not jump to negative or threat based conclusions. In cognitive therapy, it is useful to ask individuals to yoke their mind to a particularly relaxed friend or family member, and ask themselves what would that person say about this situation. What would the friend say that would lead them to approach these situations so much more easily?

CONTROL TEST

The fourth test, the Control Test, is very important. It asks if the patient is worrying about an outcome beyond their control, and if there is any point to this type of worry. A person with generalised anxiety disorder worries about her husband's business trip to New Zealand, fearing he may be killed in an earthquake. This is a classic example of a situation where worry is pointless. The individual is worrying about something beyond her control. Worrying about earthquakes does not give her any control over them. She can ask him not to go, but this will cause a range of more realistic problems such as marital strain, workplace difficulties and financial loss. Worrying about issues beyond one's control is pointless, increases distress and is generally unhelpful.

Anxious individuals are often thinking about things beyond their control. Take the example discussed above of Mary, the university student who was anxious about her examination. When she comes out of the examination, she fears she may have failed, and indeed, she may have. But the examination is complete. She cannot change the results now. Learning to let go of things that one cannot control is an important part of cognitive restructuring and cognitive therapy.

BADNESS TEST

Finally, the fifth test is the Badness Test. This is where the individual is asked, "If the thought happens to be true, is it as bad as you think?" If you feel awkward at the party tonight, is it really as bad as you think? If you fail one examination, is it really as bad as you think? This shows people that they tend to catastrophise and think that certain incidents will be disasters when, in reality, the consequences are not that bad. The badness test is very useful when the person has evidence for their negative thought or when their thought did come true. In helping the individual examine the true badness or cost of the situation, it is useful to explore the realistic consequences, both in relation to other truly terrible events and over time. For example, an individual with social anxiety stuttered while speaking at a meeting at work and worried his manager and coworkers thought he was stupid. What were the realistic consequences of his stuttering? Did his coworkers turn against him and start ignoring him? Did they ridicule him for hours or days? Did he get fired? Did he have to cancel his holiday plans? None of these consequences are likely to occur. Although he may have felt embarrassed at the time, how will he feel about this issue in a few days, a week, next month, next year, in 5 years?

Challenging the badness of the event helps the person put it in perspective, which is a very powerful way of reducing anxiety. Obviously, this method is not used when the thought would realistically be bad, e.g., "I could have a heart attack," or, "My daughter could get kidnapped."

These five tests with the accompanying probe questions are very useful in cognitive restructuring to undermine the anxious individual's thinking and reduce their anxiety.

EXAMPLE OF COGNITIVE RESTRUCTURING

A woman with OCD had become very distressed after realising that her hand was on the handrail in a bus. She said that when the bus started moving, she briefly forgot her avoidance strategies and, almost without thinking, put her hand up and touched the rail. She had become overwhelmed with the belief that she was going to get a gastrointestinal bug and become ill. There was evidence from her behaviour that this fear was present. She was taking her temperature and was very distressed about the possibility of getting sick.

The danger thought was, "I forgot what I was doing and touched the handrail on the bus. I'm sure I'll get sick from a gastrointestinal bug." She was fretting and ruminating, and had become very distressed. She was using antibacterial gargles, had started regularly taking her temperature and was unnecessarily taking paracetamol. She was avoiding going out and was resting as much as she could.

This is how the five tests could be applied.

Evidence Test

Did she really have any evidence that she would get sick from a gastrointestinal bug because she touched that surface? No, of course she did not. In cognitive restructuring, she would be pushed to become an evidence-based thinker, to learn to identify that she is fearing something in the absence of evidence. She simply has no evidence that when someone touches a handrail they contract a gastrointestinal bug. In fact, the evidence is strongly against this belief. If the majority of people touching handrails got a gastrointestinal bug and became ill, there would be health announcements about the risk, people would wear gloves whenever they touched handrails and hardly anyone would travel by public transport. People travel on buses with great regularity and regularly touch public surfaces, rails and so on without getting ill, so the weight of evidence is strongly against her proposition. The thought fails on the evidence test.

Control Test

Is she worrying about something that is beyond her control? Absolutely! She has already touched the handrail. If she gets sick, she gets sick. If she does not, she does not. But to fret about whether somehow she has picked up a gastrointestinal bug and is about to become ill in the next 24 hours is rather pointless. She cannot control that outcome. The event has occurred. The thought fails on the control test.

Externalising Test

What would her most relaxed, rational friend say? They might say that they touch handrails all the time and don't get sick and so do thousands of other people. They'd tell me I was worrying about something that was unlikely to happen, and even if it did, the worst case scenario would be that I'd be sick at home for a couple of days and would have to take a bit of time off work. It's not like I'm going to die if the worst thing happens. The thought fails on the externalising test.

Utility Test

Is there any utility to her thought? Is her thought helpful or unhelpful? It can be argued that it is completely unhelpful. It does nothing for her except to drive anxiety and avoidance; it is shutting her behaviour down. It ruined her night the previous night and is causing an enormous amount of distress. It does nothing useful for her. The thought fails on the Utility Test.

Badness Test

How bad would it really be if she contracted a vomiting bug? Despite all her worst fears, she would perhaps vomit for 24 hours, perhaps get diarrhoea, and then recover. She acknowledged that she did not fear a rapid decline to death. She acknowledged that she was catastrophising how bad this outcome would be. The thought fails on the badness test.

This is a nice example for restructuring, because it is a thought that failed the five major tests from that set of probe questions: the evidence test, the control test, the externalising test, the utility test and the badness test. She had believed in a thought for no real reason, a thought that was doing nothing for her.

ONE MAJOR MESSAGE TO BRING HOME

Cognitive therapy is really trying to bring home one major message to individuals: stop believing in the thoughts that arise in your own consciousness just because they are yours. Humans, particularly anxious individuals, have a tendency to believe in their own consciousness; that is, to believe the thoughts that arise in their own mind just because they are theirs.

In anxious individuals, those thoughts, beliefs and attitudes have been letting them down, often for decades, leading to tremendous distress and agitation, often restricting their activities and even their general living, causing a lot of misery and depression. Yet all these states have been caused by the simple mistake of believing in consciousness arising; that is, the thoughts and appraisals that arise in the human mind. Cognitive therapy is designed to undermine this tendency.

CHAPTER 36   IDENTIFYING RUMINATION AND WORRY

Michelle Moulds

IDENTIFYING RUMINATION AND WORRY

Whether a patient is worrying about the future or ruminating about the past, a number of key features signal an individual is engaging in repetitive thought. The first is perseverative thinking, where the individual becomes stuck on one idea or train of thought and replays it over and over.

Secondly, these cycles of thought contain multiple "why" questions: "Why did this happen? Why don't I feel better yet? Why do bad things always happen to me?" Although these questions are driven by the goal of reaching an answer, their abstract and vague nature means that, rather than delivering a concrete answer, they merely serve to prompt more "why" questions.

Thirdly, repetitive thinking is characterised by its negative, self-deprecating tone. For example, thoughts such as, "This is ridiculous. Why can't I pull myself together and just get over it?" or, "I'm just weak, otherwise I would be able to snap out of it."

ASSESSMENT OF WORRY AND RUMINATION

For patients who engage in rumination or worry, thorough and detailed questioning about the nature and impact of their repetitive thinking is key in order to arrive at an informed case formulation.

Clinicians should obtain details about the content of rumination or worry, the contexts in which such thinking most likely occurs, as well as the frequency and duration of rumination or worry.

Factors that maintain repetitive thinking should also be explored. For example, patients may hold positive beliefs that worry is helpful and useful. Others may ruminate to avoid directly dealing with the problem. The consequences of repetitive thinking should also be examined – both positive and negative, as well as short and long-term. Asking a patient about the consequences they perceive can elicit valuable information about unhelpful beliefs that maintain these types of thought.

It is also useful to ask patients whether they have noticed if anything helps to reduce their worry or rumination (e.g., keeping active, exercising, socialising with friends), as this may highlight useful strategies that could be further developed when treatment commences. Similarly, it is useful to ask if the patient has identified situations or cues (e.g., other people, particular mood states) that make their rumination or worry more likely to occur.

Finally, clinicians should be vigilant for clues about the function of rumination. Patients may not be able to identify possible functions of rumination or worry at the outset, but avoidance is a common function. For example, a patient may ruminate about their relationship, rather than have a difficult conversation that could result in an argument with their partner. If a patient cannot see such links at the outset, it will be important to address the issue of the function of repetitive thinking as treatment progresses.

In some cases, patients may struggle to answer these questions. Perhaps they have never thought about what triggers their rumination. Some may say that they do not have any discrete triggers – "I just worry non-stop, all the time." The clinician should elicit as much information as is possible in the assessment session.

SELF-MONITORING AND SELF-REPORTING

Self-monitoring forms that record the day, time, place and duration of worry or rumination, as well as the severity of its impact on the individual's mood, also provide critical information that will help to develop a case formulation. Monitoring should be continued throughout treatment so that patterns and changes in thinking can be examined across sessions.

Finally, the administration of self-report questionnaires to measure rumination, worry or repetitive thinking, is also an important component of the assessment. Re-administration of these measures over the course of treatment will allow both the patient and the clinician to track changes over time. Some useful measures include the Ruminative Response Scale (Treynor, Gonzalez, & Nolen-Hoeksema, 2003), the Penn State Worry Questionnaire (Meyer et al., 1990) and the Repetitive Thinking Questionnaire (McEvoy, Mahoney, & Moulds, 2010).

COMMON EXAMPLES OF REPETITIVE THINKING

Following are some common examples of repetitive thinking that are typical of anxious patients.

- "The accident was all my fault. Why didn't I leave 5 minutes earlier?"
- "Why did my boss ask to see me? What if I lose my job? How will I pay the rent?"
- "They're all laughing, I bet they're making fun of me. Why do I always say stupid things?"

Each of these examples includes "why" questions. They are abstract or vague, self-critical and catastrophic.

METACOGNITIVE BELIEFS

If rumination and worry cause distress and worsen an individual's psychological difficulties, then why do patients continue to engage in repetitive thinking?

One important factor that maintains repetitive thinking is believing that ruminating or worrying is beneficial in some way. Beliefs about thinking are called "metacognitive beliefs"; that is, cognitions about cognitions, or thoughts about thoughts. Adrian Wells' work has demonstrated the importance of these types of beliefs in keeping individuals stuck in cycles of depression and worry. These metacognitive beliefs can be both positive and negative.

Positive beliefs about rumination and worry reinforce the idea that these thinking styles are helpful. An example of a positive belief about the utility of replaying events from the past is, "Dwelling on my past mistakes helps me to understand where I went wrong." Another example is, "Worrying about things that might happen helps me to plan how to cope." Both of these examples illustrate the point that patients typically start out ruminating or worrying with good intentions, but the abstract nature of these thinking styles ultimately prevents them from reaching their goals. Specifically, vague or abstract thoughts do not help to formulate a concrete plan of action in response to a problem.

> Positive beliefs about rumination and worry reinforce the idea that these thinking styles are helpful.

Interestingly, negative metacognitive beliefs (often referred to as "worry about worry") are also problematic and similarly contribute to the persistence of repetitive thinking. An example of this type of belief is, "My worry is out of control." These beliefs further fuel repetitive thinking. While positive beliefs encourage an individual to keep thinking in this way, negative beliefs in turn prompt an individual to worry about the fact they are worrying. The outcome is paradoxical and aversive, that is, more worry.

TREATMENTS FOR RUMINATION

Treatments that directly target rumination have only relatively recently been developed and evaluated. Behavioural Activation is a treatment approach for depression that aims to increase activity by countering avoidant behaviours (such as rumination), in order to improve mood.

Another treatment, Mindfulness-Based Cognitive Therapy (MBCT), was developed with the aim of reducing rumination. MBCT was developed to teach patients who have recovered from depression strategies to interrupt the ruminative process, in order to reduce the likelihood of a depressive relapse.

Although treatment protocols that primarily address rumination for patients with anxiety disorders have not yet been trialled, a number of CBT protocols for anxiety disorders include components that target ruminative thinking. For example, treatments for social phobia developed by British experimental psychologist David M. Clark from Oxford University and his colleagues include a component in which patients are encouraged to identify anticipatory and post-event ruminative processing, and to examine the consequences of engaging in such thinking.

Similarly, the central component of evidence-based treatments for PTSD (i.e., imaginal reliving of the trauma memory) involves encouraging the patient to process their trauma memory by directly replaying the event moment by moment in imagination, while providing a direct, first person narrative of it. Importantly, this reliving process prevents patients from engaging in rumination. Ruminating along the following lines, "It's not fair, I'm a good person, why did this happen to me?" prevents emotional processing of the trauma and ultimately prolongs anxiety. In contrast, through reliving, a patient recalls the event in a concrete way, "I was scared, I thought I was going to die." Such direct recall is antithetical to rumination, and allows the trauma to be successfully processed.

Treatments that directly address rumination share a number of key features. The key focus of these treatment protocols is on the *process*, rather than the content, of thinking. That is, compared to more traditional cognitive therapy packages that teach patients to attend to and challenge the content of their unhelpful thoughts, these new approaches encourage patients to become aware of when they are engaging in the process of ruminating. By being aware of the process, patients can arrest the ruminative cycle before it takes hold, and employ alternative, more helpful strategies.

STRATEGIES TO REDUCE RUMINATION

Three key steps are involved in treatments for rumination.

Firstly, identifying the signs that they have started to ruminate (e.g., particular themes, asking unanswerable "why" questions).

Secondly, identifying their triggers for rumination, e.g., places, time, people, moods, physiological states. Anticipation of "high risk" rumination cues will help patients become aware of times and situations in which they will need to employ more adaptive responses. Implicit in these approaches is the notion that "thoughts are just thoughts". The goal, therefore, is to notice streams of ruminative thought, rather than to attend to and challenge their content.

Thirdly, exploring the function and consequences of rumination. In terms of the function, asking the patient what they would be doing if they were not engaging in rumination can be a useful way to explore the potentially avoidant function of rumination. The short- and long-term consequences of rumination should also be explored.

BEHAVIOURAL EXPERIMENTS

Another important step in these approaches is to elicit from the patient any metacognitive beliefs (positive and negative) that they possess about rumination. One powerful way to challenge such beliefs is to design behavioural experiments (see Chapter 38) to test their validity.

For example, a patient may hold the belief that, "Worrying helps me solve my problems." The clinician could encourage a patient to put this belief to the test by asking them to identify a problem and spend 5 minutes thinking about it in an abstract, vague way, such as, "What does this mean? Why did this situation arise? What if things get worse? It's hopeless, I can't do anything to change things." The patient could then be asked to write down any solutions for the problem that resulted from their worrying, and to rate their level of anxiety or mood, as well as their confidence in their capacity to solve the problem.

Next, the patient could be asked to think about the problem for another 5 minutes, but instead, focus on details such as the specific circumstances and steps they could put into place; that is, focus on "what" they could do versus "why" the problem has arisen. After that, the patient could again write down any solutions they developed, and re-rate their mood and problem-solving confidence.

The goal of this experiment is to show the patient the consequences of worrying about a problem in terms of the effect it has on their mood, their problem-solving confidence and ability to reach a solution.

TREATMENTS THAT TARGET WORRY

There are a number of CBT packages that have been developed to treat worry in patients with GAD.

Such treatments include standard CBT components such as cognitive challenging, which identify and challenge the content of worrisome thought, which is usually catastrophic.

Another CBT component is worry exposure. Similar to imaginal exposure discussed in Chapter 31, patients are guided to call to mind some of their key worries and vividly imagine the feared outcomes, replaying the scenario over and over. This can be done imaginally or the patient can write out their worry in elaborate detail and repeatedly re-read it. Although this treatment can be distressing for patients, it allows for emotional processing.

Teaching problem-solving skills is also a key component of CBT treatments for worry. Patients are taught to conceptualise their problem in a specific manner (rather than vague and catastrophic), brainstorm potential solutions, then systematically consider the advantages and disadvantages of each solution in order to select the most practical and effective.

Finally, CBT treatments for GAD also often include relaxation training, in order to reduce the arousal that is associated with worry.

RECENT DEVELOPMENTS

More recent treatments for GAD have drawn from the same principles as mentioned for rumination which focus on the process and function of worry, rather than on addressing its content. For example, Lizabeth Roemer and colleagues (Orsillo et al., 2011) developed an effective treatment for worry that included components such as mindfulness practice, strategies aimed to reduce experiential avoidance (i.e., avoidance of internal experiences and emotional states), and exercises that encouraged mindful engagement in valued actions (as opposed to engaging in worry during such activities).

Evidence that treatments employing a process or function approach to the treatment of worry in GAD serve further to highlight the overlap of rumination and worry, and speak to the value of a transdiagnostic approach that addresses common processes (such as repetitive thinking), that occur across a range of clinical disorders.

CHAPTER 37   THE EVIDENCE BASE FOR COGNITIVE THERAPY

Juliette Drobny

COGNITIVE THERAPY COMPONENTS

What is meant by cognitive therapy is not always clear cut. Although cognitive therapy typically involves altering an individual's unhelpful thoughts, the methods by which this is done vary greatly between disorders and studies alike.

Cognitive therapy may simply involve thought challenging, or cognitive restructuring, as described by in Chapter 35. Other methods incorporated in cognitive therapy involve the use of surveys or behavioural experiments, which involve collecting data to test out patients' threat-based thoughts. Some cognitive therapy packages include attention training, where individuals are trained in techniques to divert their attention away from their internal thoughts onto more external events or to simply let thoughts go, which, rather than challenging the thought, is in part designed to reduce the frequency and distress of anxiety provoking cognitions.

Cognitive therapy differs from cognitive behaviour therapy, mostly in the sense that behavioural components such as exposure therapy are not utilised.

As mentioned, some cognitive therapy packages involve behavioural experiments (see Chapter 38), which involve patients testing out their negative, threat-based thoughts, often in a real-life situation. For example, a patient with panic disorder who believes they will have a heart attack upon physical exertion may be asked to run up and down a flight of stairs for 2 minutes to test whether they do have a heart attack. A patient with OCD, who avoids using public toilets for fear of contracting a gastrointestinal bug, may be asked to use a public toilet to test whether or not they fall sick.

Unlike traditional exposure therapy, behavioural experiments are specifically designed to test patients' cognitions, and in research trials of cognitive therapy, repetition of behavioural experiments is usually not encouraged.

Bearing in mind that different studies incorporate different components of cognitive therapy, this chapter will review the evidence base for cognitive therapy across the anxiety disorders.

ABOUT THE EVIDENCE

As described in Chapter 33, the Cochrane Library was searched to obtain the highest quality independent evidence for examining the effectiveness of cognitive therapy for anxiety disorders. Where Cochrane reviews were not available, meta-analyses from the Centre of Reviews and Dissemination, or other meta-analyses, were examined. Where there were no meta-analyses, individual reports were identified that evaluated the effectiveness of cognitive therapy.

As a reminder, when interpreting effect sizes, 0.2 reflects a small effect, 0.5 reflects a medium effect and 0.8 and above represents a large effect. In short, the larger the number, the greater the effect size.

In the literature, an active treatment is often compared to a control group, such as a waitlist, a placebo or treatment as usual. A large between-group effect size indicates that the active treatment is more effective than the control group, while a small between-group effect size indicates little difference between the two groups.

PANIC DISORDER WITH AND WITHOUT AGORAPHOBIA

A meta-analysis by Sánchez-Meca et al. (2010) examined three studies comparing cognitive therapy for panic disorder with a waitlist or placebo control group. The cognitive therapy used in these studies centred around challenging catastrophic thoughts with logic, and actively discouraged participants from exposing themselves to situations or sensations known to induce panic. Behavioural experiments were not encouraged.

Interestingly, cognitive therapy without the addition of behavioural experiments was not very effective in reducing the symptoms of panic (SMD = 0.34, 95% CI = -0.25 to 0.93) or agoraphobia (SMD = -0.13, 95% CI = -0.97 to 0.71), achieving only relatively small effect sizes.

However, when cognitive therapy included behavioural experiments, effect sizes were much larger (Clark et al., 1999).

Clark and colleagues in 1999 compared cognitive therapy (which incorporated behavioural experiments to challenge patients' catastrophic panic cognitions) against a waitlist control. As Figure 37.1 shows, they found very large effects at post-treatment (ES = 2.9) which were maintained at 3-month (ES = 3.0) and 12-month follow-up (mean ES = 3.0).

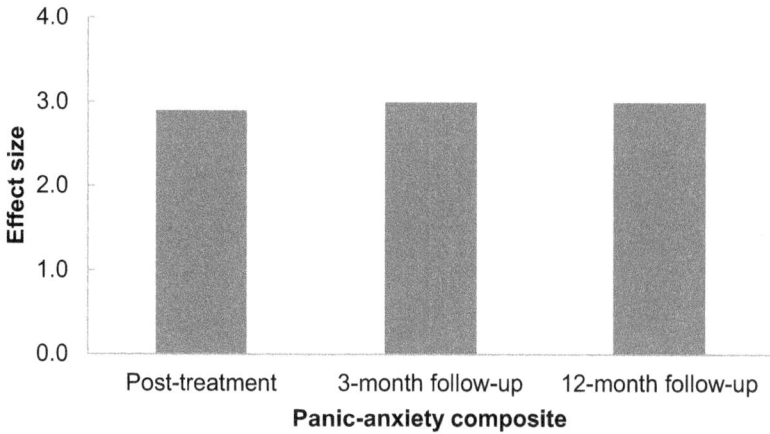

Figure 37.1   Effect sizes for cognitive therapy versus waitlist. Data adapted from Clark et al. (1999).

SOCIAL PHOBIA

A meta-analysis of cognitive-behavioural treatments for social phobia was conducted by Taylor (1996). He compared the effectiveness of cognitive therapy, exposure therapy, cognitive therapy with exposure therapy, placebo (pill and attention placebo) and waitlist (Figure 37.2). Effect sizes were calculated from pre- to post-treatment changes.

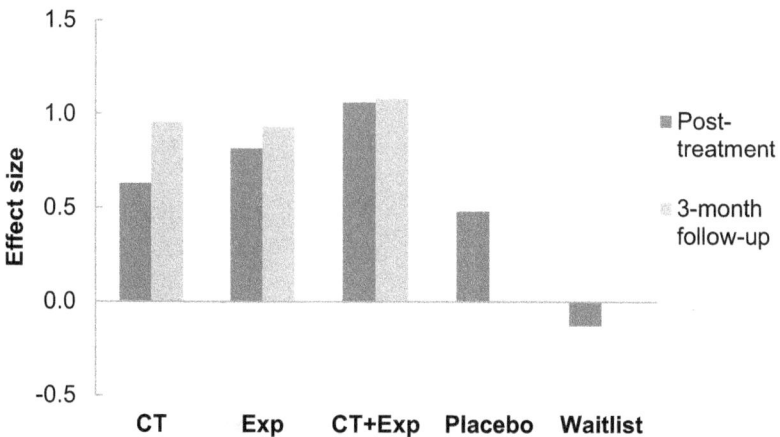

Figure 37.2   Pre to post-treatment/follow-up effect sizes across treatments. Data adapted from Taylor (1996).

At post-treatment, cognitive therapy was associated with moderate effect sizes (ES = 0.63, SD = 0.32). The exposure and cognitive therapy plus exposure treatments were associated with large effect sizes (ES = 0.82, SD = 0.25; ES = 1.06, SD = 0.34, respectively). All treatments were more effective than the waitlist ($p < .05$), however only the combined cognitive therapy plus exposure condition was more effective than placebo ($p < .05$). There were no other between group differences ($p > .05$).

At 3-month follow-up, effects of the cognitive and exposure therapies were maintained, and even tended to increase (cognitive therapy ES = 0.96, SD = 0.47; exposure ES = 0.93, SD = 0.25; cognitive therapy + exposure ES = 1.08, SD = 0.41).

Clark et al. (2006) conducted a randomised, controlled trial comparing cognitive therapy and exposure therapy against a waitlist control. In this study, cognitive therapy involved a range of cognitive techniques, including cognitive restructuring, attention training and confronting social situations as behavioural experiments to test negative predictions. The exposure condition involved repeated in vivo exposure to social situations, based on a habituation rationale. Repetition of behavioural experiments was not encouraged in the cognitive therapy condition.

As shown in Figure 37.3, both cognitive therapy and the exposure treatments were superior to waitlist for all social phobia measures, and resulted in large between group effect sizes (cognitive therapy ES = 2.63; exposure ES = 1.46). The post-treatment between group effect size for the comparison between cognitive therapy and exposure therapy was also large (ES = 1.17), indicating the superiority of cognitive therapy.

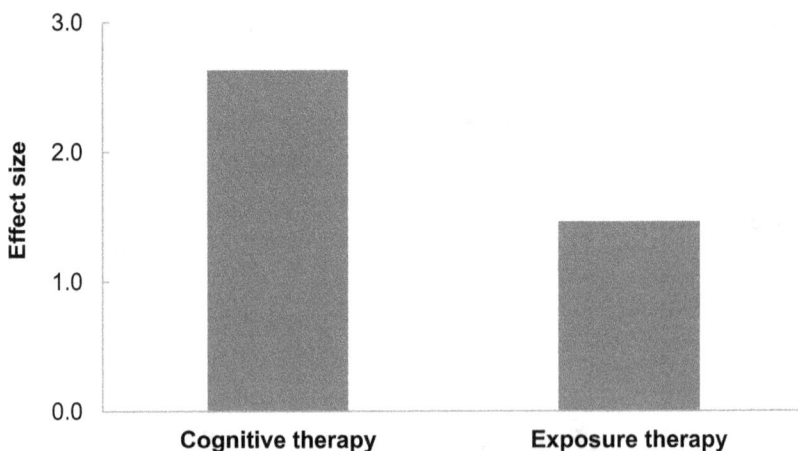

Figure 37.3   Effect size of treatment versus waitlist. Data adapted from Clark et al. (2006).

As Figure 37.4 shows, at post-treatment, 84% of cognitive therapy patients no longer met diagnostic criteria for social phobia, compared with 42% for exposure and 0% for the waitlist group. At 1-year follow-up, treatment gains were maintained, and differences between treatment outcomes persisted.

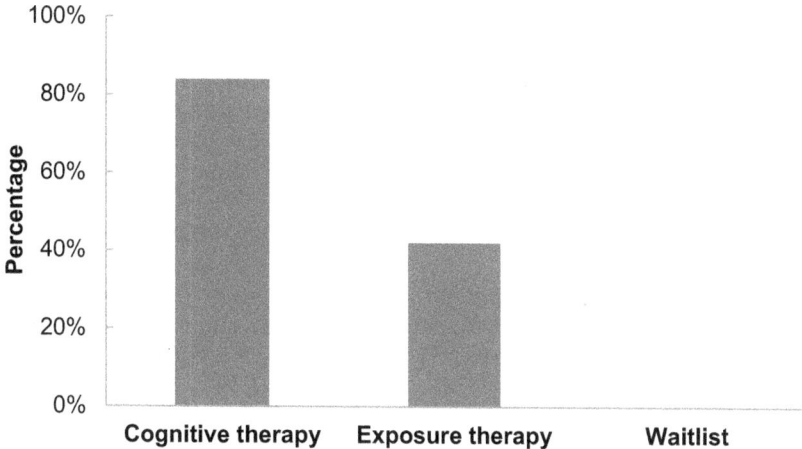

Figure 37.4   Percentage of patients no longer meeting diagnostic criteria for social phobia. Data adapted from Clark et al. (2006).

In addition, as shown in Figure 37.5, patients in the exposure therapy condition were significantly more likely to seek additional treatment outside the trial than patients receiving cognitive therapy (exposure = 44%, cognitive therapy = 6%, $p < .01$).

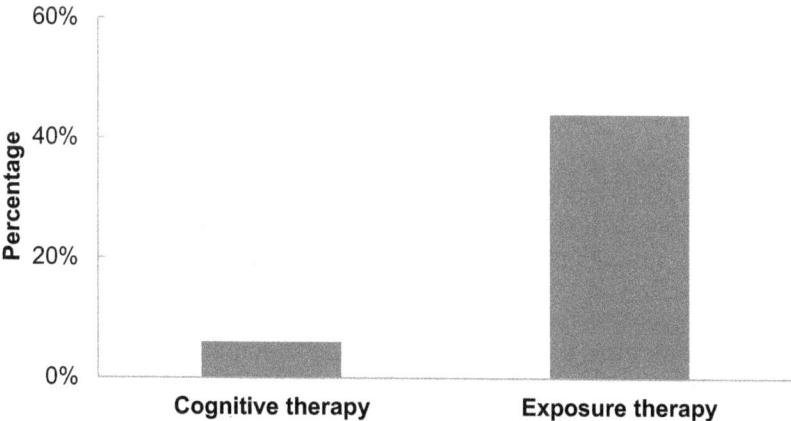

Figure 37.5   Percentage of patients receiving additional treatment. Data adapted from Clark et al. (2006).

GENERALISED ANXIETY DISORDER

For GAD, there were no meta-analyses examining cognitive therapy alone versus a no treatment control. However, a meta-analysis by Norton & Price (2007) reported the pre- to post-treatment effect sizes for a range of psychological treatments for GAD.

As can be seen from Figure 37.6, cognitive therapy alone (CT) produced large pre- to post-treatment effect sizes (ES = 2.06). What is also clear from the graph is that cognitive therapy on its own was as effective as combining it with relaxation (CT + RLX: ES = 2.08) or exposure therapy (CT + EXP: ES = 2.02) or both (CT + EXP + RLX: ES = 1.54), and was at least as effective as exposure plus relaxation (EXP + RLX: ES = 1.72). There were no significant differences in effect sizes between treatments.

The small effect sizes obtained for the post-treatment to follow-up indicate that treatment gains for cognitive therapy and other treatment combinations were maintained (CT: ES = 0.29; CT + EXP: ES = 0.17; EXP + RLX: ES = 0.11; CT + EXP + RLX: ES = 0.19).

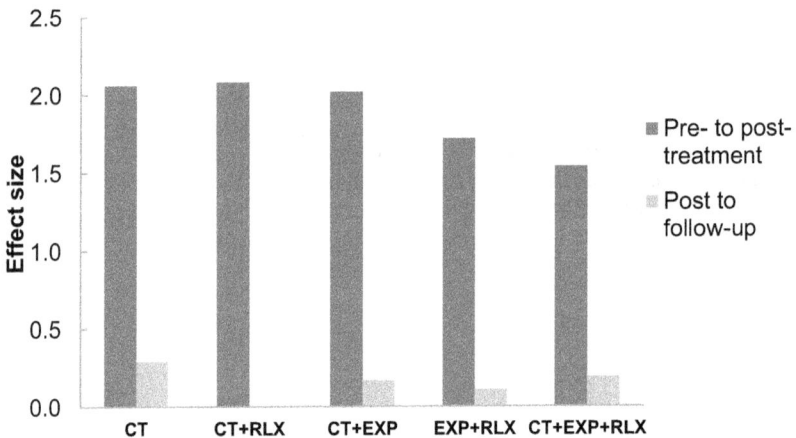

Figure 37.6   Effect sizes across treatments (Norton & Price, 2007)

A Cochrane review by Hunot et al. (2007) reviewed 5 studies comparing cognitive therapy with behavioural therapy for GAD.

Figure 37.7 indicates that at post-treatment, the cognitive therapy group showed greater clinical response than the behavioural therapy group, with 50% of those receiving cognitive therapy showing clinical response, in comparison with 31% of those treated with behaviour therapy (RR = 0.70, 95% CI = 0.56 to 0.87).

288

At 6-month follow-up, the differences in clinical response persisted between cognitive and behaviour therapy, with 58% of cognitive therapy patients achieving clinical response, in comparison to 29% of behaviour therapy patients (RR = 0.56, 95% CI = 0.40 to 0.79).

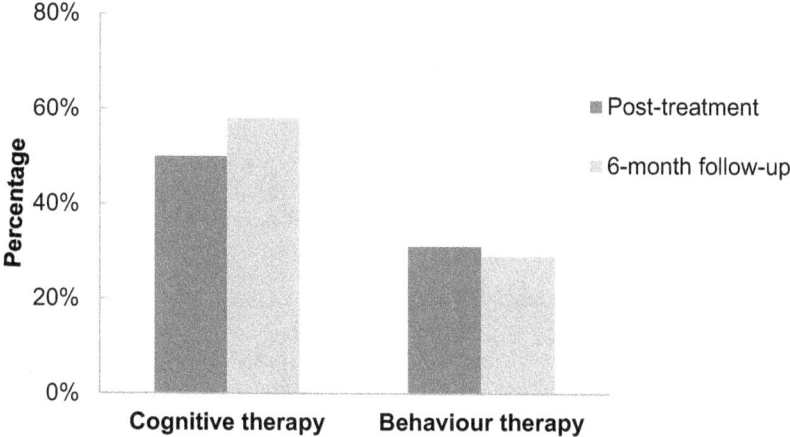

Figure 37.7   Percentage of patients achieving clinical response. Data adapted from Hunot et al. (2007).

On measures of general anxiety and worry (Figure 37.8), cognitive therapy was no more effective than behaviour therapy (Anxiety: SMD = -0.06, 95% CI = -0.40 to 0.30; Worry: SMD = 0.24, 95% CI = -0.66 to 1.14), although cognitive therapy was more effective in reducing comorbid depressive symptoms (SMD = -0.58, 95% CI = -1.01 to -1.15).

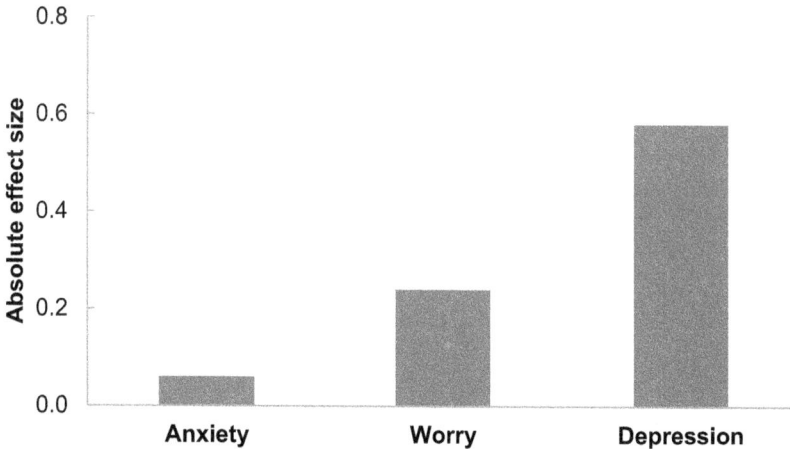

Figure 37.8   Between-group effect sizes for cognitive therapy versus behaviour therapy. Data adapted from Hunot et al. (2007).

OBSESSIVE-COMPULSIVE DISORDER

A Cochrane review by Gava et al. (2007) examined the effectiveness of cognitive therapy for OCD in comparison with treatment as usual, in two studies of 39 participants. They found cognitive therapy was more effective in reducing obsessive-compulsive symptoms (SMD = -1.21, 95% CI = -2.66 to 0.25). Interestingly, dropouts were also greater for the cognitive therapy group (OR = 2.07, 95% CI = 0.36 to 11.76).

Although there seemed to be a trend, no significant differences were reported for general anxiety (WMD = -7.70, 95% CI = -15.81 to 0.41) or depression (SMD = -1.77, 95% CI = -7.60 to 4.06). Therefore, cognitive therapy for OCD specifically targets obsessions and compulsions.

POSTTRAUMATIC STRESS DISORDER

The randomised controlled trial conducted by Bryant et al. (2008), previously discussed in Chapter 33, also investigated the effect of adding cognitive restructuring to imaginal and in vivo exposure, in comparison to imaginal exposure alone, and imaginal and in vivo exposure combined.

As noted previously, there was no difference in effect between imaginal exposure alone and imaginal exposure combined with in vivo exposure (ES = 0.01, 95% CI = -0.48 to 0.51). However, as shown in Figure 37.9, the addition of cognitive restructuring to the exposure package resulted in larger effect sizes compared with imaginal exposure alone, both at post-treatment (ES = 0.81, 95% CI = 0.27 to 1.34) and at 6-month follow-up (ES = 0.89, 95% CI = 0.35 to 1.42).

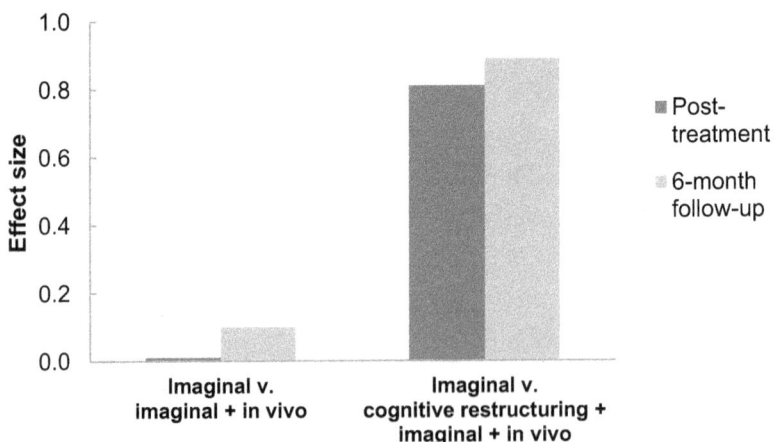

Figure 37.9 Between group effect sizes on PTSD symptoms. Data adapted from Bryant et al. (2008).

In intent to treat analyses, as shown in Figure 37.10, the cognitive restructuring plus exposure group had fewer participants with PTSD at post-treatment (CR + Imaginal + In Vivo = 35%, Imaginal Exposure = 63%, Imaginal + In Vivo Exposure = 65%) and 6-month follow-up (CR + Imaginal + In Vivo = 31%, Imaginal Exposure = 75%, Imaginal + In Vivo Exposure = 63%) than the other exposure groups (Bryant et al., 2008).

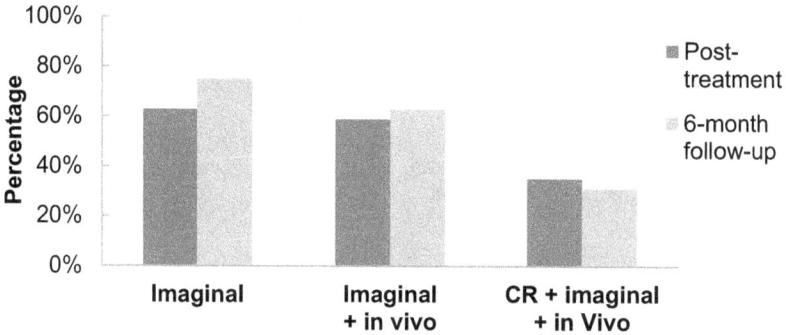

Figure 37.10   Percentage of participants with PTSD across treatment condition. Data adapted from Bryant et al. (2008).

SPECIFIC PHOBIA

Although no meta-analyses have been conducted evaluating cognitive therapy for specific phobia, six studies were reviewed by Choy, Fyer, & Lipsitz (2007). Two studies of claustrophobia found that cognitive therapy was more effective than the control condition in reducing subjective anxiety, physical symptoms and negative cognitions. Cognitive therapy also resulted in more patients achieving clinically significant change (Figure 37.11). There were no differences between cognitive therapy and in vivo exposure.

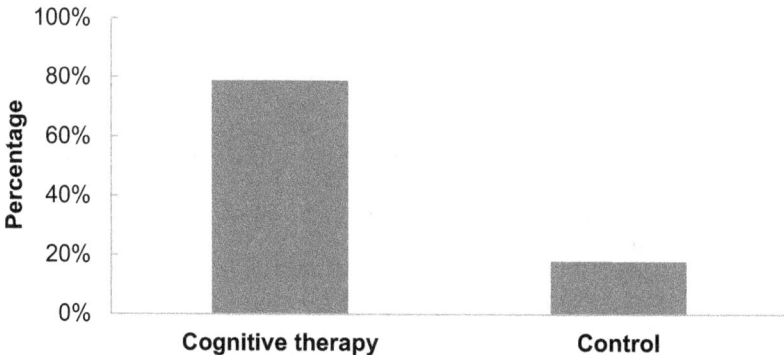

Figure 37.11   Percentage of claustrophobic patients achieving clinically significant improvement (Choy et al., 2007)

For flying phobia, the results were mixed. One study found cognitive therapy resulted in greater improvements for self-reported anxiety and physiological measures. However, another study reported that cognitive therapy was no better than a wait-list control on self-report measures.

For dental phobia, one study found that cognitive therapy led to greater reductions in subjective anxiety and negative cognitions surrounding dental treatment, compared to no treatment controls. Interestingly, another study found that cognitive therapy was as effective as nitrous oxide sedation in lowering self-reported dental anxiety.

Overall, the available evidence indicates that cognitive therapy is an effective treatment for specific phobia, and potentially a viable alternative to in vivo exposure.

MINDFULNESS- BASED THERAPY

Mindfulness-based interventions have gained popularity in recent years for helping people reduce worry and rumination. A meta-analysis by Hofmann et al. (2010) reviewed seven studies and examined the efficacy of mindfulness-based therapies for anxiety disorders.

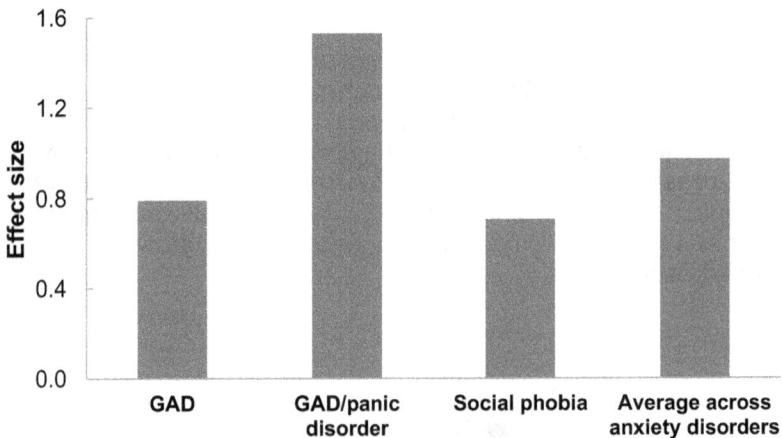

Figure 37.12   Pre- to post-treatment effect size of mindfulness based therapies across anxiety disorders (Hofmann et al., 2010)

As shown in Figure 37.12, across the different anxiety disorders, mindfulness-based therapies were associated with moderate to large pre- to post- effect sizes (GAD ES = 0.79, GAD/panic disorder ES = 1.53, social phobia ES = 0.71). The average effect size across anxiety disorders was large (ES = 0.97, 95% CI = 0.73 to 1.22).

MINDFULNESS VERSUS CBT FOR SOCIAL PHOBIA

Koszycki et al. (2007) compared mindfulness-based therapy (MBT) to cognitive-behavioural group therapy (CBGT) for social phobia.

As can be seen in Figure 37.13, patients in both groups improved. However, the CBT group showed greater pre- to post-treatment effect sizes than the mindfulness-based treatment group on clinician (fear: CBGT ES = 2.00, MBT ES = 1.48; avoidance: CBGT ES = 2.06, MBT ES = 1.40) and patient-rated (interpersonal sensitivity: CBGT ES = 1.27, MBT ES = 0.63; social interaction: CBGT ES = 1.67, MBT ES = 0.83) measures of social anxiety. Response rates (89% v. 45%) and remission rates (44% v. 9%) were also higher for patients treated with CBT than those treated with mindfulness.

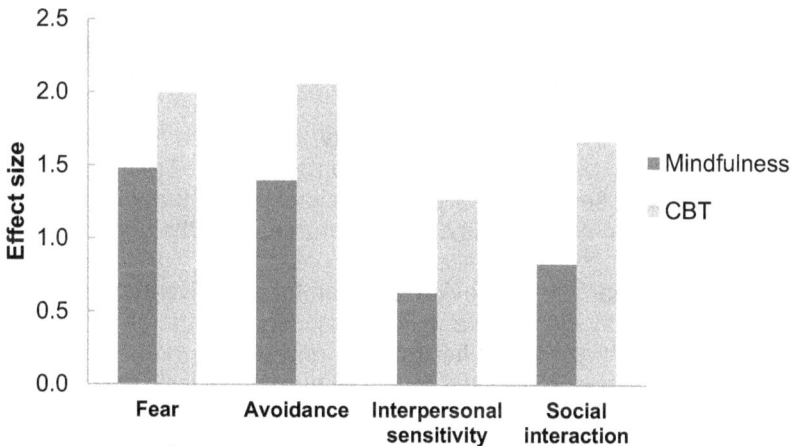

Figure 37.13   Comparison of within group effect sizes of mindfulness-based therapies and CBT for social phobia at post-treatment. Data adapted from Koszyckl et al. (2007).

Thus, although CBT remains the treatment of choice for social phobia, mindfulness-based treatments also appear to have some benefit.

PART IX SUMMARY

Based on the cognitive model of emotion, Part IX sought to build on the idea that thoughts are the drivers of emotion. Specific techniques such as thought monitoring, generating hypotheses about underlying thoughts and downward arrowing are used in therapy to elicit the thoughts that drive anxiety.

Having identified the problem thoughts that lead to negative emotions, it then becomes possible to challenge these thoughts using cognitive therapy. Challenging involves applying logical analysis to the thought, gathering evidence that either supports or negates it, questioning the usefulness and helpfulness of the thought and examining the realistic consequences. It also encourages the person not to believe in the thought simply because it arises from their own consciousness.

Part IX moved on to discuss how to identify, assess and manage repetitive thinking styles such as rumination and worry. Treatments for repetitive thinking seek to identify the unhelpful beliefs that maintain it and focus more on the process of thinking rather than the content.

Finally, Part IX examined the evidence base for cognitive therapy in the treatment of anxiety disorders and finds that cognitive therapy is an effective treatment across the full range of anxiety disorders. It is at least as effective as exposure therapy for social phobia, specific phobia and PTSD, with some suggestion it is superior for GAD. Caution is required in interpreting results of trials in the literature as there are limitations to the generalisabliity of these findings which will be discussed in detail in Chapter 40.

PART X   COGNITIVE-BEHAVIOURAL THERAPY

Paula is a 35-year-old woman with obsessions about harming others. Paula believes that if she stood behind someone on a train platform she would act on her obsession and push them in front of a train.

Her therapist set a behavioural experiment for homework where she had the task of standing behind someone on a train platform to find out if she was correct.

"I stood behind this poor guy and I was really anxious. I had the awful thought to push him in front of the train; it was like an urge, but not an urge. Then the train came and we got on it. I realised that it was just an awful thought and nothing else, and that maybe all those times when I have hung back and held onto things were just stupid. So now I recognise that it was just a thought, I know I won't do it. I've got proof that I won't act on the urge."

Cognitive behaviour therapy or CBT, as the name suggests, uses a combination of behavioural techniques (such as exposure therapy) and cognitive methods (such as thought challenging), to help identify and modify a person's unhelpful thoughts and behaviours that are contributing to, and maintaining, their negative emotional state.

Regardless of whether clinicians identify themselves more strongly as being a behavioural therapist or a cognitive therapist, most will use aspects of both cognitive and behaviour therapy in their clinical practice.

A prime example of the interplay between cognitive and behavioural techniques lies in the use of behavioural experiments. Behavioural experiments are often hotly debated. Cognitive therapists deem them a cognitive technique, as they are effective in reducing negative emotional states through changing a person's thoughts. However, behaviour therapists maintain with equal fervour that behavioural experiments are a behavioural technique, due to their reliance on the use of exposure. It is probably most useful to call them a cognitive-behavioural technique as this incorporates elements of both cognitive and behaviour therapy.

Part X will outline behavioural experiments and move on to illustrate CBT in clinical practice using a series of case studies. It will also discuss the evidence base for CBT for anxiety disorders and describe a new method of CBT delivery, namely web-based interventions.

CHAPTER 38   BEHAVIOURAL EXPERIMENTS

Rocco Crino

BEHAVIOURAL EXPERIMENTS

Although behavioural experiments incorporate elements of exposure, they are designed to test and challenge specific negative beliefs. Therefore, they are better described as a cognitive-behavioural, rather than a behavioural intervention.

Behavioural experiments are described as planned experiential activities that are based on experimentation or observation. The design of specific behavioural experiments is based on the cognitive-behavioural formulation of the individual's problem.

The purpose is to obtain new information by testing the validity of the person's belief system, constructing or testing more adaptive beliefs and contributing to the development and verification of the formulation of the individual's problem.

Behavioural experiments are a very powerful way of challenging patients' thoughts and are therefore a very effective way of reducing their anxiety and avoidance behaviours. A prime advantage of behavioural experiments is that they can be specifically tailored to the patients' unique cognitions and they get to see the results with their own eyes. In this way, the conclusions patients draw are based on their own experience. The evidence collected is real and therefore a very convincing way to change their thoughts.

ACTIVE VERSUS OBSERVATIONAL EXPERIMENTS

Although there are a variety of behavioural experiments, active experiments and observational experiments are the most commonly used.

> The purpose of behavioural experiments is to obtain new information by testing the validity of the person's belief system.

In active experiments, once a cognition or belief has been identified, the person is asked to act or behave in a way that is different from how they would usually behave. They are then asked to record what actually happens and reflect on the implications for their thinking or underlying beliefs.

Observational experiments, as the name suggests, involve the individual gathering data to test their cognition or belief. This can be done through direct observation or even conducting a survey.

For example, an individual with panic disorder may believe they must sit down if they feel dizzy or light headed, or else they will collapse. As part of an active behavioural experiment, they may be asked to test that belief by not sitting down when feeling dizzy or lightheaded in anxiety provoking situations, and record the outcome.

In another example, an individual with obsessive-compulsive disorder who fears contamination may believe they must wash their hands before eating if they have touched a public surface. As part of an observational experiment, they may be asked to test that belief by observing how many people touch handrails when leaving work for lunch, and then eat lunch without washing their hands.

In both cases, the outcome is used to challenge the person's specific underlying beliefs.

CONDUCTING A BEHAVIOURAL EXPERIMENT

There are a number of steps to take in planning and conducting a behavioural experiment.

Step 1

Clearly define the target cognition or belief.

Step 2

Plan specifically what is going to be done.

Step 3

Predict what will eventuate as a result of engaging in the experiment and rate the degree of belief in that prediction.

Step 4

Generate an alternative, rational prediction or hypothesis, and again rate the degree of belief.

Step 5

Implement the behavioural experiment and record the results in terms of the specific predictions.

Step 6

Reflect on what was learned from the experiment. Did the results support or disconfirm the individual's beliefs? Post-experimentally, the degree of belief in the initial prediction should be re-rated.

CASE STUDY: LILY

Lily is a 32-year-old woman who presented with a 10-year history of panic attacks. One of her primary concerns was a fear of losing bladder control when outside the home and when feeling anxious and panicky.

As a result, Lily engaged in a variety of safety behaviours, such as going to the toilet repeatedly before leaving home, wearing sanitary pads and making sure she knew where the toilets were located wherever she was going.

The problem was defined as avoidance of situations outside the home for fear of losing bladder control.

The target cognition was identified as: "If I am anxious or panicky then I will wet myself and I will be ridiculed."

The behavioural experiment was designed collaboratively, and involved the patient going out with a friend to the shopping centre. This setting would provoke moderate anxiety levels, and she was to remain there until the anxiety subsided. She was also instructed not to go to the toilet beforehand and not to wear any sanitary pads, both of which were safety behaviours.

Lily's prediction was that, "I will be anxious and wet myself", and she rated this as 80% likely to happen.

The alternative hypothesis was that, "My anxiety results in me focusing on my bladder and it feels full because of my attention", and she rated this belief at 30%.

The results of the experiment were that she stayed in the shopping centre for 90 minutes. She reported being anxious for some of the time, but the anxiety lessened occasionally, and got worse when she thought about it. She did not lose control of her bladder.

In noting what she had learnt from the experiment, she stated: "The anxiety makes me feel like I have got to go, but I can hold on. The less I focus on it, the less I feel I have to go."

The post-experiment rating of her original belief that she would be anxious and wet herself had reduced from 80% to 50%.

However, this single behavioural experiment clearly did not entirely change her original belief, and requires repetition in a variety of contexts, similar to standard in vivo exposure.

CHAPTER 39   CLINICAL EXAMPLES OF PSYCHOLOGICAL TREATMENTS

Rocco Crino

IMAGINAL EXPOSURE IN PTSD

Case study: Frank

Frank was a 30-year-old married father of one, who was referred for treatment for PTSD 8 months after being the sole bystander in an armed hold-up in his local suburban post office.

"Two men armed with pistols and wearing balaclavas burst into the post office yelling for everyone to stand still. One gunman pointed a gun at the postal officer and demanded the bag be filled with money. The other gunman held a gun against my eye while having his other arm around my throat, shouting and swearing that he would shoot me if I made a move. The postal officer was clearly shocked and hesitated a bit, and this seemed to enrage the gunman holding the gun to my head. He hit me with his pistol on the side of my face and head, and yelled that he would shoot me.

"I really believed that I was going to be shot in the head and I was very scared. I thought I would never see my wife and child again.

"After the bag containing money was handed over, I was thrown violently to the ground and told not to move or I would be shot. Then the robbers left. The whole event took place over a matter of minutes.

"The police and ambulance were called, and I gave a brief statement of events before being taken to hospital for my bruised face and head."

Although he returned to work and tried to live life normally, Frank continued to experience nightmares of the event, including intrusive images of the gun pointed at his eye and he avoided talking about the incident. His wife was concerned about his emotional distance from her and their son, yet he was easily moved to tears by seemingly innocuous events.

He found that being hugged around the neck, raised male voices, news reports of robberies, violent movies and police dramas were triggers of his anxiety.

Individuals with posttraumatic stress disorder try to avoid the painful memories of the traumatic experience. So an understandable rationale is critical in having the person engage with their traumatic memories.

Exposure to memories of the traumatic event in PTSD enhances the emotional processing of memories of the event. Meanwhile, avoidance strategies serve to maintain the fear of the memories, nightmares and flashbacks.

Following a comprehensive assessment and the establishment of a collaborative relationship with Frank, and only after his understanding of the rationale for conducting exposure was ensured, a series of 90 minute sessions were booked. Frank was asked to imagine and describe the events that occurred in the post office from the beginning to the end when he felt safe. The session was audio-recorded. Although Frank was asked to close his eyes and visualise the scene he was describing, he preferred to describe the events with his eyes open due to his levels of anxiety.

During imaginal exposure, the therapist gently asked the patient for specific details as to what he experienced while the event was occurring.

Questions used in imaginal exposure in PTSD include:

- What can you see?
- What can you hear?
- What can you smell?
- What are you thinking?
- How are you feeling?
- What's happening in your body?

While describing the scene, the therapist probed gently at different points as to the sensory experiences, the sights, the sounds, the smells the patient was aware of, the cognitions, emotions, and physiological sensations.

> In PTSD, avoidance strategies maintain the fear of the memories, nightmares and flashbacks.

Subjective Unit of Distress Scale or SUDS ratings were taken by the therapist throughout Frank's rendition of the events. The recording was stopped when Frank was "safe". The recording of the session was replayed, with the therapist asking Frank for SUDS ratings at various time points during the recording. This procedure is repeated several times, with the therapist asking Frank to provide SUDS ratings during each trial. After a number of exposure trials, once Frank's SUDS ratings had reduced to 50% of what they initially were, he was asked to take the tape home and listen to it on a daily basis.

For homework, Frank was asked to imagine the event happening while listening to the tape, ensuring he was very emotionally connected with the experience. He was asked to make a note of the SUDS ratings at the same time points during the recording, as he did during the therapy session. If they were extreme, for instance 9 out of 10, he was told to take a moment to remind himself where he was, what he was doing and that he was safe. Frank was instructed to listen to the tape repeatedly until the SUDS ratings reduced by 50% in each self-directed exposure session.

At the completion of each self-directed exposure session, Frank was asked to write down any salient features that were not recalled in the first rendition. The recalled features were then incorporated into subsequently recorded exposure sessions with the therapist.

As exposure sessions continued, the emphasis of the exposure shifted to the more anxiety provoking elements of the scene, such as being hit with the pistol. The process continued until all details were incorporated in the exposure recording, and anxiety about the recalled event was significantly reduced.

Once agreed upon, in vivo exposure commenced with graded exposure to avoided situations such as the post office, being hugged from behind, watching police dramas and so on.

INTEROCEPTIVE EXPOSURE IN PANIC DISORDER

Case Study: Sandy

Sandy is a 23-year-old woman who was referred for treatment of panic attacks.

She reports that her first panic attack occurred while she was attending a weekly meeting at work 6 months earlier. She worked as a fashion designer, and in the months leading up to the first attack she had been under considerable pressure to meet deadlines at work, had been skipping meals and sleep, and relied on coffee and cigarettes to keep her going.

"*My first panic attack came on when I was presenting my designs at a staff meeting. My colleagues were really concerned and called an ambulance. I was examined by the paramedics who said that they didn't think I was having a heart attack, but they took me to hospital for further testing. I stayed in hospital for 24 hours while they did various tests, all of which came back negative. They told me that I'd had a panic attack, and that I should probably consider changing my lifestyle and talk to my GP.*"

Although terrified of the experience, and unconvinced that her health was okay, Sandy returned to work the following day. She experienced another attack, precipitating another hospital admission.

She was examined at the emergency department and informed that she had had another panic attack and that her physical signs were normal. Despite repeated reassurance from her GP and cardiologist, she remained concerned about her heart and the possibility of having a heart attack.

She continued experiencing regular panic attacks, and consequently started avoiding any form of exercise or caffeine. She also ceased having sex with her boyfriend, as she had experienced a panic attack while doing so. She was referred for CBT after consulting her GP.

Following a thorough assessment, the panic cycle was presented to Sandy (Figure 39.1). She was informed that the trigger to her panic was a catastrophic misinterpretation of her physical symptoms. In her case, her pounding heart, shortness of breath and dizziness were misinterpreted as a threat of an impending heart attack.

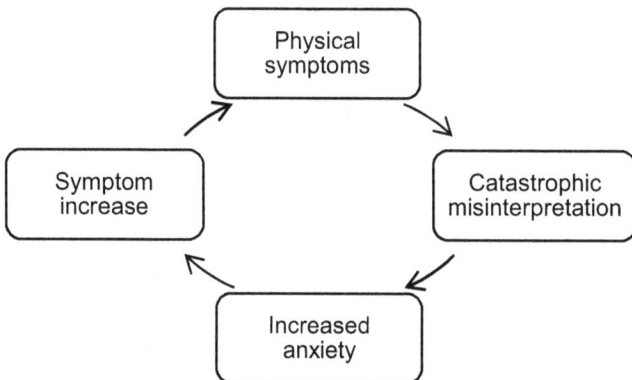

Figure 39.1 Sandy's panic cycle

This misinterpretation resulted in significantly increased anxiety, which worsened the physical symptoms she experienced, which were then further misinterpreted as something being terribly wrong, which in turn further exacerbated her anxiety and physical symptoms, culminating in a panic attack.

Various safety behaviours that Sandy engaged in (e.g., sitting down), and the avoidance of certain activities (e.g., exercise, sex), served to maintain her fear because, in her mind, they prevented the feared event, that is the heart attack, from occurring. Similarly, her avoidance behaviours also prevented disconfirmation of the catastrophic misinterpretation ("I'm having a heart attack") that was maintaining the panic cycle.

Treatment needed to focus on exposing her to the physical sensations that she feared, so they would no longer be catastrophically misinterpreted and the panic cycle could therefore be broken. Sandy reported the most troubling symptom was her pounding heart and this was the symptom on which she most wanted to work. To reduce her fear of this sensation, she was asked to run up and down a set of stairs for 1 minute without stopping. This not only exposed her to the physical sensations of a pounding heart and exposed her to exercise, a previously avoided activity, but it also allowed her to test out the likelihood of having a heart attack. Therefore, this was informally operating as a behavioural experiment.

SUDS ratings were taken at the start and at the completion of the task, and again after the physical sensation had diminished. Sandy reported her SUDS as 9 initially, 8 at completion, then 6 after the sensation settled. Consequently, when she was ready, she was asked to repeat the exercise. On second and third in-session repetitions, she reported her SUDS as 8, 7 and 5, and 6, 5, and 3, respectively. After each trial she was questioned as to whether she had had a heart attack and what she had learned about her body. This task was set as homework to be completed daily.

To address her residual avoidance behaviours, she was gradually re-exposed to caffeine and caffeinated drinks, returned to the gym and returned to normal sexual activities.

EXPOSURE PLUS RESPONSE PREVENTION IN OCD

Case Study: Jason

Jason is a 28-year-old single male who presents with a 10-year history of obsessive-compulsive disorder.

"I was mainly concerned about accidentally harming others, so I had to repeatedly check that the doors and windows were locked and that the lights and electrical appliances were off to make sure nothing bad would happen.

"I often pulled electrical plugs out of the power points for smaller items like the toaster, and I'd stand in front of larger things like the stove, to reassure myself that all the switches were in the 'off' position.

"Over time, my anxiety about electrical appliances got worse and I had to check and recheck so many times, worrying whether I'd checked it properly. It got so bad that I was checking for at least 1 hour before leaving home. I'd often be late for work because I was rechecking things over and over."

Jason finally decided to seek treatment after an incident when he was stuck at home checking and rechecking, which forced him to miss an important meeting at work.

Following a thorough assessment, the cognitive-behavioural model of OCD was discussed with Jason. This involved explaining how his response to the thoughts of possible harm reinforced the thoughts and increased their recurrence. The checking behaviours reduced the anxiety caused by the thoughts, and were further reinforced by the fact that no adverse outcomes had eventuated as a result of the checking. For as long as he continued to check and recheck, he would never learn the feared outcome would not occur.

Exposure, aimed at disconfirming the core fears, was discussed in detail and a hierarchy of triggers to thoughts and checking behaviours was constructed (Table 39.1).

In collaboration with Jason, it was agreed that exposure would commence with the clock radio and stereo. Both items were to be left plugged into their respective sockets and switched on at the power point, with no subsequent checking of these items. At the next session, Jason reported that when he left home, he was concerned that a short circuit might occur. However, this concern faded over the day, and repeated daily exposure to these tasks resulted in minimal anxiety.

Table 39.1 Hierarchy of triggers and associated SUDS ratings

Item	SUDS
Clock radio	4
Stereo	6
Refrigerator door	6
Computer at home	7
Computer at work	8
TV	7
Electric kettle	8
Iron	9
Heater	10
Stove	10

The next exposure tasks included the home computer being left plugged in and switched on. Jason was also asked not to ensure that the fridge door was closed. To challenge his fears further, he was asked to leave his clock radio or stereo playing music during the day while he was at work.

Jason successfully completed his exposure tasks on a daily basis and reported a marked reduction in SUDS ratings for the tasks over the next week. These exposure tasks were to be continued and completed repeatedly as described. In addition, the TV was also to be left plugged in with the power point switched on. He was also asked to leave his work computer on standby rather than ensure it was switched off. His SUDS ratings reduced, as displayed in Table 39.2.

Table 39.2 Reported marked reduction in SUDS ratings

Item	SUDS	
	Pre-treatment	Mid-treatment
Computer	7/8	3
Clock radio (on)	4	1
Stereo (on)	6	2
Refrigerator door	6	0

Over the following weeks, Jason worked on the harder items of the hierarchy, including the heater, kettle and stove. Although he initially found them difficult, he reported significant reductions in his SUDS ratings over a 1-week period, as a result of the self-directed exposure.

At the end of 15 exposure sessions, Jason's reported anxiety levels were relatively low. Nonetheless, the idea of continued exposure and response prevention was strongly reinforced. The rationale given for continued exposure focused on new learning that was required to replace the old.

At 6-month follow-up, Jason reported that he was still successfully resisting checking behaviours. He reported that, although the thoughts of harm were stronger at some times than at others, he maintained his determination not to go back to his old ways. He was encouraged to continue to challenge the thoughts by doing the opposite.

CHAPTER 40   EVIDENCE BASE FOR COGNITIVE-BEHAVIOURAL THERAPY

Juliette Drobny

ABOUT THE EVIDENCE

As described in Chapters 33 and 34, the Cochrane Library was reviewed to obtain the highest quality independent evidence for examining the effectiveness of cognitive behaviour therapy for anxiety disorders. Meta-analyses from the Centre of Reviews and Dissemination or other meta-analyses were examined where Cochrane reviews were not available. Individual reports were identified that evaluated the effectiveness of CBT in cases when meta-analyses were unavailable,

As a reminder, when interpreting effect sizes, 0.2 reflects a small effect, 0.5 reflects a medium effect and 0.8 and above represents a large effect. In short, the larger the number, the greater the effect size.

In the literature, an active treatment is often compared to a control group, such as a waitlist (WL), placebo or treatment as usual (TAU). A large between-group effect size indicates that the active treatment is more effective than the control group, while a small between-group effect size indicates little difference between the two groups.

OVERVIEW OF POST-TREATMENT EFFECT SIZES ACROSS THE ANXIETY DISORDERS

Figure 40.1 shows the post-treatment effect sizes for the primary outcome measures across four different anxiety disorders.

As the graph shows, when CBT is compared to either a waitlist, placebo or treatment as usual control group, the difference in effect between the two treatments is large for panic disorder, GAD and PTSD. Social phobia is associated with moderate to large effect sizes.

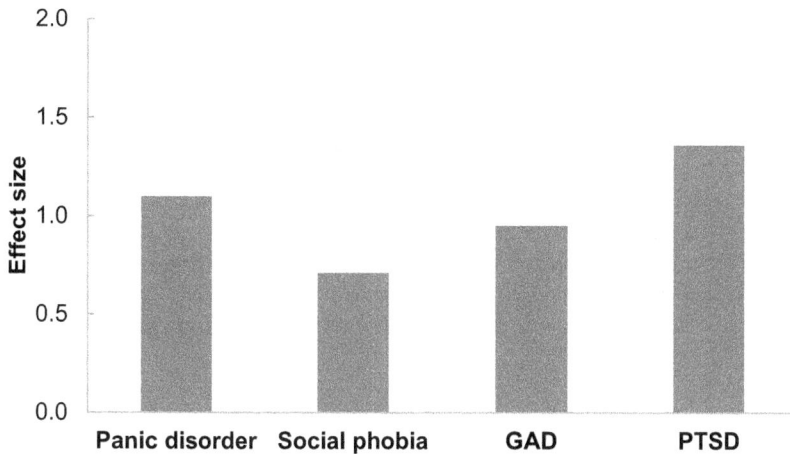

Figure 40.1 Post-treatment effect sizes (CBT v. WL/Placebo) across anxiety disorders

PANIC DISORDER WITH AND WITHOUT AGORAPHOBIA

A meta-analysis by Sánchez-Meca et al. (2010) examined the efficacy of CBT compared to a control group for panic disorder, with or without agoraphobia, across 19 studies. The control group was either a waitlist or a psychological or pill placebo. As can be seen from Figure 40.2, CBT was associated with large effect sizes. On both panic (ES = 1.29, 95% CI = 1.04 to 1.53) and agoraphobia (ES = 0.91, 95% CI = 0.62 to 1.19) measures, CBT performed around one standard deviation higher than the control group.

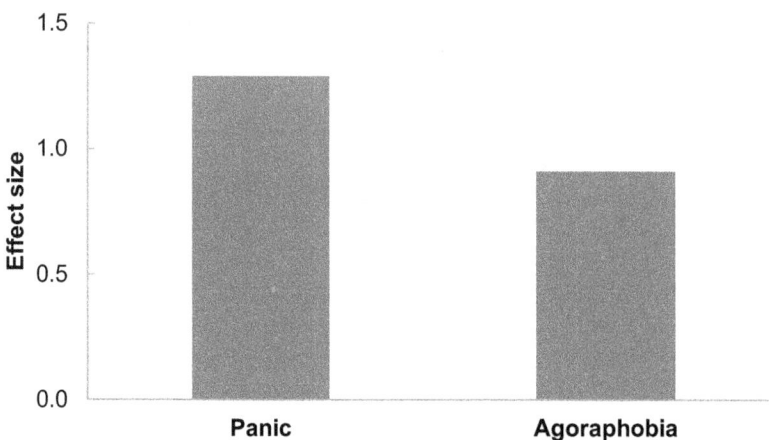

Figure 40.2 Effect sizes for CBT versus WL/Placebo. Data adapted from Sánchez-Meca et al. (2010).

SOCIAL PHOBIA

A meta-analysis by Acarturk et al. (2009) examined the effect of psychological treatments for social phobia compared to either placebo, treatment-as-usual or a waitlist control. Fourteen studies evaluated the effect of CBT. The effect size at post-treatment was 0.71, indicating a moderately large effect (ES = 0.71, 95% CI = 0.56 to 0.85). The effect size of 0.71 indicates that the mean score for the CBT group was almost three quarters of a standard deviation larger than the mean of the control group. With regard to follow-up, available results indicate that the effects of CBT for social phobia are stable over 18 months, and may even slightly increase.

However, lower effect sizes were produced for trials comprising pill placebo or treatment as usual conditions, in comparison to waitlist controls. In addition, effect sizes were smaller for participants initially meeting diagnostic criteria for social phobia, in comparison to other inclusion criteria (e.g., elevated scores on self-report measures). This indicates patients with mild disorders are more responsive to CBT than patients with more severe disorders.

GENERALISED ANXIETY DISORDER

A Cochrane review by Hunot et al. (2007) reviewed eight studies comparing CBT against treatment-as-usual or a waitlist control for GAD. As can be seen on Figure 40.3, CBT was shown to be more effective than waitlist or treatment-as-usual in reducing anxiety (SMD = -1.00, 95% CI = -1.24 to -0.77), worry (SMD = -0.90, 95% CI = -1.16 to -0.64), secondary symptoms of depression (SMD -0.96, 95% CI = -1.20 to -0.72) and quality of life (SMD 0.44, 95% CI = 0.06 to 0.82). Effect sizes were generally of a large magnitude, with more moderate effects produced for quality of life.

CBT was also more effective than supportive therapy for anxiety (SMD = -0.40, 95% CI = -0.66 to 0.14), worry (SMD = -0.55, 95% CI = -0.91 to 0.20) and depression (SMD = -0.37, 95% CI = -0.72 to 0.02), but not for quality of life (SMD = 0.30, 95% CI = -10.77 to 11.37). As can be seen, however, lower effect sizes were produced when CBT was compared with supportive therapy as opposed to waitlist or treatment-as-usual.

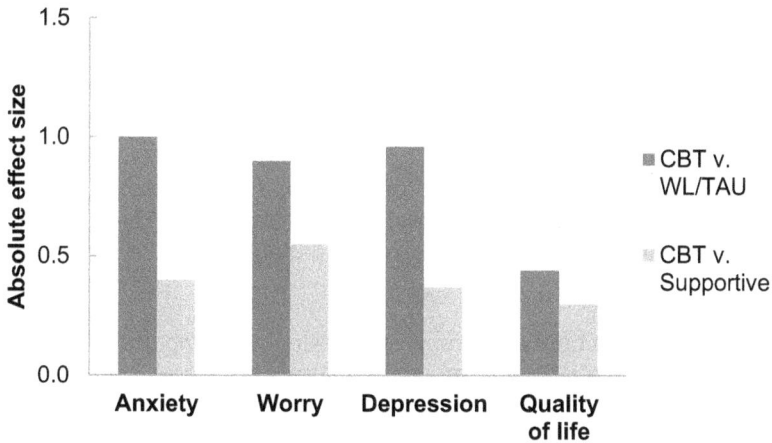

Figure 40.3 Effect sizes for CBT v. WL/TAU or supportive therapy. Data adapted from Hunot et al. (2007).

Figure 40.4 shows the percentage of patients achieving clinical response for GAD following CBT at post-treatment and 6-month follow-up. At post-treatment, significantly more people treated with CBT achieved a clinical response compared to those in the control group (46% v. 14%, RR = 0.64, 95% CI = 0.55 to 0.74).

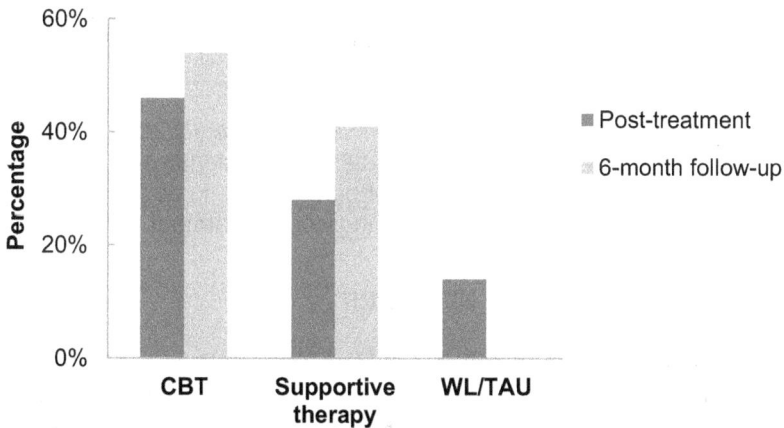

Figure 40.4 Percentage of patients achieving clinical response. Data adapted from Hunot et al. (2007).

However, there was no significant difference in clinical response between CBT and supportive therapy at either post-treatment (42% v. 28%, RR = 0.86, 95% CI = 0.70 to 1.060) or 6-month follow-up (54% v. 41%, RR 0.79, 95% CI = 0.59 to1.06), although there was a trend for CBT to be superior to supportive therapy at both time periods. Figure

40.4 also highlights the fact that treatment gains were maintained and even improved over time.

Pathological Worry in Generalised Anxiety Disorder

A meta-analysis by Covin et al. (2008) reviewed seven studies, comparing CBT with either a no treatment waitlist or placebo control group on measures of pathological worry, a cardinal feature of GAD in the DSM-5.

They found a large between-group effect size, indicating that CBT was significantly more effective at reducing pathological worry than placebo or no treatment (ES = -1.15, range = -0.06 to 2.47).

Effect sizes were larger for younger adults than older adults (younger adults ES = -1.69; older adults ES = -0.82). In addition, when treatment format was analysed, results showed that individual treatment yielded larger effect sizes than group treatment (individual ES = -1.72; group ES = -0.91).

Results of follow-up assessments revealed that benefits of treatment were maintained at 6 and 12-month follow-up, and those treated with group CBT continued to improve at 12-months follow-up.

Dropout Rates in Cognitive Behaviour Therapy for Generalised Anxiety Disorder

The review by Hunot et al. (2007) also examined predictors of attrition from CBT in GAD. They found older patients were significantly more likely to drop out of treatment than younger patients. In addition, dropout rates were higher for Group CBT than individual treatment.

OBSESSIVE-COMPULSIVE DISORDER

A Cochrane review by Gava et al. (2007) reviewed five studies, with 130 participants, comparing CBT versus treatment as usual. As can be seen on the visual analogue scale in Figure 40.5, patients receiving CBT showed significantly greater reductions in obsessive-compulsive symptoms, compared to patients receiving treatment-as-usual (WMD = -7.73, 95% CI = -9.92 to -5.55). In addition, those receiving CBT demonstrated significantly better quality of life (WMD = -10.50, 95% CI = -20.74 to -0.26) than those receiving usual care.

Obsessive-compulsive disorder

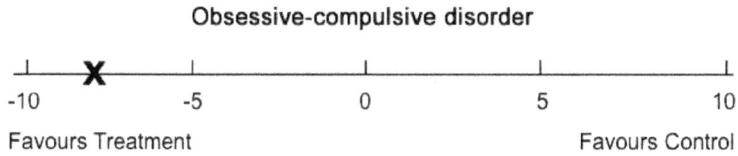

-10   -5   0   5   10

Favours Treatment   Favours Control

Quality of life

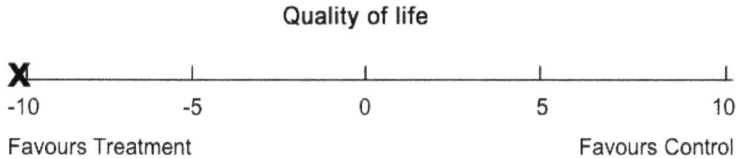

-10   -5   0   5   10

Favours Treatment   Favours Control

Figure 40.5   Reduction in obsessive-compulsive symptoms and improvement of quality of life with CBT versus TAU. Data adapted from Gava et al. (2007).

However, as Figure 40.6 shows, the same study showed that there were no significant differences between CBT and controls on measures of anxiety (SMD = -0.38, 95% CI = -0.97 to 0.21), depression (SMD = -0.34, 95% CI = -0.70 to 0.02) or dropout (OR = 0.88, 95% CI = 0.35 to 2.18).

Anxiety

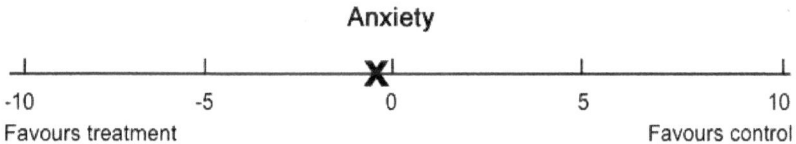

-10   -5   0   5   10

Favours treatment   Favours control

Depression

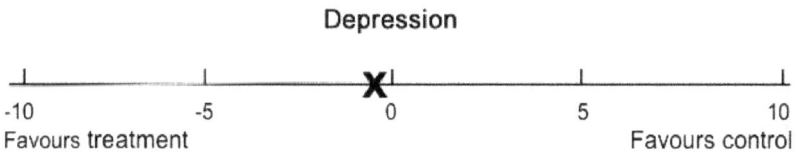

-10   -5   0   5   10

Favours treatment   Favours control

Dropouts

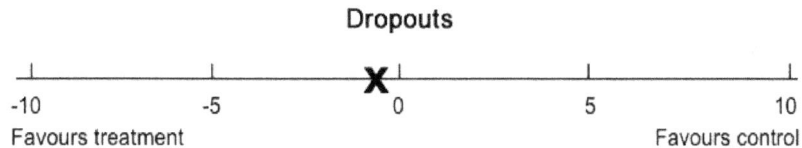

-10   -5   0   5   10

Favours treatment   Favours control

Figure 40.6   Anxiety, depression and dropout with CBT versus TAU. Data adapted from Gava et al. (2007).

POSTTRAUMATIC STRESS DISORDER

A Cochrane review by Bisson & Andrew (2007) reviewed 14 studies of 649 participants, comparing the efficacy of trauma focused CBT with waitlist or treatment-as-usual, on symptoms of PTSD, anxiety and depression. They also examined the efficacy of other PTSD treatments, including eye-movement desensitisation reprocessing (EMDR) and stress management.

Figure 40.7 displays the effect sizes for the three treatment groups in comparison to the control groups for measures of PTSD, anxiety and depression. At post-treatment, the CBT group performed significantly better than the waitlist or usual care control groups on measures of PTSD symptoms (SMD = -1.40, 95% CI = -1.89 to -0.91). Similarly, both the EMDR (SMD = -1.51, 95% CI = -1.87 to -1.15) and stress management groups (SMD = -1.14, 95% CI = -1.62 to -0.67) performed better than the control groups.

Strong effect sizes were also found on secondary symptoms of anxiety (CBT SMD = -0.99, 95% CI = -1.2 to -0.78; EMDR SMD = -1.10, 95% CI = -1.45 to -0.76; stress management SMD = -0.77, 95% CI = -1.23 to -0.31) and depression (CBT SMD = -1.26, 95% CI = -1.69 to -0.82; EMDR SMD = -1.48, 95% CI = -1.84 to -1.12; stress management SMD = -0.73, 95% CI = -1.12 to -0.33). Interestingly, there were no significant differences between the three treatment groups on any of these measures at post-treatment.

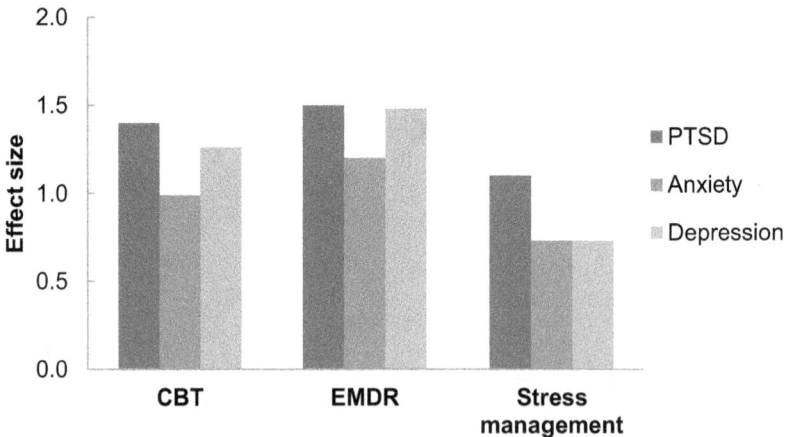

Figure 40.7   Post-treatment effect sizes for treatment versus WL/TAU. Data adapted from Bisson & Andrew (2007).

However, at 2 to 5-month follow-up, CBT was superior to stress management on measures of PTSD symptoms, but not for general anxiety and depression. No differences emerged between CBT and EMDR at follow-up on any measure.

In a meta-analysis, Bradley et al. (2005) reported the percentage of patients no longer meeting criteria for PTSD across CBT, EMDR, a supportive control group and a waitlist control. As displayed in Figure 40.8, CBT and EMDR treatments resulted in relatively high rates of patients no longer meeting PTSD criteria in analyses of treatment completers (CBT = 70%, EMDR = 65%). Lower rates were seen for the supportive therapy control (39%) and waitlist (16%) groups. In intention-to-treat analyses, rates decreased somewhat, particularly for the CBT group (CBT = 54%, EMDR = 60%, Supportive control = 36%, Waitlist = 14%).

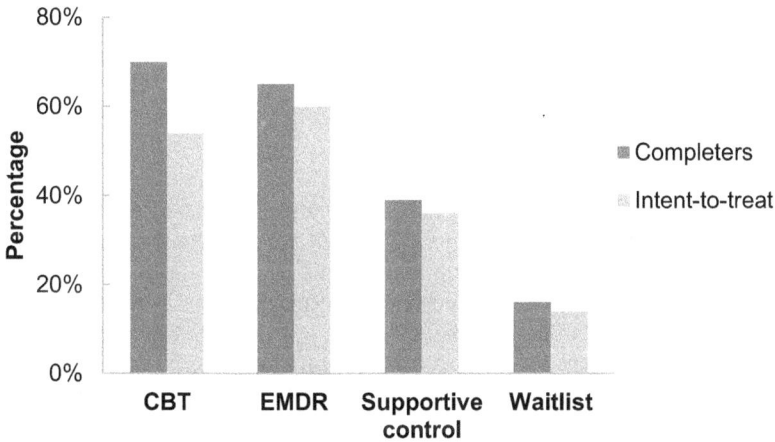

Figure 40.8 Percentage of patients no longer meeting diagnostic criteria for PTSD across treatment conditions. Data adapted from Bradley et al. (2005).

Bradley et al. (2005) also compared the percentage of patients no longer meeting criteria for PTSD between exposure therapy, cognitive therapy and CBT across treatment completers and intent-to-treat samples. Figure 40.9 shows that all treatments resulted in similar rates of improvement. In treatment completer samples, the percentages no longer meeting criteria for PTSD across treatments were exposure = 68%, cognitive therapy = 56% and CBT = 70%. In intent-to-treat analyses, percentages were exposure = 53%, cognitive therapy = 46% and CBT = 54%.

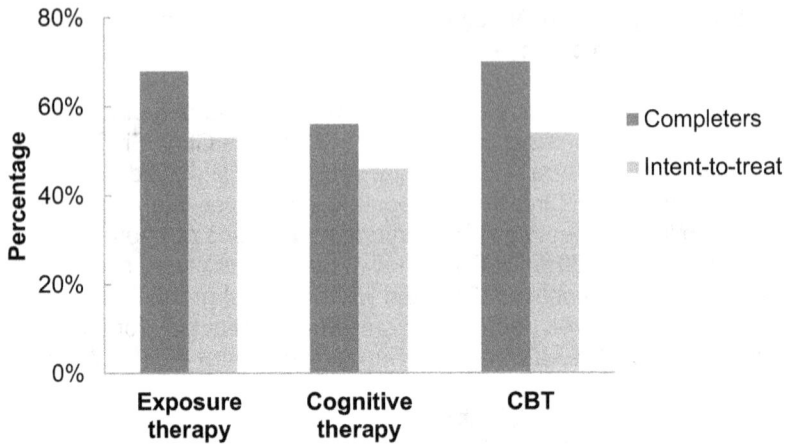

Figure 40.9 Percentage of patients no longer meeting diagnostic criteria for PTSD across treatment conditions. Data adapted from Bradley et al. (2005).

SPECIFIC PHOBIA

Choy et al. (2007) reviewed three studies examining the effect of combining cognitive therapy with in vivo exposure, in the treatment of specific phobias. One study of claustrophobic patients found that adding cognitive therapy to in vivo exposure was more effective in reducing phobic anxiety than in vivo exposure alone. In another study comparing CBT versus in vivo exposure for small animal phobia, CBT was as effective as in vivo exposure, with both treatments producing large effects. In a study of individuals with a flying phobia, CBT was as effective as behaviour therapy. Each treatment produced large reductions in flight anxiety, which were clinically significant. Importantly, improvements were maintained at 12-months follow-up.

Wolitzky-Taylor et al. (2008) published a meta-analysis of psychological treatments for specific phobias. They examined 18 studies of 961 participants, comparing exposure-based treatments with a waitlist control. They found that exposure-based treatments, which included cognitive components, were associated with a large effect size (ES = 1.05, 95% CI = 0.91-1.20).

Five studies, comprising 316 participants, compared exposure-based treatments to placebo treatment. Compared to placebo, exposure was associated with a moderate effect size (ES = 0.48, 95% CI = 0.25 to 0.80). This study included follow-up data, and as can be seen in Figure 40.10, the superiority of exposure treatment was stronger at follow-up (ES = 0.80, 95% CI = 0.50 to 1.09). Finally, five studies compared pure exposure treatments with exposure augmented with cognitive techniques. As can be seen, exposure with cognitive therapy did not outperform exposure therapy alone, either at post-treatment (ES = 0.17, 95% CI = -0.09 to 0.44) or follow-up (ES = 0.14, 95% CI = -0.21 to 0.49).

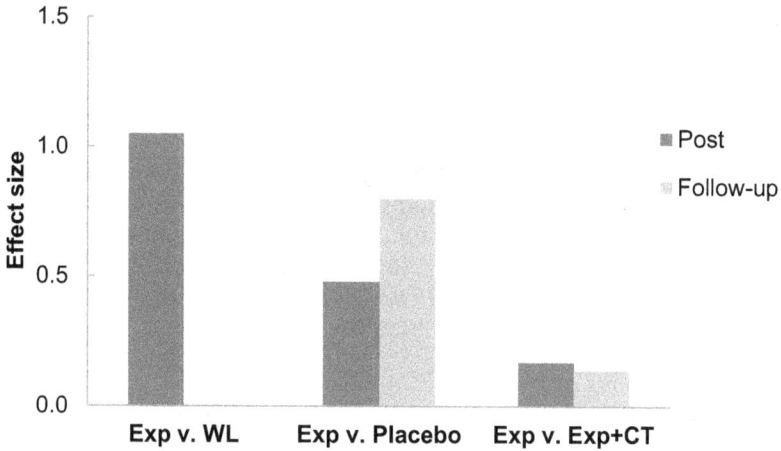

Figure 40.10   Effect sizes for exposure versus other treatments. Data adapted from Wolitzky-Taylor et al. (2008).

SUMMARY OF EVIDENCE FROM META-ANALYSES

In summary, evidence from meta-analyses indicates CBT is more effective than waitlist, placebo or treatment-as-usual in the treatment of all anxiety disorders. Only a few meta-analyses have compared CBT to other psychological treatments. In GAD, CBT was more effective than supportive counselling. However, for PTSD, general stress management was almost as effective as CBT, and there was no difference between CBT and EMDR. For specific phobias, CBT was no more effective than behaviour therapy, such as in vivo exposure.

IMPORTANT FACTORS TO CONSIDER WHEN INTERPRETING THE LITERATURE

Although the evidence reviewed above indicates that CBT is an efficacious treatment for anxiety disorders, caution is needed when interpreting these findings.

Firstly, most studies reported data for treatment completers only, with very few studies including intention-to-treat analyses. This means the true effectiveness of CBT is likely to be lower for the general population, as data from treatment dropouts and non-starters were not included in analyses. This was illustrated in the meta-analysis of psychological treatments for social phobia by Acarturk et al. (2009), in which the effect size for intention to treat analyses was around half of that obtained for analyses restricted to treatment completers.

A second issue in CBT comparison studies concerns the nature of the control group. Some studies use a no treatment control or waitlist, while others use a placebo condition or treatment-as-usual. Many of the meta-analyses reviewed here combine these different control conditions together as one control group, which can obscure the interpretation of findings. Typically, effect sizes are larger when CBT is compared with a waitlist. But when CBT is solely compared with treatment-as-usual, between-group differences often reduce to non-significant levels. Therefore, when interpreting the effect sizes comparing CBT with control conditions, it is important to determine what proportion of the control group is comprised of waitlist controls versus treatment-as-usual conditions.

It is also important to realise that while CBT is shown to be effective in reducing anxiety symptoms, this does not mean patients are "cured". The majority of patients treated with CBT will go on to experience residual anxiety symptoms, and many require additional treatment over time.

Related to this is the question of what is meant by improvement or successful outcome. Improvement rates markedly decrease when more conservative outcome criteria are applied. To illustrate this point, Brown & Barlow (1995) re-analysed the 2-year follow-up data for patients with panic disorder treated with CBT. When improvement was defined as no panic attacks in the last month, 75% of patients were classified as having improved. However, when the definition of improvement involved meeting criteria for high end-state functioning and no further requirement for treatment, the percentage of patients classified as having successful outcomes reduced to 48%. When even more stringent criteria of "no panic attacks in the last year" and "no further need for treatment" were applied at 3-month and 2-year follow-up, successful outcome rates reduced to 21%. So, the effectiveness of CBT is, in part, influenced by how improvement is defined.

What about the long-term effectiveness of CBT? For ethical reasons, there are no randomised controlled trials with a long-term follow-up period. However, studies investigating the long-term effects of CBT have found that patients tend to maintain their gains, although symptoms tend to wax and wane over time.

CBT is effective in reducing anxiety symptoms, but this does not mean patients are "cured".

A final point is that participants included in clinical trials evaluating CBT are not necessarily representative of patients in real world community settings. Often there are strict inclusion criteria where participants are excluded if they have comorbid depression, a history of substance abuse, psychosis, suicidality, personality disorder, neurological conditions and so on. Highlighting this point, a randomised controlled trial conducted by Clark et al. (2006) for social phobia excluded 54 of 116, or 47% of participants meeting criteria for social phobia, for many of the reasons cited above.

Such strict inclusion criteria limit the generalisability of findings, and provide an upper limit to the efficacy of CBT for anxiety disorders. Effect sizes are likely to be lower for the more complex patients seen in real world clinical settings. That is, CBT is likely to be less effective in the real world. Indeed, in their meta-analysis of psychotherapy for PTSD, Bradley et al. (2005) found that the number of exclusion criteria reported in studies was positively correlated with pre- to post-treatment effect sizes. Put another way, this means that studies adopting more liberal inclusion criteria yielded weaker effects.

Overall, the available evidence indicates that CBT is an effective treatment for anxiety disorders; in fact, it is the most effective psychological treatment available to date. However, there is considerable room for improvement.

Chapter 45 will discuss the effect of combining CBT with pharmacotherapy as a means of improving treatment outcome.

CHAPTER 41   WEB-BASED TREATMENTS FOR ANXIETY: AVAILABILITY AND EVIDENCE BASE

Helen Christensen

WHY USE THE INTERNET

As Part I explained, anxiety disorders are common, costly and debilitating. This, combined with low rates of treatment sought and a shortage of therapists, makes anxiety disorders a major health problem. Research shows that many patients do not feel comfortable approaching their GP for assistance with anxiety, and prefer the anonymity that is offered by the internet. Furthermore, health patients are increasingly turning to the internet for health-related information and direct assistance for their health needs. The *Pew Internet & American Life Project* reported that 75% of internet users have searched for health-related information online. Of these, 23% have searched for information about depression, anxiety, stress or mental health conditions. As such, researchers and policy makers are now turning to the internet for innovative and effective solutions for mental health treatment.

ADVANTAGES OF WEB-BASED PROGRAMS

From the Individual's Perspective

Web-based programs have a number of advantages over traditional face-to-face therapy approaches. From the patient's perspective, web-based programs can overcome many of the barriers to help-seeking, such as:

- geographical barriers
- financial barriers
- attitudinal barriers.

> 75% of internet users have searched for health-related information online.

People from rural areas, or those in developing countries often have little or no access to mental health services. Web-based programs offer faster access to treatment, avoiding delays associated with waiting lists. Traditional face-to-face treatments such as CBT can be very expensive. In contrast, web-based programs are often free or very low cost. The stigma associated with seeking professional help, or the belief that the person does not have the time to attend therapy sessions, can interfere with seeking help. Web-based programs can reduce these barriers.

As previously mentioned, web-based treatments offer increased anonymity through lack of face-to-face contact, and the ability to use the program in a convenient location such as the privacy of the individual's own home.

They are also more flexible so that, unlike face-to-face treatments, patients can access the program 24 hours a day. Patients are also free to alter the pace of treatment, with the potential to work at a faster pace than what is traditionally offered in face-to-face therapy.

From a Population Perspective

In addition, web-based programs have particular advantages from a population perspective, such as lower cost of service delivery due to the reduction in therapist contact, reduced demands on the clinical workforce, being able to be disseminated world-wide and offer low cost solutions, and increased access to hard-to-reach groups such as young people, men, armed forces personnel and those who have previously had stigmatising or disempowering experiences with traditional methods.

DISADVANTAGES OF WEB-BASED PROGRAMS

Despite the advantages, there are a number of disadvantages associated with web-based treatments, such as:

- low engagement
- lack of adherence
- lack of practitioner acceptance
- safety concerns.

It can be difficult to engage people with early intervention and prevention based programs. Further research is needed to understand factors associated with help seeking. Dropout rates can be quite high. However, these do not differ significantly from face-to-face therapy, where dropout rates can be as high as 70%. Some practitioners believe that web-based programs offer ineffective or inadequate doses. Some believe they prevent access to "proper" treatment or result in exposure to unregulated environments. There are numerous poor quality sites on the internet, and it can be difficult for patients to discriminate between high quality and low quality sites.

WHAT KINDS OF WEB-BASED PROGRAMS ARE THERE

Various types of web-based programs are available. These often vary in the intensity of information or interaction provided. They include:

- automated self-help on open access websites
- interactive screening
- guided assistance through help lines
- full virtual clinic experience.

Often, these types of sites are augmented with differing levels of therapist support. Some programs offer no therapist support, while others include automated reminders or motivational emails. Some offer non-professional support, and some offer therapist support via email, SMS, phone or live chat, or the support of a general practitioner.

THE BEACON PORTAL

A useful website indicating the quality of mental health websites available is the Beacon Portal (beacon.anu.edu.au).

Beacon is an open access website that provides information about a range of web interventions used in the prevention or treatment of mental and physical health disorders.

Beacon reviews a broad range of web-based programs for the treatment of a large number of conditions, including generalised anxiety disorder, obsessive-compulsive disorder, panic disorder, posttraumatic stress disorder, and social anxiety.

EVIDENCE BASE OF WEB-BASED INTERVENTIONS FOR ANXIETY DISORDERS

In a review of the efficacy of internet interventions for anxiety disorders, Christensen, Griffiths & Farrer (2009) reviewed 16 published randomised controlled trials of CBT-based internet interventions for anxiety disorders. Of these studies, five targeted panic disorder, five social phobia, four posttraumatic stress disorder, and two unspecified anxiety disorder. An additional two studies targeted both depression and anxiety. Almost all of the anxiety trials employed some level of therapist input.

All of the interventions yielded positive results on at least one measure, regardless of the type of control group they employed, except for the non-therapist arm of one social phobia study. The effect size differences of all anxiety programs ranged from 0.29 to 1.74, with most exceeding 0.65. The effect sizes reported here are consistent with controlled effect sizes reported for face-to-face treatment (see Chapter 40).

The findings of this review clearly demonstrate that the internet can be an effective medium for the delivery of interventions designed to reduce the symptoms of anxiety conditions. Web-based interventions can be used as a self-help application for patients, or as an adjunct to usual care.

With regard to long-term outcome, Carlbring et al. (2009) investigated the long-term effects of a web-based program for social phobia. At 30-month follow-up, the treatment showed large effect sizes. A 3-year follow-up of a web-based treatment for panic symptoms also showed similarly strong effects.

THIS WAY UP ® Social Phobia Course

An example of an effective web-based intervention for social phobia is THIS WAY UP ® Social Phobia Course (previously known as the Shyness Program) from the University of New South Wales and St Vincent's Hospital Sydney (www.thiswayup.org.au/clinic/courses/courses-we-offer/social-phobia). This online CBT program incorporates psycho-education, exposure and behavioural experiments, cognitive challenging and relapse prevention. Users are asked to participate in an online forum to promote further learning and support. Access to a therapist by email is available if users need further help.

The program has produced large effect sizes. Randomised controlled trials have found that the program resulted in a significant reduction in primary measures of social phobia, compared to waitlist controls, with a mean between-group effect size of 1.04. Secondary measures of general anxiety, depression, psychological distress and disability also reduced. Participants were satisfied with the program, regardless of whether support was provided through a clinician or forum (Titov et al., 2008).

The Brave Program

An example of an effective Generalised Anxiety Disorder web-based program is the Brave Program developed by the University of Queensland and Griffith University (brave4you.psy.uq.edu.au).

This is an online CBT-based intervention used to treat childhood anxiety. It focuses on developing skills to manage anxiety, such as the recognition of its physiological signs, relaxation strategies and cognitive training including self-talk and restructuring, exposure, problem-solving and empowerment. Automated feedback is provided following exercises, and each family is assigned a therapist, who provides feedback through weekly emails.

The efficacy of the site has been tested in two randomised controlled trials using child samples. Compared to a waitlist control, the program resulted in significant improvements in clinical ratings of severity and global assessments of functioning at post-test. The percentage of children not meeting DSM-IV criteria for anxiety disorders increased from 30% post-test to 75% at 6-month follow-up (March, Spence, & Donovan, 2009).

Panic STOP!

An example of an effective CBT web-based treatment for Panic Disorder is the "Panic STOP!" program (previously known as panic online) developed by Swinburne University (www.anxietyonline.org.au).

This site uses the treatment methods and principles of CBT, such as controlled breathing, changing thinking, and exposure to stimuli or events. It is designed to assist the user in understanding and mastering strategies effective in reducing the impact of panic disorder. The program includes interactions via email with therapists who assist with questions about the program and provide support and feedback.

Compared to an information control, this program was found to significantly reduce panic symptoms and cognitions, lower negative affect and improve physical health at post-treatment and 3-month follow-up (Klein et al., 2006).

ROLE OF THERAPIST CONTACT

Internet-based mental health services do not necessarily aim to compete with or decrease access to face-to-face treatment. Rather, for many users it is likely that web-based services will simply be the first step towards accessing more traditional therapist-based services.

Most researchers agree that guided help online by a non-professional leads to the same effect sizes as web interventions guided by a health professional, such as a psychiatrist or psychologist. So it appears that therapist contact is not essential.

What is less clear is the effect of guided help versus non-guided help. With regards to the effect of therapist support, Spek et al. (2007) conducted a meta-analysis of web-based interventions for anxiety and depression examining the effect of therapist support. They found large effect sizes for studies with therapist support (ES = 1.00, 95% CI = 0.75 to 1.24), and only small effects for studies without therapist support (ES = 0.26, 95% CI = 0.08 to 0.44).

However, when looking at frequency of therapist contact, it appears that increasing the frequency offers little benefit. Klein et al. (2009) randomly allocated patients with panic disorder to receive the web-based treatment, Panic Online, with email contact from a psychologist either once a week or three times a week. Both conditions were effective, with no significant differences between groups.

So it appears that web-based CBT interventions are effective, particularly if they contain some level of therapist input.

PART X SUMMARY

Cognitive behaviour therapy aims to help individuals reduce their emotional distress through modifying unhelpful thinking styles and behavioural responses. Having discussed Behaviour Therapy in Part VIII and Cognitive Therapy in Part IX, Part X began with a discussion of behavioural experiments, a powerful therapeutic technique involving an interplay of cognitive and behavioural mechanisms. Although exposure techniques are incorporated in behavioural experiments, they are designed to test out and challenge maladaptive cognitions. The rationale for utilising behavioural experiments in the treatment of anxiety disorders and the steps involved in designing and implementing these experiments is described. Secondly, Part X provided case examples highlighting the use of different CBT methods across anxiety disorders, including imaginal exposure in PTSD, interoceptive exposure in panic disorder, and exposure plus response prevention in OCD.

Part X went on to present the empirical evidence supporting the effectiveness of CBT in the treatment of anxiety disorders. It indicates that there is good support for CBT being more efficacious than control or placebo conditions in the treatment of all anxiety disorders. However, there are numerous methodological limitations of the literature which cast doubt on the generalizability of the findings to real world clinical populations.

Part X concluded with a discussion of web-based interventions for anxiety disorders. Advantages of this treatment modality include reduced geographical, financial and attitudinal barriers, increased anonymity, flexibility and convenience. Disadvantages, however, include the potential for poor engagement, reduced adherence and safety concerns. Examples of web-based programs currently operating are provided. Finally, the evidence for web-based treatments is presented which strongly suggests they are effective when they contain a level of therapist support.

PART XI   PHARMACOTHERAPY

Throughout history people have used various substances to alleviate their distress, including their anxiety and fear. Often these substances were herbal preparations and drinks containing alcohol. This was the origin of modern pharmacotherapy for anxiety disorders.

Ever since substances started to be used to alleviate anxiety and distress, there has been some discomfort and ambivalence about doing so. Many people have a dilemma over whether it is "right" to use external agents to make their emotional suffering bearable.

In some cultures and under certain social circumstances, use of substances has been seen as a sign of weakness, and people have been encouraged to endure their difficulties so they would emerge stronger afterwards. Hence the saying, "What doesn't kill you, makes you stronger."

These dilemmas are often present today. Some patients with anxiety disorders are hesitant to use medications for a range of reasons.

Medication treatment of anxiety disorders so often elicits strong views, and polarises both patients and clinicians. While some tend to see medications as a panacea and have unrealistic expectations of them, others exhibit overt antagonism to this kind of treatment.

Ethical issues have also been raised, as physicians often find themselves prescribing medications that may be perceived as "addictive", which has even led to them being labelled "drug dealers".

It has been difficult to find the middle ground between these extreme views, and appraise pharmacotherapy realistically for what it is. To this date, getting the balance right has been the greatest challenge to medication treatment of anxiety disorders.

Anxiolytic agents have been around for several thousand years, and there is no reason to believe that they will disappear now. Regardless of one's personal preference, it is likely that there will always be patients keen to be treated with these medications. As the clinician's task is to respect patients' treatment preferences, it is sensible to explore with the patient their motivation to take medication and discuss with them whether this is appropriate. This will contribute to making the pharmacotherapy of anxiety disorders safer.

CHAPTER 42   HOW TO USE MEDICATIONS TO TREAT ANXIETY DISORDERS

Vladan Starcevic

WHEN TO USE MEDICATIONS FOR ANXIETY DISORDERS

When treatment options are considered for patients with anxiety disorders, it is important to understand when particular treatments should be used. With regards to pharmacotherapy, there are certain clinical situations suggesting that treatment with medication might be beneficial.

A common such situation is when patients present with severe symptoms of anxiety and high levels of distress, and indicate that they need quick alleviation of their suffering and relief from symptoms. This is particularly common in people who have panic attacks, to whom it may seem as if relief cannot come soon enough. The rationale for using medications in these situations is that they work faster than other treatments.

Another situation in which medications are likely to be used is when the particular disorder is more severe, and associated with greater disability. This is because, in general, the more severe the anxiety disorder, the greater the perceived need for pharmacotherapy.

Pharmacotherapy is often chosen if another psychiatric condition co-occurs with the anxiety disorder, or if there is a history of co-occurrence with such a condition. Most commonly, this condition is depression or another mood disorder for which pharmacotherapy may be effective.

Some patients are not interested in undergoing psychological treatments. There may be many reasons for this. Some people are not particularly "psychologically minded", and may believe that all they need is for their "chemical imbalance" in the brain to be corrected. Others are not motivated to undergo psychological treatments because these may seem to be too arduous, or patients may think that in the course of such treatments they would first have to experience and endure more anxiety, distress, or discomfort before they can feel better.

Finally, several practical issues may play a role in the choice of pharmacotherapy. Medications are generally more widely available than specific and effective psychological treatments, they may cost less and they are easier to administer.

DISCUSSION WITH PATIENTS

A decision to use medication in the treatment of anxiety disorders should be a result of discussion and collaboration between the physician and the patient. It is very important that the physician explains to the patient why the medication is indicated, what to expect from this treatment, when benefits are likely to be experienced, what side effects may occur and how long the treatment is likely to last.

GOALS AND EXPECTATIONS

Patients should be informed that the main goals of pharmacotherapy are alleviation of anxiety and distress by controlling the symptoms, especially physical symptoms, prevention of complications and improvement in functioning. All other changes that may occur, for example changes in the patterns of behaviour and thinking, are secondary to these primary effects of medications. Therefore, this is what patients may expect from pharmacotherapy.

Patients also need to understand that the goals of pharmacotherapy are achievable whilst they are taking medications. Once they cease the medication, treatment gains may be maintained or they may disappear, and patients may experience a return of their symptoms and their anxiety, i.e., a recurrence of their anxiety disorder.

PROS AND CONS

When compared to psychological treatments, pharmacological treatment has both advantages and disadvantages. Perhaps the main advantage of pharmacotherapy is that its effects become apparent more quickly than the effects of psychological treatments. This is especially the case with benzodiazepines, although antidepressants may sometimes work more quickly than psychological therapy. Also, medications may have more obvious or more prominent effects on physical symptoms and symptoms of tension.

> The main advantage of pharmacotherapy is that its effects become apparent more quickly than the effects of psychological treatments.

The disadvantages of pharmacological treatment include possible side effects of medications, dependence on some agents used in long-term treatment of anxiety disorders, a relatively passive attitude towards treatment, and perhaps a greater risk of recurrence after treatment has been ceased.

ACHIEVING REMISSION

The aim of pharmacological treatment is remission – having few or no symptoms, whereby the patient's functioning has returned to normal. That means that it is not enough to achieve response, i.e., some improvement with a decrease in symptoms, because the presence of residual symptoms may increase the risk of recurrence after the cessation of medication.

The key to achieving remission is finding the dose that is effective for the particular patient, while taking into account any side effects of the medication. If the symptoms become less prominent with a low dose of medication, but have not abated, the dose should be increased, provided the patient can tolerate it. There is no need to increase the dose if the patient has practically no symptoms, even with a lower dose.

The medication should be taken for four to ten weeks to determine whether it is effective. If intolerable side effects develop at the beginning of treatment, the medication should be stopped. If there is no improvement at all after four to ten weeks of treatment with the highest possible dose, another medication should be considered. If there is some improvement, various augmentation strategies can be used to help achieve remission. These usually entail addition of another medication or the combination of medication with psychological treatment.

MAINTAINING REMISSION

Once the remission has been achieved, the medication should be taken continuously, every day for at least six months. In clinical practice, this period of maintenance treatment usually lasts one to two years. The effectiveness of pharmacotherapy of anxiety disorders usually does not diminish over time. It is unclear whether the duration of maintenance treatment is associated with the risk of recurrence after the cessation of medication.

CESSATION OF PHARMACOTHERAPY

The majority of patients want to stop taking the medication at some point. When this should happen varies considerably from one person to another, but it is a critical moment in the pharmacological treatment of anxiety disorders. This is mainly because recurrence rates after the cessation of medication can be high.

Cessation can be considered at least 6 months to 1 year after the remission has been achieved. Patients should not be pressured to stop the medication if they feel that they are not ready for it. While people may have different notions as to what it means to be ready for medication cessation, it usually implies that they feel comfortable enough to face anxiety without relying on the medication.

Just as the timing of the medication cessation should be discussed and negotiated with the patient, so should the rate at which the medication is discontinued. This means that some patients may go through the process of discontinuation in several weeks, whereas others will need several months or even longer. This also depends on the type of medication; for example, antidepressants are tapered more quickly than benzodiazepines. As a rule, medications should never be ceased abruptly, but after a gradual and careful decrease in the dose. This is because both antidepressants and benzodiazepines are often associated with various symptoms upon their discontinuation; the constellation of these symptoms is referred to as "discontinuation syndrome". Although these symptoms are rarely severe, the distress associated with them suggests that they should be avoided.

GENERAL PHARMACOTHERAPY PROCEDURES

When considering using medication for anxiety disorders, a nine-step general procedure should be followed to ensure their safe use and to maximise the benefit.

Step 1

Assess the patient and ascertain whether pharmacological treatment might be useful. This is done during the initial encounter with the patient.

Step 2

Discuss pharmacological treatment with the patient if it seems that this approach is suitable and the patient indicates that he or she is interested in taking medication. This involves providing the patient with all the relevant information, such as the reasons for and goals of pharmacological treatment, the chosen medication(s), possible side effects, the expected onset of therapeutic benefit, and the likely course and duration of treatment. At this point, the patient should be encouraged to ask questions about the treatment and he or she should be given adequate explanations.

Step 3

It is important to ensure that the patient understands what medication treatment entails, and that he or she agrees to it.

Step 4

The patient commences taking the medication. This may happen on the day of the assessment or at some point in the near future, depending on the patient's particular circumstances.

Step 5

Monitor the patient's response and any side effects of the medication(s). This is often the critical stage of pharmacological treatment, because some patients have difficulty enduring their symptoms and distress or they may experience significant side effects, the result of which is that they stop treatment. Therefore, it is important to be in close contact with patients during the first few weeks of treatment, encouraging them to ring their clinician in case of need, and scheduling frequent appointments with them (e.g., once a week).

Step 6

Make any adjustments to the pharmacological treatment, depending on the patient's response and side effects. This usually occurs after several weeks of treatment and entails changes in the dose, changing a medication and/or adding another one.

Step 7

Ascertain whether the patient has achieved remission – a state with a few or no symptoms, and a return to normal functioning. Some patients may remit fairly quickly, after a few weeks, whereas others need to be treated for several months to only achieve treatment response.

Step 8

Ensure that the patient has been maintaining remission by monitoring his or her state.

Step 9

Consider medication cessation, when this becomes appropriate – at least 6 months after the remission has been achieved. The decision about cessation of pharmacotherapy should be made after assessing the patient and discussing with them as to what this step entails (e.g., how it should be done, what to expect, etc.). Medication should not be ceased without the patient's full agreement.

CHAPTER 43   MEDICATIONS THAT WORK AND HOW TO CHOOSE BETWEEN THEM

Vladan Starcevic

EFFICACY OF MEDICATION

A number of medications have been found to be efficacious across the anxiety disorders. Efficacy implies an ability of the pharmacological agent to bring about a remission, with remission being defined as a state with very few or no symptoms and a return to normal functioning. In contrast, response is conceptualised as a 50% reduction in symptoms. Because obsessive-compulsive disorder is more difficult to treat, efficacy in the context of this condition usually means response, and response here refers to a more modest improvement – only a 25-35% decrease in symptoms.

The efficacy of the pharmacological agent is established when there is a statistically significant difference in favour of the medication, between remission (or response) rates with medication and remission (or response) rates with placebo.

Various instruments, or outcome measures, have been developed to ascertain whether remission has been achieved. An example of such an instrument is the Hamilton Rating Scale for Anxiety, which is usually used to determine the efficacy of medications in generalised anxiety disorder. A very low score on this instrument indicates remission.

EFFICACY VERSUS EFFECTIVENESS

The efficacy of medications for anxiety disorders has been investigated in numerous randomised, double-blinded, placebo-controlled studies. These studies often have strict inclusion and exclusion criteria. For example, patients with certain co-occurring conditions such as depression, substance abuse and dependence, severe personality disorders and many medical illnesses are usually excluded. Also, women of childbearing age are not included unless they use strict methods of contraception. Therefore, conditions under which these controlled studies are conducted are often not representative of patients and treatments in real world conditions. For the same reason, the efficacy of medications established in these studies does not necessarily translate to their effectiveness – a term that implies therapeutic effects in real world conditions. It is important to bear this in mind, as there are very few effectiveness studies.

MEDICATIONS EFFICACIOUS IN ANXIETY DISORDERS

Several groups of medications have been identified as efficacious in treating various anxiety disorders. Groups that are efficacious for at least one anxiety disorder include several types of antidepressants and benzodiazepines (BDZ), which act mainly as anxiolytics or antianxiety agents. The efficacy has been demonstrated for the following antidepressants:

- selective serotonin reuptake inhibitors (SSRIs)
- serotonin and noradrenaline (norepinephrine) reuptake inhibitors (SNRIs)
- tricyclic antidepressants (TCAs)
- classical monoamine oxidase inhibitors (MAOIs).

MEDICATIONS ARE NOT EFFICACIOUS FOR ALL ANXIETY DISORDERS

The medications mentioned above are not efficacious for all anxiety disorders.

Selective serotonin reuptake inhibitors are efficacious for panic disorder, generalised anxiety disorder, social anxiety disorder, and obsessive-compulsive disorder. They are also efficacious in the treatment of posttraumatic stress disorder.

Venlafaxine, a serotonin and noradrenaline reuptake inhibitor, has shown efficacy in treating panic disorder, generalised anxiety disorder, and social anxiety disorder. It may also be efficacious for posttraumatic stress disorder. Duloxetine, another serotonin and noradrenaline reuptake inhibitor, is efficacious for generalised anxiety disorder. Imipramine, which is a tricyclic antidepressant, is efficacious in the treatment of panic disorder and generalised anxiety disorder, whereas clomipramine, a tricyclic antidepressant with predominantly serotonergic effects, is efficacious for obsessive-compulsive disorder and panic disorder. Classical monoamine oxidase inhibitors, especially phenelzine, have been efficacious in treating social anxiety disorder, but they have also shown some efficacy in treating panic disorder. Benzodiazepines have an established efficacy for panic disorder, generalised anxiety disorder and social anxiety disorder.

EVIDENCE FOR PANIC DISORDER

Table 43.1 shows the results of two systematic reviews of pharmacological treatments of panic disorder with and without agoraphobia. They show that when compared to placebo, selective serotonin reuptake inhibitors, tricyclic antidepressants imipramine and clomipramine, and benzodiazepines alprazolam and clonazepam are approximately equally efficacious in the treatment of panic disorder.

Table 43.1 Systematic reviews of pharmacological treatments of panic disorder with and without agoraphobia

Comparison	Effect size for "anxiety"	Number needed to treat (NNT) estimates
SSRIs v. placebo	0.41	All SSRIs: NNT = 8, 95% CI = 6 to 11 Paroxetine: NNT = 5, 95% CI = 3 to 7 Citalopram: NNT = 5, 95% CI = 3 to 11 Sertraline: NNT = 8, 95% CI = 5 to 20
TCAs v. placebo	0.41	All TCAs: NNT = 6, 95% CI = 5 to 8 Imipramine: NNT = 6, 95% CI = 4 to 8 Clomipramine: NNT = 7, 95% CI = 4 to17
BDZ v. placebo	0.40	Alprazolam: NNT = 5, 95% CI 4 to 7 Clonazepam: NNT = 5, 95% CI 4 to 7

Note. NNT = number needed to treat. Data adapted from Mitte (2005) and von Knorring et al. (2005).

EVIDENCE FOR GENERALISED ANXIETY DISORDER

One systematic review of antidepressant medications for generalised anxiety disorder (Table 43.2) shows that antidepressants are more efficacious than placebo (Kapczinski et al., 2003).

Table 43.2 Results of a systematic review of antidepressant medications for generalised anxiety disorder

Comparison	Result
Overall antidepressants v. placebo	NNT = 6, 95% CI = 5 to 9
Paroxetine v. placebo	NNT = 6.72, 95% CI = 3.9 to 24.7
Venlafaxine v. placebo	NNT = 5, 95% CI = 3.58 to 8.62
Imipramine v. placebo	NNT = 4, 95% CI = 3 to 14

Note. Response rate was 54% with antidepressants and 38% with placebo. NNT = number needed to treat. Data adapted from Kapczinski et al. (2003).

EVIDENCE FOR SOCIAL ANXIETY DISORDER

A systematic review of all randomised controlled trials of the pharmacotherapy for social anxiety disorder (Table 43.3) demonstrated the efficacy of medication treatment, with the selective serotonin reuptake inhibitors being most consistently efficacious. Medications were found to be efficacious in both short-term and long-term treatment (Stein et al., 2009a).

Table 43.3 Results of a systematic review of all randomised controlled trials of the pharmacotherapy for social anxiety disorder

Comparison	Result
Medication v. placebo	Change in symptom severity: WMD = -18, 95% CI = -25.17 to -10.83
All medication groups v. placebo	Short-term treatment response: RR of non-response = 0.64, 95% CI = 0.57 to 0.73
Maintenance trials	Treatment response: RR of non-response = 0.62, 95% CI = 0.50 to 0.77
Relapse prevention trials	RR of relapse = 0.33, 95% CI = 0.22 to 0.49
SSRIs v. reversible MAOIs	SSRIs more efficacious than reversible MAOIs (e.g., moclobemide, brofaromine)

Note. Data adapted for Stein et al. (2009a).

EVIDENCE FOR OBSESSIVE-COMPULSIVE DISORDER

One meta-analysis of controlled pharmacotherapy trials in obsessive-compulsive disorder has found the efficacy of clomipramine and several selective serotonin reuptake inhibitors (Ackerman & Greenland, 2002). It also reported that there were no significant differences in efficacy between clomipramine and three of the selective serotonin reuptake inhibitors: fluoxetine, fluvoxamine, and paroxetine.

EVIDENCE FOR POSTTRAUMATIC STRESS DISORDER

A systematic review of all randomised controlled trials of the pharmacotherapy for posttraumatic stress disorder demonstrated the efficacy of medication treatment, with selective serotonin reuptake inhibitors being the most efficacious agents (Stein et al., 2009b).

OTHER MEDICATIONS FOR ANXIETY DISORDERS

A number of other medications have also been found to be efficacious for various anxiety disorders. They are usually used in patients who are resistant to standard pharmacotherapy with antidepressants and/or benzodiazepines. The strength of evidence for their efficacy varies, and while they may be useful in some conditions and in some clinical situations, they lack efficacy in others. These medications are shown in Table 43.4.

Table 43.4   Alternative pharmacotherapy for anxiety disorders

Medication	Usage
Second-generation antipsychotics (e.g., quetiapine, risperidone, olanzapine)	In conjunction with antidepressants for obsessive-compulsive disorder and posttraumatic stress disorder; evidence of efficacy for quetiapine monotherapy in generalised anxiety disorder
Pregabalin	Strong evidence of efficacy in the treatment of generalised anxiety disorder
Hydroxyzine	Efficacious in the treatment of generalised anxiety disorder
Buspirone	Efficacious in the treatment of generalised anxiety disorder
Beta-blockers (e.g., propranolol, atenolol)	In combination with antidepressants for generalised anxiety disorder and social anxiety disorder (especially performance-type social anxiety)
Mirtazapine	Useful for some patients with posttraumatic stress disorder and generalised anxiety disorder
Prazosin	Efficacy in treating nightmares as part of posttraumatic stress disorder
Anticonvulsants and mood stabilisers	In combination with antidepressants for posttraumatic stress disorder

In addition, various other medications have been used to treat anxiety disorders, either as monotherapy or in combination with other agents. Their efficacy remains to be established through controlled trials.

EVIDENCE FOR PHARMACOTHERAPY AUGMENTATION

Ipser et al. (2006) performed a systematic review of 28 short-term, randomised controlled trials of medication versus placebo augmentation, in the treatment of patients with anxiety disorders who failed to respond adequately to first-line pharmacotherapy.

Of these trials, 20 investigated antipsychotic augmentation of serotonin reuptake inhibitors in patients with obsessive-compulsive disorder who were unresponsive to serotonin reuptake inhibitors alone. Results showed overall superiority of various medications over placebo as augmentation strategy in treatment-resistant anxiety disorders (Table 43.5).

Table 43.5   Results of a systematic review of medication augmentation in the treatment of anxiety disorders

Comparison	Result
Medication v. placebo (9 studies)	Responder status: RR = 3.16, 95% CI = 1.08 to 9.23
Medication v. placebo (14 studies)	Reduction in symptom severity: SMD = -0.87, 95% CI = -1.37 to -0.36

Note. Data adapted from Ipser et al. (2006).

EVIDENCE FOR AZAPIRONES

Another systematic review (Chessick et al., 2006) was performed to ascertain the efficacy of azapirones in generalised anxiety disorder. Buspirone is the main medication in this group of drugs, which act on the 5-HT1A receptors. The review included 36 short-term trials (lasting 4–9 weeks, except for one trial where the duration was 14 weeks), which randomly allocated patients to azapirones and/or placebo, benzodiazepines, antidepressants, psychotherapy, or kava kava. Azapirones were superior to placebo (NNT = 4.4, 95% CI = 2.16 to 15.4).

However, they may be less efficacious than benzodiazepines, and the review could not determine whether azapirones were superior to antidepressants, kava kava or psychotherapy. Azapirones also did not appear as well tolerated as benzodiazepines.

SIDE EFFECTS OF MEDICATIONS

Establishing efficacy of the pharmacotherapy is only one side of the coin. The other is tolerability of the medications, which is just as important a consideration when making a decision about using pharmacological agents. Also, side effects are a common reason for patients to stop taking the medication.

Tolerability of medication is just as important a consideration as efficacy of the pharmacotherapy.

Unfortunately, it is practically impossible to predict with great certainty whether a particular patient will develop specific side effects of a particular medication unless he or she took that medication in the past. With this uncertainty in mind, it is best to inform patients of the most common side effects, stay in contact with them after they have started the medication, and ask them specifically whether they are experiencing any side effects. It is important for clinicians to know how troubled patients are by the side effects, as this will help them take appropriate action. Likewise, patients need to know which side effects are transient and which ones are likely to persist.

SPECIFIC SIDE EFFECTS

The most common side effects of the selective serotonin reuptake inhibitors are nausea, upset stomach, diarrhoea, headache, dizziness and insomnia (Table 43.6). These side effects may be particularly prominent at the beginning of treatment and usually abate with continued pharmacotherapy. They are generally unpredictable, and patients differ tremendously in their tendency to experience and ability to tolerate the side effects of the selective serotonin reuptake inhibitors. Thus, some individuals report virtually no side effects, whereas others describe this treatment as "the worst ever experience".

Table 43.6 Common side effects of the selective serotonin reuptake inhibitors (SSRIs) and venlafaxine

Medication	Side effect
SSRIs	Nausea, upset stomach, diarrhoea, headache, dizziness, insomnia Increased anxiety or agitation Sexual dysfunction Weight gain (in some cases and with some SSRIs)
Venlafaxine	Lower doses: side effects similar to those of SSRIs Higher doses: hypertension, in addition to side effects typical of SSRIs

Another side effect of the selective serotonin reuptake inhibitors, which may be observed during the first few weeks of treatment, is an increase in anxiety or agitation, often referred to as "jitteriness syndrome" or "activation syndrome". Patients may find it particularly difficult to tolerate increase in anxiety or agitation, and it is therefore a frequent reason for premature cessation of the medication. This side effect commonly occurs in patients with panic disorder and in others who are troubled by somatic symptoms, possibly because of their intolerance, fear or misinterpretation of these symptoms. One way of preventing increased anxiety or agitation is to commence treatment with a very low dose, then gradually increase it. The other option is to commence a selective serotonin reuptake inhibitor with a benzodiazepine from the beginning of treatment, then gradually discontinue a benzodiazepine after 6 to 12 weeks of treatment, while continuing treatment with a selective serotonin reuptake inhibitor.

The most troublesome potential long-term side effect of the selective serotonin reuptake inhibitors are various problems with sexual functioning. Sexual dysfunction usually takes the form of delayed or inhibited ejaculation in men and anorgasmia in women, and is one of the common reasons for premature cessation of pharmacological treatment.

Weight gain has generally not been a problem with the selective serotonin reuptake inhibitors, but there have been reports that some of these medications, especially paroxetine, may be associated with weight gain.

When used in lower doses, venlafaxine has a side effect profile similar to that of the selective serotonin reuptake inhibitors. In higher doses, it may be associated with high blood pressure.

Tricyclic antidepressants generally produce more side effects than selective serotonin reuptake inhibitors, and these include anticholinergic symptoms such as dry mouth, blurred vision, constipation and urinary hesitancy, in addition to sedation, weight gain, postural hypotension, tachycardia, sexual dysfunction and lowering of the seizure threshold (Table 43.7). In view of their side-effect profile and specific organ toxicity, tricyclic antidepressants are contraindicated in patients with cardiac arrhythmias, enlarged prostate, glaucoma and epilepsy.

Table 43.7 Common side effects of tricyclic antidepressants (TCAs), classical monoamine oxidase inhibitors (MAOIs) and benzodiazepines

Medication	Side effects
TCAs	Dry mouth, blurred vision, constipation, urinary hesitancy, sedation, weight gain, postural hypotension, tachycardia, sexual dysfunction, lowering of the seizure threshold
Classical MAOIs	Hypotension, insomnia, agitation, weight gain, sexual dysfunction
Benzodiazepines	Sedation, impaired psychomotor coordination, memory problems, falls in elderly

The use of classical monoamine oxidase inhibitors is limited by their unfavourable side-effect profile (e.g., hypotension, insomnia, agitation, weight gain and sexual dysfunction), potentially dangerous interactions with numerous medications and the necessity of avoiding all food that contains tyramine (e.g., many types of cheese) to prevent an abrupt and large increase in blood pressure.

Benzodiazepines are generally well tolerated. Their main side effect is sedation, which usually occurs at the very beginning of treatment or immediately after the dose has been increased. Tolerance to the sedative effects of benzodiazepines develops quickly, which means that the initial dose that caused sedation usually ceases to do so within a few days of continued administration.

Another common side effect is impaired psychomotor coordination, which calls for caution when patients drive, operate heavy machinery or perform complex tasks such as flying planes. Both sedation and impaired psychomotor performance become more prominent if the person also drinks alcohol and they may be particularly troublesome in the elderly, because of their association with falls and fractures. It follows that elderly patients should use benzodiazepines with caution and preferably at the lowest possible dose. Some people complain of having difficulty remembering what happened in the period of up to several hours after they took a benzodiazepine – this is commonly referred to as anterograde amnesia.

CHOICE OF PHARMACOTHERAPY WHEN THERE IS NO DIFFERENCE IN EFFICACY

How do clinicians go about choosing medications for anxiety disorders?

As with other conditions and clinical situations, these choices result mainly from consideration of the medications' efficacy and tolerability, but there are additional factors that influence the decision in anxiety disorders (Table 43.8).

As already noted, in some anxiety disorders such as panic disorder and generalised anxiety disorder, substantial differences in efficacy between various medications have not been observed. Therefore, a number of factors may play a crucial role in determining which medication is used.

- If the onset of efficacy is an important consideration, benzodiazepines have an advantage over antidepressants because they work faster.
- In terms of the side effects, benzodiazepines are generally better tolerated than selective serotonin reuptake inhibitors and venlafaxine, and in turn, selective serotonin reuptake inhibitors and venlafaxine are usually better tolerated than tricyclic antidepressants.

- When patients with anxiety disorders present with other mental disorders, especially depression, or if they have a history of depression, antidepressants are a more logical choice.
- If there is a relatively high risk of suicide, benzodiazepines and selective serotonin reuptake inhibitors have an advantage, because they are relatively safe in overdose. Cases of lethal outcome of an overdose with venlafaxine have been reported, while tricyclic antidepressants are usually lethal in overdose.
- If patients have a history of alcohol or other substance use disorders, benzodiazepines should generally be avoided, because they may then be more likely to be misused.

Table 43.8 Factors that influence the decision about medication use in anxiety disorders

Factors	SSRIs	Venlafaxine	TCAs	BDZ
Speed of therapeutic response	0	0	0	+++
Side effect profile/tolerability	++	+/++	0	+++
Presence of other mental disorders, especially depression and history of depression	+++	+++	+++	0
Safety in overdose	+++	+	0	+++
History of alcohol or other substance abuse/dependence	+++	+++	+++	0

Note. +++ = Clear advantage. ++ = Some/relative advantage. + = Minimal advantage. 0 = No advantage.

Sometimes a few other factors may play a role, for example cost and drug interactions. However, almost all of these medications exist in a generic form and do not differ substantially in terms of cost. Care should be taken not to combine selective serotonin reuptake inhibitors, venlafaxine or tricyclic antidepressants with classical monoamine oxidase inhibitors. Furthermore, these groups of antidepressants should generally not be combined with each other, while some selective serotonin reuptake inhibitors such as fluoxetine and fluvoxamine should not be taken together with a number of cholesterol-lowering agents and other psychiatric medications.

When all these factors are taken into consideration, selective serotonin reuptake inhibitors are usually the first-line medication in the treatment of most anxiety disorders.

CHAPTER 44   BENZODIAZEPINES AND ANXIETY DISORDERS

Vladan Starcevic

BENZODIAZEPINES: HISTORICAL AND SOCIAL CONTEXT

Benzodiazepines (BDZs) were introduced in the early 1960s. They have been called "sedatives" and "minor tranquilisers". More precisely, benzodiazepines have been classified as anti-anxiety medications or "anxiolytics", and they remain the prototypical medications in this group. They have also been used for other purposes: as hypnotics (to alleviate sleep disturbance), anticonvulsants (in the treatment of epilepsy), muscle relaxants and to induce anaesthesia.

Benzodiazepines quickly became very popular for a variety of reasons. The most succinct explanation for their rise entails the societal need for substances with calming effects. Throughout the centuries, this need has been met mainly with alcohol. In the decade prior to the introduction of benzodiazepines, barbiturates and meprobamate were often used to alleviate anxiety and distress. However, they were both associated with dependence, and barbiturates were lethal in overdose. Being much safer than alcohol, barbiturates and meprobamate, benzodiazepines were described as "one of the twentieth century's greatest inventions". Small wonder, then, that diazepam, the quintessential benzodiazepine, was the most widely prescribed medication of any kind in the Western world between 1968 and 1987.

What caused a decreased enthusiasm for benzodiazepines?

In a nutshell, it is the fact that they are habit-forming – a characteristic often referred to as "dependence" or "addictiveness". Benzodiazepines have thus become controversial in the treatment of anxiety disorders and they have divided doctors into those who emphasise problems with their use and avoid them and others who continue to prescribe them, albeit often reluctantly, if not secretively. Benzodiazepines are also a common reason for the rift between patients who believe they are useful and doctors who refuse to prescribe them because of their "addictiveness."

CONTINUING POPULARITY OF THE BENZODIAZEPINES

Despite the fact that benzodiazepines are not considered to be a first-line pharmacotherapy option for anxiety disorders, there are several reasons for their ongoing use and popularity among both the patients and doctors who prescribe them.

First, benzodiazepines are consistently effective for relieving anxiety, tension and various physical symptoms of anxiety. This is particularly apparent in an acute setting, for example, an emergency department.

Second, the great advantage of benzodiazepines over antidepressants is that they work quickly – the onset of their anti-anxiety action occurs within minutes after their administration. Again, this is very useful in an acute setting, where patients usually ask for quick alleviation of their distress.

Third, benzodiazepines are usually well tolerated, often with fewer side effects than antidepressants. Side effects, which were discussed in detail in Chapter 43, relatively rarely appear to be a reason for stopping these medications.

Fourth, benzodiazepines are safe in an overdose, if not taken in combination with some other medications. This is of particular importance when pharmacotherapy is considered for suicidal or depressed patients.

Fifth, benzodiazepines can be administered on an "as-needed" (prn) basis, because they work quickly. Such use is popular with those patients who prefer not to take these medications on a regular, long-term basis.

Finally, there has been some disappointment with antidepressants in the treatment of anxiety disorders, and this has probably also contributed to the popularity of benzodiazepines. These problems include antidepressants' slow onset of therapeutic action, their occasionally severe side effects and inconsistent or unreliable effectiveness in some cases.

> The great advantage of benzodiazepines over antidepressants is that they work quickly.

EVIDENCE OF EFFICACY

Panic Disorder

Two large 8-week, randomised, double-blinded, placebo-controlled trials of alprazolam, a high-potency benzodiazepine, demonstrated that it was superior to placebo in treating panic disorder (Ballenger et al., 1988; Cross-National Collaborative Panic Study Second Phase Investigators, 1992). In one of these studies, 55% of patients taking alprazolam were panic-free after 8 weeks of treatment, compared to 32% of patients taking placebo (Ballenger et al., 1988).

In addition, alprazolam was found to be equally efficacious as imipramine, a tricyclic antidepressant, with a distinct advantage of alprazolam being its quicker onset of action (Cross-National Collaborative Panic Study Second Phase Investigators, 1992).

Generalised Anxiety Disorder

Table 44.1 shows the results of two meta-analyses of pharmacological treatments of generalised anxiety disorder. Mean effect size for benzodiazepines was comparable to that for other medications in one study (Mitte et al., 2005). It was comparably lower in the other meta-analysis (Hidalgo et al., 2007). In both studies, however, mean effect sizes for benzodiazepines were higher than mean effect sizes for selective serotonin reuptake inhibitors.

Table 44.1   Results of two meta-analyses of pharmacological treatments of generalised anxiety disorder

Meta-analysis	Medication	Mean effect size
Mitte et al. (2005)	Venlafaxine	0.33
	Benzodiazepines	0.32
	Buspirone	0.30
	Paroxetine	0.20
Hidalgo et al. (2007)	Pregabalin	0.50
	Hydroxyzine	0.45
	Venlafaxine	0.42
	Benzodiazepines	0.38
	SSRIs	0.36

Social Anxiety Disorder

Controlled studies have also established the efficacy of two benzodiazepines, clonazepam and bromazepam, in short-term treatment of social anxiety disorder, as demonstrated in Table 44.2.

Table 44.2   Studies suggesting efficacy of benzodiazepines for social anxiety disorder

Medication	Result
Clonazepam v. placebo	A 10-week double-blind, placebo-controlled trial (Davidson et al., 1993) Responder rate: 78% (clonazepam) v. 20% (placebo)
Bromazepam v. placebo	A 12-week randomised, double-blind, placebo-controlled trial (Versiani et al., 1997) Bromazepam superior to placebo on all outcome measures

BENZODIAZEPINE DEPENDENCE

Benzodiazepine dependence is the most controversial aspect of the benzodiazepine use.

When benzodiazepines are used over longer periods of time, which may mean just a few months, a physiological adaptation occurs at the receptor and neurotransmitter level to the continuous presence of these medications.

If benzodiazepines are then suddenly stopped, this triggers a reaction, which is called a withdrawal or abstinence syndrome. From a clinical perspective, dependence means that care must be taken when stopping a benzodiazepine – it does not imply abuse, drug-seeking or lack of benefit.

This type of dependence has sometimes been referred to as "therapeutic" or "non-addictive", to distinguish it from dependence that occurs in the context of true substance addiction.

BENZODIAZEPINE ABUSE

Benzodiazepines can certainly be abused. Abuse refers to a pattern of indiscriminate use, often with a tendency to increase the dose. Such a pattern is rarely seen among people suffering from anxiety disorders and most commonly occurs in conjunction with other substance abuse. According to the *American Psychiatric Association Task Force Report on*

Benzodiazepines, "Benzodiazepines are not drugs of abuse, although benzodiazepine abuse is common among people who are actively abusing alcohol, opiates, cocaine or sedative hypnotics" (Salzman, 1991, p.152).

Thus, patients with anxiety disorders who use benzodiazepines on a long-term basis and who have developed physical dependence on these medications but have very few or no symptoms and are functioning well, are not abusing benzodiazepines. Likewise, patients with anxiety disorders who have no tendency to abuse alcohol or other drugs usually need not worry that they will end up abusing benzodiazepines.

BENZODIAZEPINE DEPENDENCE VERSUS ADDICTION TO SUBSTANCES

Despite the distinctions suggested in the previous text, benzodiazepines are still commonly regarded as "addictive". This continues to contribute to their negative image. Therefore, it is important to clarify how benzodiazepine dependence differs from addiction to substances such as alcohol, heroin or cocaine (Table 44.3).

Table 44.3   Distinction between benzodiazepine dependence and addiction to substances

Distinction criteria	Benzodiazepine dependence	Addiction to substances
Tolerance	No *	Yes
An all-encompassing preoccupation with and/or craving for the substance	No	Yes
Compulsive drug-seeking behaviour	No	Yes
Adverse health and/or social consequences	No	Yes
Withdrawal symptoms upon abrupt cessation	Yes	Yes

Note. * Most of the evidence suggests that patients with anxiety disorders do not develop tolerance to anxiolytic effects of benzodiazepines during long-term treatment.

Addiction can be considered to exist if several criteria have been met. First, the person exhibits tolerance. This means a need to increase the dose of the substance to produce the same initial effect.

Furthermore, there is an intense craving for and/or preoccupation with the addictive substance, the person engages in compulsive drug-seeking behaviour, there are adverse health and/or social consequences of the substance use and withdrawal symptoms occur upon abrupt discontinuation of the substance. Of these characteristics of addiction, benzodiazepines are clearly associated only with withdrawal symptoms upon their abrupt discontinuation.

The association between benzodiazepines and tolerance to their anxiolytic effect has been debated, and there have been reports of patients who needed to increase the dose in order to continue experiencing the initial anti-anxiety effect.

However, several studies have shown that, during long-term treatment with benzodiazepines, the vast majority of patients with anxiety disorders who have no substance abuse issues do not exhibit a tendency to increase the dose. Studies have also reported no loss of therapeutic benefit of benzodiazepines over their long-term use, suggesting, therefore, that no tolerance develops to the anxiolytic effects of benzodiazepines.

BENZODIAZEPINE WITHDRAWAL SYNDROME

From a practical perspective, benzodiazepine use remains controversial largely because of the fear of withdrawal syndrome. Benzodiazepine withdrawal syndrome (Table 44.4) consists of symptoms that are often vague, difficult to describe and non-specific. These symptoms may be difficult to distinguish from recurrence of an anxiety disorder.

Table 44.4   Benzodiazepine withdrawal syndrome

Non-specific symptoms	Relatively specific symptoms
Increased anxiety	Hypersensitivity to light, sound,
Restlessness	smell, or taste
Insomnia	Feeling of things moving as if being
Nausea	on a boat
Stomach cramps	Distorted body image
Flu-like symptoms	Suspiciousness
Numbness or tingling sensations	Feeling confused
Unsteady gait	Depersonalisation
Muscle cramps	Derealisation
Involuntary muscle movements	Disturbances of perception
Irritability	Ringing in the ears
Feeling depressed or weak	Seizures (rare)
Tiredness	

There are also a number of relatively specific symptoms, although they are not always present. Seizures are the most serious withdrawal symptom, but they occur rarely. Withdrawal symptoms do not last very long, usually from several days to two weeks. They leave no consequences and often disappear without treatment.

While benzodiazepine withdrawal syndrome is not a pleasant experience, it is rarely life-threatening.

However, it is often portrayed in an exaggerated manner, as the worst experience one can have. This only intensifies patients' fears, and some continue taking benzodiazepines only to avoid a withdrawal, not because they really think they need the medication. In these situations, patients may believe that they cannot stop taking the medication, which only reinforces the notion that they are "addicted".

PREVENTING BENZODIAZEPINE WITHDRAWAL SYNDROME

Benzodiazepine withdrawal syndrome should be neither overestimated nor underestimated. As with many other health-related issues, the best approach to the benzodiazepine withdrawal syndrome is its prevention.

The key to a successful prevention of the benzodiazepine withdrawal symptoms is a gradual and careful decrease in the dose of benzodiazepines before they are ceased. The patient should not feel forced into a benzodiazepine taper, and the taper needs to be individualised. In other words, the patient needs to feel ready for gradual medication cessation, and it is crucial to be flexible about the duration of taper and not to set time limits. Hence the benzodiazepines can be discontinued over a broad range of periods – in the course of only several weeks or over as long as one year.

The taper should ideally proceed under a physician's supervision; not only is the physician best placed to suggest the pace at which the dose is to be decreased, but they should be there to monitor the patient's progress and provide support. This support is especially important when some of the withdrawal symptoms occur during taper or when the patient becomes ambivalent about continuing the taper.

Finally, some techniques of cognitive-behavioural therapy have been effective in facilitating discontinuation of the benzodiazepines. These techniques may be used when patients find it particularly difficult to complete the taper.

SAFE LONG-TERM USE OF BENZODIAZEPINES

Benzodiazepines can be used safely and effectively over long periods of time. There are several rules that should be followed, with the goal of minimising the risks and maximising the benefits in the course of treatment with these agents.

First, there should be a careful consideration of the type of patients who might benefit from benzodiazepines. For example, people with current or past substance use problems should generally be considered unsuitable for treatment with benzodiazepines, because of their propensity to misuse dependence-producing agents.

Second, the side effects of benzodiazepines should be carefully monitored and any adjustment in dosage should be made accordingly.

Finally, and as already mentioned, prevention of the withdrawal syndrome is particularly important. This entails a gradual and individualised taper, supportive psychological measures and when necessary, specific techniques of cognitive-behavioural therapy.

Some patients may vehemently resist cessation of benzodiazepines. In such cases, it is pointless to antagonise patients by insisting that they stop benzodiazepines "no matter what". While the clinician should not abandon efforts to persuade patients that continued treatment may not be necessary, refusing to prescribe benzodiazepines or using other coercive measures is only likely to lead to more difficulties. It is fortunate that benzodiazepines may be taken for many years without adverse consequences, as there is no evidence that they cause permanent tissue damage.

CHAPTER 45   COMBINING MEDICATIONS AND COGNITIVE-BEHAVIOURAL TREATMENTS

Vladan Starcevic

WHY COMBINE MEDICATIONS WITH COGNITIVE-BEHAVIOURAL THERAPY

Both medications and cognitive-behavioural therapy (CBT) have advantages and disadvantages. The rationale for combining them in anxiety disorders is that they might act in a complementary fashion and thereby lead to better outcomes. For example, medication treatment may reduce incapacitating levels of anxiety or panic in patients who have commenced CBT, and thereby enhance the latter. Conversely, patients initially treated with medications may benefit from decreased avoidance behaviour resulting from the addition of an exposure-based therapy. Combining the two approaches has an intuitive appeal and is the likely reason for the apparent popularity of combined treatment in clinical practice. Therefore, the issue of combined treatment and potential problems associated with it deserves a closer scrutiny.

POTENTIAL PROBLEMS WITH COMBINATION TREATMENT

Whenever the two treatments are combined, the fundamental question is about the benefit of such a combination. In other words, does a combination of pharmacotherapy and CBT achieve better results than either treatment alone? If it does, there is justification for its use; if it does not, pharmacotherapy alone or CBT alone may be sufficient. It is this issue that has generated the most controversy.

Furthermore, instead of potentiating each other's effects, medications and CBT may not work synergistically. In particular, it has been suggested that medications may interfere with CBT: if treatment progress primarily entails coping better with anxiety and learning that anxiety is not dangerous, this can be achieved only if patients confront anxiety-provoking situations and symptoms without the facilitating effects of the concomitantly administered medication. In other words, according to the CBT approach, anxiety is necessary for the successful outcome of exposure to anxiety-eliciting situations.

It has been argued that by decreasing anxiety, medications may promote passivity and reduce motivation for participation in CBT. If this is correct, patients may not fully benefit from CBT, a result which becomes apparent especially during and after long-term treatment.

During the concomitant administration of pharmacotherapy and CBT, there is no precise way of knowing what proportion of improvement is due to medication and what proportion is a result of CBT. If patients attribute progress to the medication more than to learning new skills through CBT and personal mastery, they may run a risk of recurrence once the medication has been ceased. The recurrence may then be a consequence of patients' difficulty in developing a sense of ownership of their treatment gains.

Medications may also interfere with the acquisition of new skills through CBT, because of the "state-dependent" learning of these skills. That is, the skills learned while patients are taking a medication cannot be applied to other situations (in which they were not originally learned); also, patients may not be able to use these skills if medication is no longer taken. However, there has been mixed support for the existence of state-dependent learning, and, more broadly, for the interference of medications with learning that occurs during CBT.

It is also possible for some medications, especially benzodiazepines, to interfere with memory, so that material presented and discussed in the course of CBT sessions may not be well remembered if a benzodiazepine has been taken just prior to these sessions.

Finally, medications may serve as "safety devices" when taken in the course of CBT. That means that the mere presence of medications provides a sense of safety as patients attempt to cope with anxiety, and this may interfere with their reliance on the newly learned skills in managing anxiety. When, for example, patients carry medications whilst doing their exposure tasks in the course of CBT, this behaviour is often referred to as "safety behaviour". The use of medications as "safety devices" perpetuates a notion that anxiety and its physical symptoms are dangerous and should be best dealt with by suppression. When the medication is ceased, patients may then feel unprotected and fully exposed to the perceived danger of their symptoms and anxiety.

COMBINATION TREATMENT: RESEARCH FINDINGS

Most combination treatment studies have been conducted in panic disorder and obsessive-compulsive disorder, with very few being conducted in other anxiety disorders. The most consistent finding across the studies and the disorders is that combination treatment is more efficacious than pharmacotherapy alone, and that it is associated with a lower likelihood of relapse after the treatment has been ceased. Combination treatment may also be more efficacious than CBT alone, but this has not been reported consistently. When the combination treatment works better than CBT, the difference in efficacy is usually observed over the short-term treatment period. It appears that this advantage of combination treatment tends to decrease or even disappear over the long-term treatment and especially after the cessation of pharmacotherapy, leading to reports of equal long-term efficacy of combination treatment and CBT, or even greater efficacy of CBT.

These findings call for efforts to conduct large and better-designed studies of combination treatment, especially in view of the cost-effectiveness issues and the fact that combination treatment is popular in clinical practice, preferred by some patients and clinicians, and often endorsed by experts and treatment guidelines.

Panic Disorder

A systematic review of all controlled studies compared combined treatments to psychotherapy alone and antidepressant treatment alone, for panic disorder with and without agoraphobia (Furukawa et al., 2009). Twenty-one of 23 studies involved behaviour therapy or CBT. This review demonstrated advantages of combined treatment over either monotherapy in the short-term, but failed to show its superiority over behaviour therapy or CBT in the long run (Table 45.1).

Table 45.1 Results of a systematic review of controlled studies that compared combined treatments to psychotherapy alone and antidepressant treatment alone for panic disorder with and without agoraphobia

Phase	Results
Acute phase treatment	Combined therapy v. antidepressants alone: RR = 1.24, 95% CI = 1.02 to 1.52
	Combined therapy v. psychotherapy (CBT) alone: RR = 1.17, 95% CI = 1.05 to 1.31
After the acute phase	As long as the medication was continued: Combined therapy > antidepressants alone Combined therapy > psychotherapy (CBT) alone
After termination of the acute phase and during continuation treatment	Combined therapy v antidepressants alone: RR = 1.61, 95% CI = 1.23 to 2.11
	Combined therapy v psychotherapy (CBT) alone: RR = 0.96, 95% CI = 0.79 to 1.16

Note. Data adapted from Furukawa et al. (2009).

Another study reached a different conclusion about the value of long-term medication treatment in patients with panic disorder with and without agoraphobia (van Apeldoorn et al., 2010). This study compared the efficacy of CBT alone, treatment with a selective serotonin reuptake inhibitor (SSRI) alone, and treatment with a combination of CBT and an SSRI over a one-year period and for up to a one-year follow-up after treatment discontinuation. Patients treated with an SSRI alone and with CBT+SSRI were faster to show treatment gains in comparison with those treated with CBT alone, and there were no significant differences between treatment modalities at the end of the one-year follow-up. The most important finding was that SSRIs, whether administered alone or in combination with CBT, were associated with the maintenance of treatment gains in panic disorder to the same extent as CBT for up to one year after treatment discontinuation.

Social Anxiety Disorder

One randomised, double-blind, placebo-controlled study compared cognitive-behavioural group therapy (CBGT), phenelzine (a classical MAO inhibitor) and combined CBGT and phenelzine, in 128 patients with social anxiety disorder (Blanco et al., 2010). After 12 and 24 weeks of treatment, combined treatment was superior to either treatment alone and to placebo in terms of the rates of response and remission (Table 45.2).

Table 45.2 Results of a double-blind comparison of cognitive-behavioural group therapy (CBGT), phenelzine, placebo and combined CGBT and phenelzine

Treatment	Response rate at Week 12 ($p = 0.001$)	Remission rate at Week 24 ($p = 0.001$)
CBGT	52.9%	23.5%
Phenelzine	48.6%	25.7%
Placebo	33.3%	14.8%
CBGT + phenelzine	78.1%	53.1%

Note. Data adapted from Blanco et al., (2010).

Obsessive-compulsive Disorder (OCD)

In obsessive-compulsive disorder, only a few controlled trials compared the efficacy of combined treatments with monotherapy with medication or with exposure and response prevention. The latter is the most widely used form of behavioural therapy for obsessive-compulsive disorder.

As shown in Table 45.3, after 12 weeks of treatment in one of these trials (Foa et al., 2005), all active treatments were more efficacious than pill placebo.

However, there was no difference in efficacy between the combination of exposure and response prevention and clomipramine and exposure and response prevention administered alone; also, both of these were superior to treatment with clomipramine alone.

Another trial (van Balkom et al.,1998) compared cognitive therapy alone, exposure and response prevention alone, fluvoxamine (a selective serotonin reuptake inhibitor) plus cognitive therapy, fluvoxamine plus exposure and response prevention and absence of treatment in patients with obsessive-compulsive disorder who were on a waiting list. In this study, there were no groups receiving fluvoxamine alone or a pill placebo, and in patients receiving a combined treatment, psychological therapy was commenced after 8 weeks of treatment with fluvoxamine. All four active treatments were superior to the wait-list condition, but did not differ significantly between themselves.

Table 45.3 Comparisons of pharmacotherapy alone, exposure and response prevention (ERP) alone, cognitive therapy (CT) alone and combination treatments in OCD

Clinical trail	Result
Foa et al. (2005)	ERP + clomipramine = ERP > clomipramine > pill placebo (122 participants)
van Balkom et al. (1998)	ERP = CT = ERP + fluvoxamine = CT + fluvoxamine > wait-list (117 participants)

Posttraumatic Stress Disorder (PTSD)

One systematic review reported results of comparisons between combined treatment and psychological therapy (prolonged exposure or a cognitive-behavioural intervention) alone and selective serotonin reuptake inhibitors administered alone for posttraumatic stress disorder (Hetrick et al., 2010). Only four studies were included.

There was no evidence that significant differences existed between the outcome in patients receiving combined interventions and the outcome in those treated either with psychological therapy alone or pharmacotherapy alone (Table 45.4).

Table 45.4 Results of a systematic review comparing combined treatments with psychological treatment alone and pharmacotherapy alone in PTSD

Comparison	Result
Combined treatment v. prolonged exposure or CBT alone	Mean difference = 2.44 95% CI = -2.87 to 7.35
Combined treatment v. SSRIs alone	Mean difference = -4.70 95% CI = -10.84 to 1.44

Note. Data adapted from Hetrick et al. (2010).

COMBINATION TREATMENT: RESEARCH DIFFICULTIES

Establishing efficacy of combination treatment in anxiety disorders has been difficult for a number of reasons. Such studies are complex and require a collaboration of researchers with different orientations, who also use different methodology, including different outcome criteria. With regards to control conditions, pharmacological studies use pill placebos, whereas psychological placebos have been difficult to develop, and various approaches have been used, e.g., waitlist and "treatment-as-usual". Furthermore, there are uncertainties about the optimal design of these studies. For example, should medications and CBT be administered together from the very beginning of treatment, or should one treatment modality follow the other, and under what circumstances? The interpretation of findings of the studies examining the efficacy of combination treatment can be difficult and can be influenced by researcher allegiance issues. Last, but certainly not the least, it is generally more difficult to find funding for studies of this kind.

For these and other reasons, the number of studies investigating the efficacy of combination treatment in anxiety disorders has been relatively small. Moreover, their findings have often been conflicting, or difficult to reconcile with clinical practice.

HOW CAN COMBINATION TREATMENT BE USED TO MAXIMISE ITS POTENTIAL BENEFIT

Situations when combination treatment may be useful include:

- greater severity of the disorder
- presence of a psychiatric condition besides the anxiety disorder
- partial response to only one treatment modality
- intolerable levels of anxiety or distress at the beginning of CBT, which may interfere with continuation of CBT.

It is crucial to combine medications and CBT in a manner that makes clinical sense.

This means that patients understand the rationale for using combined treatment, because they might have been receiving conflicting messages about the value of different treatments and different underlying models of their anxiety disorder. While patients need to know what the global treatment plan is at the beginning of treatment and should agree to it, they should also be prepared for treatment changes that may need to be introduced (including addition of another treatment modality), depending on their progress.

Patients should also be discouraged from using medication as a safety device. For example, it would not be useful for patients to carry the medication in their purse or pockets whilst undergoing exposure.

Finally, the clinician should not favour one type of treatment, and suggest indirectly that he or she does not value the other treatment as much. In other words, combination treatment is more likely to work if the clinician has a positive attitude toward all of its components and emphasises that they may all contribute to a favourable outcome.

PART XI SUMMARY

Part XI has shown that medications continue to play a role in the treatment of anxiety disorders. Their use does not exclude the use of psychological therapy and vice versa, as both have advantages and disadvantages. The key issue here is to ascertain, as much as possible, which patients might benefit from which type of treatment, and then institute that treatment in full collaboration with the patient and in a way that would improve the outcomes.

Part XI has also emphasised an effective use of medications. This can be done first through a clear understanding of what medications can do and of the goals of pharmacotherapy for anxiety disorders. Secondly, the ways in which medications are administered and ceased often play a crucial role in determining the outcome of pharmacological treatment. Thirdly, the recognition and management of the side effects of medications helps to ensure their appropriate, safe and effective use. For the most part, medications that are used for anxiety disorders include several types of antidepressants and benzodiazepines. Their effectiveness and side effects were presented in an effort to provide a balanced view that takes into account both their advantages and disadvantages. This should assist clinicians in discussing pharmacotherapy treatment options with their patients and in making decisions about the appropriate course of treatment.

Extreme views about the benefit, or lack of benefit, of the pharmacotherapy for anxiety disorders should be abandoned, and medications need to be considered and evaluated in light of both the available evidence and the needs of individual patients. In this regard, the role of benzodiazepines in the treatment of anxiety disorders has been assessed critically, and more light has been shed on the reasons for their continued use and popularity. A careful and safe use of benzodiazepines is likely to be of more benefit than their vilification or prohibition. More broadly, practical and rational considerations should replace various myths about pharmacological treatment.

Finally, Part XI has discussed the common practice of combining pharmacotherapy and cognitive-behavioural therapy in the treatment of anxiety disorders. The studies of combined treatment have been difficult to conduct and have produced some conflicting evidence, calling for more refined research efforts. In the meantime, clinicians should be flexible in their practice and administer this combination, when indicated, in the way that is more likely to lead to better outcomes.

PART XII   REVIEW AND PUTTING IT ALL TOGETHER

The previous chapters have explained that anxiety disorders are a significant public health problem, with one in five people presenting with an anxiety disorder sometime in their life. Table XII.1 summarises the key content in all previous chapters.

Table XII.1   Summary of all previous chapters

Chapters	Key content
1–6	The classification of anxiety orders, their epidemiology, comorbidity and effect upon the individual
7–9	The normal stress response, how that manifests itself as anxiety symptoms and how these symptoms arise from the normal physiological responses of the body. The initial response is rapid and acts in concert with other fast acting mediators to increase vigilance and concentration. The slower mode of response helps the body adapt to stress, learn the lessons and commit them to memory, and prepare us for future stress.
10–12	The biological aetiology of anxiety disorders. The genetic basis of the disorders has been explained, as well as the epigenetic interaction with environmental and developmental factors. There is proof of the concept that the gene-environment interactions do exist. They seem to matter and they are useful for prediction.
13–15	The factors operative early in the development of an individual. These are linked to both childhood and later anxiety. As can be learned from attachment theory, all forms of anxiety disorders other than discrete animal phobias are related to the availability of an attachment figure or absent attachment comforts in childhood. Parental control through over-protection or rejection would increase the likelihood of serious separations.
16–19	The fundamental neurobiology of anxiety. Every therapy session with an anxious patient directly impacts on the neurocircuitry of anxiety, and in this sense, every clinician influences how the patient's brain is managing anxiety. This book has explained how neurobiological processes lead to the development of anxiety disorders, how they underpin the maintenance of these conditions, and most importantly, how they can facilitate effective pharmacology and psychotherapy treatment.

20-24	The cognitive basis for anxiety disorders. This is essential for an understanding of the individual's patterns of thinking, the underlying schemas, as well as their biases. They facilitate and perpetuate the maladaptive ways that people think about their worries. When people go to a clinician in a state of anxiety, they tend to believe that events are the driver of emotions and that events occur to them, and then they find themselves in situations, and that these situations, events and activities drive their emotion. When the clinician understands the cognitive model, their task is to make sure that those people with anxiety disorder understand that it is their thoughts or beliefs that are the real driver of emotion.
25–29	Interview techniques. Effective interview techniques are essential, in order to communicate effectively with patients and understand their current cognitive state. This will further help the clinician elicit the signs and symptoms of anxiety disorders and factors that may predispose, or lead to the maintenance of the disorders. When conducting an interview, it is important to keep in mind that some medical disorders may present as anxiety disorders. This includes substance abuse. During the diagnostic process, structured diagnostic instruments play a critical role, although the choice of instrument will depend on the needs of the assessment.
30–41	Evidence-based techniques for the treatment of anxiety disorders. The behavioural techniques in the treatment of anxiety disorders are widely used. Exposure therapy is central, and was adumbrated in the introduction to the use of cognitive techniques. Panic disorder and obsessive-compulsive disorder were used as templates, and brought together in cognitive-behavioural therapy. The effectiveness of these treatments and the newer web-based therapies for anxiety disorders were then reviewed.
42–45	Medication as treatment for anxiety disorders. While some patients tend to see medications as a panacea and have unrealistic expectations of them, others exhibit overt antagonism to this kind of treatment. Health professionals should be able to explain to their patients about the adverse effects of medication, the rationale and pitfalls of their use and how they might be combined with cognitive-behavioural techniques.

In the final part of this book, we will provide you with a discussion on the debate as whether to use psychological treatments or pharmacotherapy.

CHAPTER 46   PSYCHOTHERAPY OR PHARMACOTHERAPY

Philip Boyce

EVIDENCE-BASED TREATMENTS

How does a clinician decide about what type of treatment will be required for a particular patient?

There is good evidence, based on randomised clinical control trials, for the efficacy of psychological treatments, including cognitive-behavioural therapy and exposure-based therapy, as well as for the effectiveness of pharmacological treatments, particularly the serotonin reuptake inhibitors.

But how is the strength of this evidence determined?

Previous chapters on treatment evidence have explained that the strength of the evidence was reported as the numbers needed to treat, the effect sizes, relative risks, or probability of improvement.

EFFICACY

An important consideration when evaluating these clinical trials is that these are efficacy trials.

Efficacy refers to the beneficial effects of a treatment under experimental conditions. It is important to keep this in mind when evaluating treatments because the patient visiting a clinician may be nothing like the patients who are seen in clinical trials.

Patients seen in clinical trials are selected to have no complications or confounding factors that can influence the experimental study testing the difference between a drug and placebo. This means that many of the patients routinely seen in clinical practice would be excluded from these trials, particularly patients with comorbid medical or psychiatric conditions, and those who misuse substances or alcohol, or have a personality disorder or a complex illness.

EFFECTIVENESS

Such patients could be evaluated by effectiveness trials, which test the beneficial effects of treatment under clinical or real life conditions. These trials test treatments on the sort of patients routinely seen by clinicians.

Unfortunately, there are not many clinical effectiveness trials for the anxiety disorders that are useful for guiding treatment. Instead, the data from the efficacy trials can be used to make informed decisions about which treatment is most appropriate for the patient.

A GUIDING PRINCIPLE

A guiding principle in planning the management for a patient with an anxiety disorder is to fit the treatment to the patient; not the other way around. Often a therapist has one particular therapeutic approach and every patient will be treated using that particular modality, regardless of the patient's problem.

THE PROCRUSTEAN BED

The patient should not be forced into a Procrustean bed.

Procrustes, the son of Poseidon, was a mythological Greek character. He kept a house by the side of the road and offered hospitality to travellers, to whom he gave a meal and a night's rest in his special bed. He told his visitors that this bed had a unique property, in that its length exactly matched whoever lay upon it.

What Procrustes did not say was that, if his guests were too short for the bed, they would be stretched. If too long for the bed, they would have their limbs shortened with an axe.

POINTS TO CONSIDER

In making decisions about the most appropriate treatment for a patient, a number of things need to be taken into account. In particular, the clinician should consider the issues related to the particular patient they are seeing, and balance the patient's illness against their own experience and skills, as well as looking at the pros and cons, or advantages and disadvantages, of the particular treatment. The pragmatic issues of access to treatment and cost also need to be considered.

ISSUES RELATED TO TREATMENT CHOICE

The treatment should be tailored to the patient, rather than having the patient shoehorned into a particular form of a treatment. This means that specific aspects of the patient need to be taken into account.

The Patient's Age

This is important in determining the optimal treatment. For example, medication would not be used for a child as a first-line treatment.

The Patient's Life Circumstances

An example of this would be for women who may be pregnant, when the clinician must consider the risk of exposing the developing foetus to medications. Similarly, if a mother is breastfeeding, the risk of the medication passing through breast milk must be considered.

The Patient's "Mental Health Literacy"

This is critical, as it relates to the person's knowledge and understanding of their disorder and their treatment choices. In this day of the internet, many patients will have some knowledge and expectation of what treatments are available.

The Patient's Motivation

This is linked to their understanding of their disorder. Patients who are not motivated to improve or change are often not good subjects for psychological treatment. It may be that they benefit more from pharmacotherapy.

The Patient's Preference

This is, perhaps, the most important issue in deciding treatment, and needs to be carefully evaluated in the patient's assessment.

The patient should always be told about treatment options. There are many people who do not want to take medications, and offering them pharmacotherapy only, would not be appropriate.

By contrast, there are those who have a preference for "being cured" by taking a tablet, and do not want to put in the work required of a psychological treatment.

OTHER FACTORS THAT INFLUENCE TREATMENT DECISIONS

Aspects of the patient's anxiety disorder that might influence treatment decisions should also be considered.

As discussed in the chapters on the particular types of treatment, there is no "one size fits all" treatment for the anxiety disorders. The treatment one might consider for OCD would not be the same as for a simple phobia. This applies as much for the psychological treatments as it does for the drug treatments.

The severity of the disorder and the amount of associated distress and disability need to be taken into account. When patients have severe and disabling disorders, pharmacotherapy may, in the first instance, be more appropriate than psychological treatments.

Many patients with anxiety disorder have other psychiatric disorders and medical conditions in addition to their anxiety disorder. This will clearly have an impact on the type of treatment the clinician chooses for the patient, particularly as they may already be on other medications.

When they are on other medications, the impact of those medications on the treatment of anxiety must be considered. A classic example of this is the effect of benzodiazepines on memory, and how this can affect psychological treatments.

If the patient is on treatments for a medical condition, there may be drug interactions to take into account if they are to be put on a serotonin reuptake inhibitor.

The clinician's experience, knowledge and skill set is important, as conducting psychological treatments requires training, clinical experience and good counselling skills. For those without such clinical experience, psychological treatment should be applied only if there is appropriate supervision of their therapy.

Psycho-education can be provided for patients, provided the clinician has sufficient knowledge about the conditions to be able to explain the various treatment options to them. Pharmacotherapy also requires experience and knowledge, particularly for dealing with the side-effects of medication, interactions with other medications and the treatment outcomes that could be expected for the patient.

An important aspect of treatment applies to the ability of the patient to get access to the clinician. Trying to provide psychological treatments for a patient when access is only available every two or three months is not going to lead to a good outcome.

In considering the treatments, the advantages and disadvantages of each should be examined.

Patients can expect to get relief from their anxiety in a few weeks if they take medication. Pharmacological treatments are very helpful for patients who are not psychologically minded, or are not motivated to work the psychological treatments. Medications are helpful if the clinician is inexperienced in providing psychological treatment; they are cheaper (in the short term) than psychological treatments and they are also more time efficient, an important consideration in primary care where there are excessive demands on the clinician.

The disadvantages of pharmacological treatments are the side effects that accompany medications, and the fact that the patient will be required to take the medication every day, or suffer a relapse. More important is the fact that they will not learn the skills in dealing with their anxiety, and are at risk of relapsing when the medication is ceased.

Another important consideration is that if there is a good response to the medication, a patient may develop the belief that they have an illness that can be "cured" by a pill. This attribution can lead to the patient being unwilling to take responsibility for dealing with their own anxiety.

The advantages of the psychological treatment are that the patient will learn skills in dealing with their own anxiety. These are lifelong skills, and after the conclusion of treatment they can be used again, should the person be confronted with stressful events that could trigger another episode of their anxiety disorder. These skills give the patient empowerment and a sense of control of themselves. An important aspect of psychological treatments is that they do not have any major side-effects or interactions with other medications, or interfere with a developing foetus or breastfeeding mothers.

The disadvantages of the treatments are the time they take to have an effect. It can take several weeks to a few months for some people to respond to psychological treatment. If the patients are very disabled by their anxiety, this can be a problem. They also take up considerable therapist time.

Initially, these treatments also cost more. While this may be seen as a disadvantage, over time, with their relapse prevention potential, they are more cost-effective than medication.

PUTTING IT TOGETHER

All these issues should be considered before discussing an appropriate treatment plan with the patient. It is critically important that the pros and cons of each type of treatment are discussed with the patient.

Perhaps the most important aspect in determining the treatment is that pharmacotherapy on its own is never appropriate. It needs to be combined with some psychological intervention as well. It is no good for someone to be treated for agoraphobia with medication if they do not expose themselves to situations by which they previously felt threatened, otherwise they will never be able to overcome their agoraphobia.

If pharmacotherapy brings symptoms under control, this is an ideal time to teach the patient skills in managing their own anxiety. It is also essential that they overcome their anxiety-induced avoidance of particular situations. If psychological treatments are combined with pharmacotherapy, the risk of relapse when medication is taken away will be significantly reduced.

REFERENCES

Acarturk, C., Cuijpers, P., van Straten, A., de Graaf, R. (2009). Psychological treatment of social anxiety disorder: a meta-analysis. *Psychological Medicine, 39*(2), 241-254.

Andrews, G., Henderson, S., & Hall, W. (2001). Prevalence, comorbidity, disability and service utilisation: overview of the Australian National Mental Health Survey. *British Journal of Psychiatry, 178,* 145-153.

Andrews, G., Sanderson, K., & Beard, J. (1998). Burden of disease. Methods for calculating disability from mental disorder. *British Journal of Psychiatry, 173,* 123-131.

Australian Bureau of Statistics. (2008). *National Survey of Mental Health and Wellbeing: Summary of Results 2007.* Canberra: Australian Bureau of Statistics.

Australian Institute of Health and Welfare. (2010). *Australia's health 2010.* Canberra: AIHW.

Ballenger, J. C., Burrows, G. D., DuPont, R. L., Lesser, I. M., Noyes, R., Pecknold, J. C., Rifkin, A., Swinson, R. P. (1988). Alprazolam in panic disorder and agoraphobia: results from a multicenter trial. I. Efficacy in short-term treatment. *Archive of General Psychiatry, 45*(5), 413-422.

Bisson, J., & Andrew, M. (2007). Psychological treatment of post-traumatic stress disorder (PTSD). *Cochrane Database of Systematic Reviews 2007*(3), Art. No.: CD003388.

Blanco, C., Heimberg, R. G., Schneier, F. R., Fresco, D. M., Chen, H., Turk, C. L., Vermes, D., Erwin, B. A., Schmidt, A. B., Juster, H. R., Campeas, R., Liebowitz, M. R. (2010). A placebo-controlled trial of phenelzine, cognitive behavioral group therapy, and their combination for social anxiety disorder. *Archives of General Psychiatry, 67*(3), 286-295.

Bradley, R., Greene, J., Russ, E., Dutra, L., Westen, D. (2005). A multidimensional meta-analysis of psychotherapy for PTSD. *American Journal of Psychiatry,162*(2), 214-227.

Brown, T. A., & Barlow, D. H. (1995). Long-term outcome in cognitive–behavioral treatment of panic disorder: clinical predictors and alternative strategies for assessment. *Journal of Consulting and Clinical Psychology, 63*(5), 754-765.

Bryant, R., Moulds, M., Guthrie, R., Dang, S., Mastrodomenico, J., Nixon, R., Felmingham, K., Hopwood, S., Creamer, M. (2008). A randomized controlled trial of exposure therapy and cognitive restructuring for posttraumatic stress disorder. *Journal of Consulting and Clinical Psychology ,76*(4), 695-703.

Bruce, S. E., Yonkers, K. A., Otto, M. W., Eisen, J. L., Weisberg, R. B., & Pagano, M. (2005). Influence of psychiatric comorbidity on recovery and recurrence in generalized anxiety disorder, social phobia, and panic disorder: a 12-year prospective study. *American Journal of Psychiatry, 162*, 1179-1187.

Bouchard, T. J. (1984). Twins reared together and apart: what they tell us about human diversity. In S. W. Fox (Ed.), *Individuality and Determinism: Chemical and Biological Bases.* New York: Plenum Press.

Camp, N. J., Lowry, M. R., Richards, R. L., Plenk, A. M., Carter, C., Hensel, C. H., Abkevich, V., Skolnick, M. H., Shattuck, D., Rowe, K. G., Hughes, D. C., & Cannon-Albright, L. A. (2005). Genome-wide linkage analyses of extended Utah pedigrees identifies loci that influence recurrent, early-onset major depression and anxiety disorders. *American Journal of Medical Genetics Part B: Neuropsychiatric Genetics, 135B*(1), 85-93.

Carlbring, P., Nordgren, L. B., Furmark, T., & Andersson, G. (2009). Long-term outcome of internet-delivered cognitive-behavioural therapy for social phobia: a 30-month follow-up. *Behaviour Research and Therapy, 47*(10), 848-850.

Caspi, A., McClay, J., Moffitt, T. E., Mill, J., Martin, J., Craig, I. W., et al. (2002). Role of genotype in the cycle of violence in maltreated children. *Science, 297*(5582), 851-854.

Chessick, C. A., Allen, M. H., Thase, M. E., Batista Miralha da Cunha, A. A. B. C., Kapczinski, F. F. K., Silva de Lima, M., dos Santos Souza, J. J. S. S. (2006). Azapirones for generalized anxiety disorder. *Cochrane Database of Systematic Reviews, 3*, CD006115.

Choy, Y., Fyer, A. J., Lipsitz, J. D. (2007). Treatment of specific phobia in adults. *Clinical Psychology Review, 27*(3), 266-286.

Christensen, H., Griffiths, K. M., & Farrer, L. (2009). Adherence in Internet interventions for anxiety and depression: Systematic review. *Journal of Medical Internet Research, 11*(2), e13.

Clark, D. M., Ehlers, A., Hackmann, A., McManus, F., Fennell, M., Grey, N., Waddington, L., Wild, J. (2006). Cognitive therapy versus exposure and applied relaxation in social phobia: a randomized controlled trial. *Journal of Consulting and Clinical Psychology, 74*(3), 568-578.

Clark, D. M., Salkovskis, P. M., Hackmann, A., Wells, A., Ludgate, J., Gelder, M. (1999). Brief cognitive therapy for panic disorder: a randomized controlled trial. *Journal of Consulting and Clinical Psychology, 67*(4), 583-589.

Covin, R., Ouimet, A. J., Seeds, P. M., & Dozois, D. J. A. (2008). A meta-analysis of CBT for pathological worry among clients with GAD. *Journal of Anxiety Disorders, 22*(1), 108-116.

Cross-National Collaborative Panic Study Second Phase Investigators. (1992). Drug treatment of panic disorder: Comparative efficacy of alprazolam, imipramine, and placebo. *British Journal of Psychiatry, 160*, 191-202.

Davison, J., Potts, N., Richichi, E., Krishnan, R., Ford, S., Smith, R., Wilson, W. (1993). Treatment of social phobia with clonazepam and p lacebo. *Journal of Clinical Psychopharmacology, 13*(6), 423-428.

Dodd, J., & Role, L. W. (1991). The autonomic nervous system. In E. R. Kandel, J. H. Schwartz & T. M. Jessell (Eds.), *Principles of Neural Science* (3rd ed., pp. 761-775). East Norwalk: Appleton & Lange.

Etkin, A., & Wager, T. D. (2007). Functional neuroimaging of anxiety: a meta-analysis of PTSD, social anxiety disorder, and specific phobia. *American Journal of Psychiatry, 164*(10), 1476-1488.

Feder, A., Nestler, E. J., & Charney, D. S. (2009). Psychobiology and molecular genetics of resilience. *Nature Reviews Neuroscience, 10*(6), 446-457.

Felmingham, K., Kemp, A., Williams, L., Das, P., Hughes, G., Peduto, A., et al. (2007). Changes in anterior cingulate and amygdala after cognitive behavior therapy of posttraumatic stress disorder. *Psychological Science, 18*(2), 127-129.

Foa, E. B., Liebowitz, M. R., Kozak, M. J., Davies, S., Campeas, R., Franklin, M. E., et al. (2005). Randomized, placebo-controlled trial of exposure and ritual prevention, clomipramine, and their combination in the treatment of obsessive-compulsive disorder. *American Journal of Psychiatry, 162*(1), 151-161.

Flint, J., Corley, R., DeFries, J., Fulker, D., Gray, J., Miller, S., & Collins, A. (1995). A simple genetic basis for a complex psychological trait in laboratory mice. *Science, 269*(5229), 1432-1435.

Fullerton, J. M., Willis-Owen, S. A. G., Yalcin, B., Shifman, S., Copley, R. R., Miller, S. R., et al. (2008). Human-mouse quantitative trait locus concordance and the dissection of a human neuroticism locus. *Biological Psychiatry, 63*(9), 874-883.

Furukawa, T., Watanabe, N., Churchill, R. (2009). Combined psychotherapy plus antidepressants for panic disorder with or without agoraphobia. *Cochrane Database of Systematic Reviews 1*, CD004364.

Gava, I., Barbui, C., Aguglia, E., Carlino, D., Churchill, R., De Vanna, M., et al. (2007). Psychological treatments versus treatment-as-usual for obsessive-compulsive disorder (OCD). *Cochrane Database of Systematic Reviews, 2*, Art. No.: CD005333.

Guastella, A. J., Richardson, R., Lovibond, P. F., Rapee, R. M., Gaston, J. E., Mitchell, P., & Dadds, M. R. (2008). A randomized controlled trial of d-cycloserine enhancement of exposure therapy for social anxiety disorder. *Biological Psychiatry, 63*(6), 544-549.

Hetrick, S.E., Purcell, R., Garner, B., Parslow, R. (2010). Combined pharmacotherapy and psychological therapies for post traumatic stress disorder (PTSD). *Cochrane Database of Systematic Reviews 7*, CD007316.

Hidalgo, R., Tupler, L., Davidson, J. (2007). An effect-size analysis of pharmacologic treatments for generalized anxiety disorder. *Journal of Psychopharmacology, 21*(8), 864-872.

Hofmann, S.G., Sawyer, A.T., Witt, A.A., Oh, D. (2010). The effect of mindfulness-based therapy on anxiety and depression: a meta-analytic review. *Journal of Consulting and Clinical Psychology, 78*(2), 169-183.

Hoyer, J., Beesdo, K., Gloster, A. T., Runge, J., Höfler, M., Becker, E. S. (2009). Worry exposure versus applied relaxation in the treatment of generalized anxiety disorder. *Psychotherapy and Psychosomatics, 78*(2), 106-115.

Hudson, J. L., & Rapee, R. M. (2008). Familial and social environments in the etiology and maintenance of anxiety disorders. In M. M. Antony & M. B. Stein (Eds.), *Oxford Handbook of Anxiety and Related Disorders* (pp. 173-189). Oxford, New York: Oxford University Press.

Hunot, V., Churchill, R., Teixeira, V., Silva de Lima, M. (2007). Psychological therapies for generalised anxiety disorder. *Cochrane Database of Systematic Reviews 1*, CD001848.

Ipser, J., Carey, P., Dhansay, Y., Fakier, N., Seedat, S., Stein, D. (2006). Pharmacotherapy augmentation strategies in treatment-resistant anxiety disorders. *Cochrane Database of Systematic Reviews 4*, CD005473.

Issakidis, C., & Andrews, G. (2002). Service utilisation for anxiety in an Australian community sample. *Social Psychiatry and Psychiatric Epidemiology, 37*(4), 153-163.

Ito, L. M., de Araujo, L. A., Tess, V. L., de Barros-Neto, T. P., Asbahr, F. R., Marks, I. (2001). Self-exposure therapy for panic disorder with agoraphobia: randomised controlled study of external v. interoceptive self-exposure. *The British Journal of Psychiatry 178*(4), 331-336.

Joels, M., & Baram, T. Z. (2009). The neuro-symphony of stress. *Nature Reviews Neuroscience, 10*(6), 459-466.

Kapczinski, F., Silva de, L. M., dos Santos Souza, J., Batista Miralha da Cunha, A., Schmitt, R. (2003). Antidepressants for generalized anxiety disorder. Cochrane Database of Systematic Reviews 2, CD003592.

Kessler, R. C., Chiu, W. T., Demler, O., Walters, E. E. (2005). Prevalence, severity, and comorbidity of 12-month DSM-IV disorders in the national comorbidity survey replication. *Archives of General Psychiatry, 62*(6), 617-627.

Klein, B., Richards, J. C., & Austin, D. W. (2006). Efficacy of internet therapy for panic disorder. *Journal of Behavior Therapy and Experimental Psychiatry, 37*(3), 213-238.

Klein, B., Austin, D., Pier, C., Kiropoulos, L., Shandley, K., Mitchell, J., et al. (2009). Internet-based treatment for panic disorder: Does frequency of therapist contact make a difference? *Cognitive Behaviour Therapy, 38*(2), 100-113.

Koszycki, D., Benger, M., Shlik, J., Bradwejn, J. (2007). Randomized trial of a meditation-based stress reduction program and cognitive behavior therapy in generalized social anxiety disorder. *Behaviour Research and Therapy, 45*(10), 2518-2526.

Kushner, M. G., Kim, S. W., Donahue, C., Thuras, P., Adson, D., Kotlyar, M., et al. (2007). D-cycloserine augmented exposure therapy for obsessive-compulsive disorder. *Biological Psychiatry, 62*(8), 835-838.

LeBlanc, J., Cote, J., Jobin, M., & Labrie, A. (1979). Plasma catecholamines and cardiovascular responses to cold and mental activity. *Journal of Applied Physiology, 47*(6), 1207-1211.

Ledgerwood, L., Richardson, R., & Cranney, J. (2003). Effects of D-cycloserine on extinction of conditioned freezing. *Behavioral Neuroscience, 117*(2), 341-349.

March, S., Spence, S., & Donovan, C. (2009). The efficacy of an internet-based cognitive-behavioral therapy intervention for child anxiety disorders. *Journal of Pediatric Psychology, 34*(5), 474-487.

Maron, E., Hettema, J. M., & Shlik, J. (2010). Advances in molecular genetics of panic disorder. *Molecular Psychiatry, 15*(7), 681-701.

McEvoy, P. M., Grove, R., & Slade, T. (2011). Epidemiology of anxiety disorders in the Australian general population: findings of the 2007 Australian National Survey of Mental Health and Wellbeing. *Australian and New Zealand Journal of Psychiatry, 45*(11), 957-967.

McEvoy, P. M., Mahoney, A. E. J., & Moulds, M. L. (2010). Are worry, rumination, and post-event processing one and the same?: Development of the repetitive thinking questionnaire. *Journal of Anxiety Disorders, 24*(5), 509-519.

Meyer, T. J., Miller, M. L., Metzger, R. L., & Borkovec, T. D. (1990). Development and validation of the Penn State Worry Questionnaire. *Behaviour Research and Therapy, 28*(6), 487-495.

Mitte, K. (2005). A meta-analysis of the efficacy of psycho- and pharmacotherapy in panic disorder with and without agoraphobia. *Journal of Affective Disorders, 88*(1), 27-45.

Mitte, K., Noack, P., Steil, R., Hautzinger, M., (2005). A meta-analytic review of the efficacy of drug treatment in generalized anxiety disorder. *Journal of Clinical Psychopharmacology, 25*(2), 141-150.

Mosing, M. A., Gordon, S. D., Medland, S. E., Statham, D. J., Nelson, E. C., Heath, A. C., Martin, N. G., & Wray, N. R. (2009). Genetic and environmental influences on the co-morbidity between depression, panic disorder, agoraphobia, and social phobia: a twin study. *Depression and Anxiety, 26*(11), 1004-1011.

Nemeroff, C. B. (1998). The neurobiology of depression. *Scientific American, 278*(6), 42-49.

Norton, P. J., Price, E. C. (2007). A meta-analytic review of adult cognitive-behavioral treatment outcome across the anxiety disorders. *The Journal of Nervous and Mental Disease, 195*(6), 521-531.

Nutt, D., & Ballenger, J. (2005). *Anxiety Disorders: Panic Disorder and Social Anxiety Disorder.* Melbourne: Blackwell Publishing Asia Pty Ltd.

Orsillo, S. M., Roemer, L., & Segal, Z. V. (2011). *The Mindful Way through Anxiety: Break Free from Chronic Worry and Reclaim Your Life.* New York City: The Guilford Press.

Rentz, T. O., Powers, M. B., Smits, J. A. J., Cougle, J. R., Telch, M. J. (2003). Active-imaginal exposure: examination of a new behavioral treatment for cynophobia (dog phobia). *Behaviour Research and Therapy, 41*(11), 1337-1353.

Ressler, K., Rothbaum, B., Tannenbaum, L., Anderson, P., Graap, K., Zimand, E., et al. (2004). Cognitive enhancers as adjuncts to psychotherapy: use of d-cycloserine in phobic individuals to facilitate extinction of fear. *Archives of General Psychiatry, 61,* 1136-1144.

Roy-Byrne, P. P., Davidson, K. W., Kessler, R. C., Asmundson, G. J. G., Goodwin, R. D., Kubzansky, L., Lydiard, R. B., Massie, M. J., Katon, W., Laden, S. K., Stein, M. B. (2008). Anxiety disorders and comorbid medical illness. *General Hospital Psychiatry, 30*(3), 208-225.

Salzman, C. (1991). The APA Task Force report on benzodiazepine dependence, toxicity, and abuse. *American Journal of Psychiatry 148*(2), 151-152.

Sanchez-Meca, J., Rosa-Alcazar, A. I., Marin-Martinzez, F., Gomez-Conesa, A. (2010). Psychological treatment of panic disorder with or without agoraphobia: a meta-analysis. *Clinical Psychology Review, 30,* 37-50.

Shea, S. A., & White, D. P. (2008). Disorders of Ventilatory Control. In L. Goldman & D. A. Ausiello (Eds.), *Cecil Medicine* (23rd ed., pp. 609). Philadelphia: Saunders Elsevier.

Slade, T., Johnston, A., Teesson, M., Whiteford, H., Burgess, P., & Pirkis, J. (2009). *The Mental Health of Australians 2: Report on the 2007 National Survey of Mental Health and Wellbeing.* Canberra: Department of Health and Aging.

Smoller, J. W. (2011). Who's afraid of anxiety genetics? *Biological Psychiatry, 69*(6), 506-507.

Smoller, J. W., Block, S. R., & Young, M. M. (2009). Genetics of anxiety disorders: the complex road from DSM to DNA. *Depression and Anxiety, 26*(11), 965-975.

Spek, V., Cuijpers, P., Nyklicek, I., Riper, H., Keyzer, J., Pop, V. (2007). Internet-based cognitive behaviour therapy for symptoms of depression and anxiety: a meta-analysis. *Psychological Medicine, 37*(3), 319-328.

Stein, D. J., Ipser, J. C., van Balkom, A. J. (2009). Pharmacotherapy for social anxiety disorder. *Cochrane Database of Systematic Reviews 1,* CD001206.

Stein, D. J., Ipser, J. C., & McAnda, N. (2009). Pharmacotherapy of posttraumatic stress disorder: a review of meta-analyses and treatment guidelines. *CNS Spectrums, 14*(1 Suppl 1), 25-31.

Taylor, S. (1996). Meta-analysis of cognitive-behavioral treatments for social phobia. *Journal of Behavior Therapy and Experimental Psychiatry, 27*(1), 1-9.

Teesson, M., Slade, T., Mills, K. (2009). Comorbidity in Australia: findings of the 2007 National Survey of Mental Health and Wellbeing. *Australian and New Zealand Journal of Psychiatry, 43*(7), 606-614.

The Wellcome Trust Case Control Consortium. (2007). Genome-wide association study of 14,000 cases of seven common diseases and 3,000 shared controls. *Nature, 447*(7145), 661-678.

Titov, N., Andrews, G., Schwencke, G., Drobny, J., & Einstein, D. (2008). Shyness 1: distance treatment of social phobia over the internet. *Australian and New Zealand Journal of Psychiatry, 42*(7), 585-594.

Treynor, W., Gonzalez, R., & Nolen-Hoeksema, S. (2003). Rumination Reconsidered: A Psychometric Analysis. *Cognitive Therapy and Research, 27*(3), 247-259.

van Apeldoorn, F.J., Timmerman, M.E., Mersch, P.P.A., van Hout, W.J.P.J., Visser, S., van Dyck, R., den Boer, J.A. (2010). A randomized trial of cognitive-behavioral therapy or selective serotonin reuptake inhibitor or both combined for panic disorder with or without agoraphobia: treatment results through 1-year follow-up. *Journal of Clinical Psychiatry, 71*(5), 574-586.

van Balkom, A., de Haan, E., van Oppen, P., Spinhoven, P., Hoogduin, K., & van Dyck, R. (1998). Cognitive and behavioral therapies alone and in combination with fluvoxamine in the treatment of obsessive-compulsive disorder. *Journal of Nervous and Mental Disease, 186*(8), 492-499.

Versiani, M., Nardi, A.E., Figueira, I., Mendlowicz, M., Marques, C. (1997). Double-blind, placebo-controlled trials with bromazepam. *Jornal Brasileiro de Psiquiatria, 46*(3), 167-171.

Visscher, Peter M., Brown, Matthew A., McCarthy, Mark I., & Yang, J. (2012). Five Years of GWAS Discovery. *The American Journal of Human Genetics, 90*(1), 7-24.

von Knorring, L., S, T., Pettersson, A. (2005). Treatment of anxiety syndrome. A systematic literature review. Summary and conclusions by the SBU. *Lakartidningen, 102*(47), 3561-3562, 3565-3566, 3569.

Yerkes, R. M., & Dodson, J. D. (1908). The relation of strength of stimulus to rapidity of habit-formation. *Journal of Comparative Neurology and Psychology, 18*, 459-482.

Wolitzky-Taylor, K. B., Horowitz, J. D., Powers, M. B., Telch, M. J. (2008). Psychological approaches in the treatment of specific phobias: A meta-analysis. *Clinical Psychology Review, 28*(6), 1021-1037.

INDEX

placebo control, 252, 261, 284, 312

polymorphisms, 91, 92, 94, 393

poor concentration, 38

positive reinforcement, 234

post-event processing (PEP), 183, 188, 189, 190, 194, 373

postsynaptic receptor, 150

posttraumatic stress disorder, 15, 25, 31, 32, 34, 35, 38, 120, 134, 149, 183, 217, 290, 301, 314, 322, 335, 337, 338, 356, 369, 370, 375

predictive validity, 223

predisposing factor, 201

prefrontal, 59, 63, 74, 77, 78, 146, 147, 148, 150, 151, 156

presynaptic neuron, 150

prevalence, 28, 43, 44, 45, 46, 47, 48, 49, 82, 83, 84, 85, 90, 97, 109, 117, 214, 218, 220, 393

prn, 345

probability bias, 174

psychomotor coordination, 341, 342

psychopathology, 31, 35, 38, 41, 42, 129, 131, 165, 167 p

sycho-stimulant, 219

pulse rate, 65, 67

p-value, 95, 251

rational emotive therapy, 167

reactive attachment disorder, 34

recurrence, 25, 173, 305, 329, 330, 331, 349, 353, 369

re-experiencing symptom, 26

reinforcement, 161, 233, 234, 235

reinforcer, 233

relaxation training, 242

reliability, 221, 222, 224, 225, 226, 227, 229, 251

remission, 142, 293, 330, 331, 332, 333, 334, 355

respiratory rate, 59, 69

response, 2, 3, 4, 6, 7, 10, 11, 12, 23, 24, 33, 34, 44, 57, 58, 59, 60, 61, 62, 63, 65, 66, 68, 73, 76, 77, 78, 79, 88, 97, 119, 120, 121, 122, 129, 134, 135, 143, 147, 151, 155, 158, 160, 162, 169, 183, 186, 209, 216, 221, 233, 236, 238, 239, 240, 244, 249, 255, 259, 261, 278, 288, 289, 305, 307, 311, 326, 330, 332, 334, 337, 343, 355, 356, 357, 360, 366, 392, 394

restlessness, 3, 38

reticular formation, 68

rumination, 182, 183, 184, 185, 186, 194, 276, 279, 280, 375

safety behaviour, 21, 236, 249, 250, 353

safety seeking behaviour, 10

Schedule for Affective Disorders and Schizophrenia (SADS), 224, 225

schema, 165

second-generation antipsychotic, 338

secure attachment, 131

sedative, 15, 344

selective mutism, 32, 118

selective serotonin reuptake inhibitor (SSRI), 335, 341, 355, 356

self-monitoring, 277

semi-structured interview, 221

separation, 15, 28, 32, 111, 113, 117, 118, 129, 132, 201

separation anxiety disorder, 15, 28, 29, 32, 111, 117, 118

serotonin, vi, 33, 34, 41, 59, 101, 121, 150, 156, 335, 336, 337, 338, 340, 341, 342, 343, 346, 355, 356, 362, 365, 376

serotonin and noradrenaline (norepinephrine) reuptake inhibitor, 335

sexual dysfunction, 340, 341

APPENDIX 1   RELATED COURSEWORK AT THE UNIVERSITY OF SYDNEY

SHORT COURSES (NON-AWARD COURSES)

The Discipline of Psychiatry, the Brain and Mind Research Institute, and the Centre for Eating and Dieting Disorders at Sydney Medical School, the University of Sydney, offer a range of related online and face-to-face short courses to complement your use of this book (Table A1.1)

Table A1.1   Short courses in mental health

Course	Find more information at
Anxiety Disorders: The Foundations (Online)	sydney.edu.au/cce/course/anxd
Managing Anxiety Disorders in Primary Care	sydney.edu.au/cce/course/adgp
Mood Disorders: The Foundations (Online)	sydney.edu.au/cce/course/mdcf
Perinatal Mental Health: An Introduction (Online)	sydney.edu.au/cce/course/pmhc
Agomelatine in the Management of Depression (Online)	sydney.edu.au/cce/course/amdc
Understanding and Treating Hoarding Disorder	sydney.edu.au/cce/course/uthd
DSM-5: Common Mental Disorders	sydney.edu.au/cce/course/dsm5
Interpersonal Psychotherapy: Level A	sydney.edu.au/cce/course/ipta
Eating Disorder (Online)	cedd.cadre.com.au
Foundations of Leadership & Policy in Mental Health	sydney.edu.au/bmri/courses/continuing -professional-development/policy-and- leadership.php
Suicide Prevention	sydney.edu.au/bmri/courses/continuing -professional-development/suicide- prevention.php
Nicotine Addiction & Smoking Cessation	sydney.edu.au/bmri/courses/continuing -professional-development/smoking- cessation.php

Note. For an up-to-date list of all available short courses in mental health, visit sydney.edu.au/medicine/future-students/courses/short-courses

MENTAL HEALTH SUPERVISION PROGRAM (ONLINE)

Want high quality supervision and guidance for your practice in mental health? Join this innovative, cost effective and convenient online supervision program at the University of Sydney!

The Mental Health Clinical Supervision Program is designed to support mental health professionals such as psychologists, clinical psychologists, GPs, psychiatrists, psychiatry registrars, social workers, mental health nurses and counsellors in their clinical practice.

With a membership in the Program, you will be able to:

- submit up to six clinical cases in every 90-day period for supervision
- receive detailed written responses and instructions from your supervisors
- access a wide range of cases submitted by your peer supervisees
- join live online conferences (webinars) and learn about interesting topics highlighting the Program
- download and watch recordings of past webinars at your convenience
- save 10% off regular price when enrolling in any Psychiatry short courses (sydney.edu.au/cce/courses/health-nutrition/psychiatry).

Supervision aims to support mental health professionals in their clinical practice through enhancing their skills and knowledge along with encouraging reflection of their own practice. The Program will help you deliver a high quality professional service to your patients or clients and advance as a leader and/or an expert in your organisation. It provides the opportunity for reflection and processing of your personal beliefs, attitudes and feelings about your practice and your patients or clients, as well as allowing for discussion of therapeutic challenges, diagnostic uncertainties and ethical considerations.

In this way, supervision enhances your capacity to practise in ways that promote good mental health for yourself and reduce the risk of professional burnout. Ultimately, your participation in the Program will ensure that therapy is being delivered in a safe, effective and ethical manner, thus protecting and maximally benefiting your patients or clients.

Find more information about a membership in this Program at sydney.edu.au/cce/course/mhcs or call +61 2 8999 9608.

AWARD COURSES

So you are ready to develop a multidisciplinary understanding of mental disorders from the lab bench to the clinic and beyond? Sydney Medical School and Faculty of Science offer postgraduate award courses in the areas of psychiatry, psychotherapy, brain and mind sciences, and clinical psychology. Options of graduate certificate and graduate diploma are also available within the master's degrees.

Master of Medicine (Psychiatry)

The Master of Medicine (Psychiatry) is tailor-made for psychiatry trainees. It has been accredited by the Royal Australian and New Zealand College of Psychiatrists (RANZCP) as a Formal Education Course, and is aligned with its new competency-based fellowship program.

It will help you develop a sophisticated understanding of the neuro-scientific basis of psychiatry and expertise in critical appraisal and research design. You will learn how to translate research into clinical practice and develop interdisciplinary clinical and research professional networks. Facilitated by experts, sessions will be presented in small groups and supported by online learning technology.

The course includes an elective capstone experience in an area of advanced study. Options include a research project which may be used to fulfil RANZCP requirements or a range of coursework units.

This master's degree is delivered by the Brain and Mind Research Institute (BMRI), one of Australia's leading neuro-psychiatric institutes. The BMRI supports world leaders in mental health, neuroscience and neurology, and unites patients, support groups and frontline carers with scientists and clinicians.

Find more information at: sydney.edu.au/courses/psychiatry
Ask a question at: sydney.edu.au/courses/ask_a_question

Master of Medicine (Psychotherapy)

Psychotherapy covers a range of techniques used to improve an individual's mental health. Psychotherapists treat conditions including personality disorders, generalised anxiety disorder, dysthymia and chronic depression.

Our courses equip clinicians with the skills and experience to treat people who suffer from psychological disorders. Our students learn to apply psychodynamic principles in a variety of clinical settings and gain competency in psychodynamic concepts. Many go on to publish in the field and participate in scientific conferences. Students who complete this program will be eligible to gain professional recognition with the Australian and New Zealand Association of Psychotherapy and the Psychotherapy and Counselling Federation of Australia.

Find more information at: sydney.edu.au/courses/psychotherapy
Ask a question at: sydney.edu.au/courses/ask_a_question

Master of Brain and Mind Sciences

This course prepares you for a career in mental health and neuroscience. It focuses on the inter-disciplinary research that underpins the University of Sydney's Brain and Mind Research Institute. We cover areas such as substance abuse, clinical depression, dementia and psychosis, at both the fundamental neuroscience level and in the clinic.

This course is designed to:

- give you a solid understanding of basic neuroscience, clinical applications and interventions
- explore mental illness from both the basic and clinical research perspectives rather than as disparate scientific disciplines, empowering you to form meaningful collaborations and improve research outcomes.

The core units of study focus on fundamental neuroscience and its research, and their impact in a clinical setting, while electives allow for study into more specialised areas of brain and mind science such as brain and mind disorders of youth, ageing, genetics and suicide.

We offer our programs through the University of Sydney's Brain and Mind Research Institute which is home to clinics focused on Parkinson's disease, multiple sclerosis, dementia, youth mental health and sleep disorders, all of which are tied to clinical research programs. There are numerous laboratories undertaking basic science research, such as genetics, Alzheimer's disease and behavioural neuroscience. Our courses are taught by leading Australian mental health researchers and you will have opportunities for research alongside them.

Find more information at: sydney.edu.au/courses/brain-mind-sciences
Ask a question at: sydney.edu.au/courses/ask_a_question

Master of Clinical Psychology

Psychology is the scientific study of human behaviour and mental processes, investigating the way we behave as individuals and as social beings, interrogating the way we act and the way we think, and exploring our interaction with the physical world and with each other.

Clinical psychology can be studied as either a standalone coursework program, the Master of Clinical Psychology (MCP), or as a postgraduate double degree incorporating coursework and research, the Master of Clinical Psychology and Doctor of Philosophy (MCP and PhD). The MCP and PhD provides psychology graduates with clinical and doctorate-level research training in clinical psychology that is consistent with international standards of professional psychology.

The programs adopt a scientific and evidence-based approach to clinical psychology. The treatment model is based on a cognitive-behavioural approach, and the introduction of alternative models of therapy in the second year ensures both a depth and breadth to your clinical training.

The MCP and PhD involves 4.5 years of full-time study and includes three components: academic coursework, supervised clinical placements and research.

Qualified clinical psychologists provide you with supervised clinical practice in an internal on-campus psychology clinic, as well as a variety of external teaching hospitals and clinics. The programs include a minimum of 1200 hours of clinical placement experience. The research component in the MCP and PhD requires you to produce a Doctor of Philosophy (PhD) research thesis.

Find more information at:
sydney.edu.au/courses/master-of-clinical-psychology
Ask a question at: sydney.edu.au/courses/ask_a_question

APPENDIX 2   RELATED RESEARCH OPPORTUNITIES AT THE UNIVERSITY OF SYDNEY

UNDERSTANDING SOCIAL PROBLEMS IN YOUTH MENTAL HEALTH

To improve cognitive-behavioural interventions and develop a better understanding of the interaction between biological and psychological processes. The BMRI allows for front-line community-based research and the provision of quality treatment for hundreds of individuals across many mental health conditions, with over a thousand youth aged 12 to 30 accessing our services every year. The BMRI consists of interrelated and integrated out-patient community treatment clinics across inner Sydney and western Sydney, with specialist centres included (Anxiety Clinic, Centre for Autism Research and Evaluation). We use a wide variety of neuroscience technology (e.g., Genotyping, PET, EEG, Chronobiology, eye-tracking) with a multi-disciplinary team of neuroscientists, neurologists, psychiatrists, general practitioners, clinical psychologists, nurses, social and youth workers, to facilitate the development of research and psychobiological treatment approaches. This base provides a unique environment to conduct trials that have real community relevance while also integrating a range of potential neurobiological assessments/interventions.

Clinical Psychology Interventions and Translational Neuroscience

This research showed that oxytocin increases gaze to the eye-region of human faces and enhances encoding of positive social information. This research has laid some of the experimental foundation for future clinical treatment applications for a range of disorders. We are now currently evaluating whether oxytocin can be used to treat a range of mental health problems that are primarily associated with a difficulty in developing social-relationships (e.g., autism, schizophrenia, substance misuse/dependence).

Identifying Markers of Social Anxiety Disorder and How They Change Following Successful Cognitive-Behavioural Treatment

This research focuses on using fear-conditioning, cognitive attention tasks, decision making, hormonal and autonomic measures from young patients with social anxiety disorder to determine how these markers change over the course of cognitive-behavioural treatment programs and are unique to the development of social anxiety disorder. Social anxiety disorder is one of the most common mental health problems in young people and we conceptualise it as a gateway disorder that substantially increases risk for chronic and persistent mental ill-health over the course of a lifetime. This project will, therefore, substantially advance our knowledge of what marks the disorder in young people and how these markers change following successful treatment. This base provides a unique environment to conduct trials that have real community relevance while also integrating a range of potential neurobiological assessments/interventions.

Social Anxiety: Treatment and Assessment

We currently run an active CBT group program to treat social concerns in young people and we wish to identify markers of response. We currently use a range of assessments (startle response, conditioning, attention b ias assessment/modification) to assess markers of response, and you can develop unique assessments to understand social anxiety disorder or to assess change subsequent to CBT therapy. We also offer a novel treatment project utilizing advances in attention bias modification that will be co-supervised by Colin Macleod (UWA).

Using Human Psychopharmacology Assessments to Identify Unique Markers of Mental Ill-Health and Treatment Response

This research focuses on using plasma hormonal assessments to determine relationships of peripheral hormone levels and a range of mental health outcomes. This is primarily a psychopharmacology PhD and could explore how hormones and other potential markers of mental health problems, or change following intervention, in a range of clinical patient populations. The Youth Mental Health Clinic of the BMRI assesses over 1000 young people with mental health problems each year and provides treatment to patients with a range of mental health concerns (anxiety, depression, psychosis, addiction). This base provides a unique environment to conduct trials that have real community relevance while also integrating a range of potential neurobiological assessments/interventions.

Supervisor: Associate Professor Adam Guastella
Program type: Masters/PhD
Find more information at:
sydney.edu.au/research/opportunities/opportunities/714
Ask a question at: sydney.edu.au/courses/ask_a_question

THE NATURE AND TREATMENT OF OBSESSIVE-COMPULSIVE DISORDER

Obsessive-compulsive disorder (OCD) is the fourth most common psychiatric condition with a lifetime prevalence of up to 3.1%. The disorder can begin in childhood and is a chronic and disabling condition, the symptoms of which are time consuming, distressing, and often bizarre. OCD frequently leads to isolation, family dysfunction, difficulty forming and maintaining relationships, and unemployment. OCD is also associated with an increased risk of developing other psychological disorders, such as depression, drug or alcohol abuse and phobic disorders. The World Health Organisation ranks OCD as 20th among all causes of burden of disease, in recognition of the extreme financial and social cost of the disorder to the community. The proposed research aims to investigate the treatment of OCD, the cognitive mediation of OCD, and the relevance of negative life events such as unwanted sexual experiences in the onset of this condition. The treatment involves a newly developed cognitive therapy approach that targets expectancies of harm. The research is conducted in randomised, controlled trials and involves a comparison of new approaches with standard psychological treatments. The research also examines the relationship between change in distorted cognitions and symptom reduction in people whose focus of concern is either checking or washing/contamination. The research has the potential to dramatically reduce the significant social and economic burden cause by OCD and contribute to our understanding of the etiology of this condition

Supervisor: Dr Mairwen Jones
Program type: PhD
Find more information at:
sydney.edu.au/research/opportunities/opportunities/173
Ask a question at: sydney.edu.au/courses/ask_a_question

BRAIN STRUCTURAL CHANGES IN OBESITY AND THEIR EFFECT ON COGNITION AND MOOD DISORDERS

Obesity is independently associated with significant cognitive dysfunction. Converging evidence shows that there are underlying structural brain changes that occur in obesity that may form the basis for this. The goal of this project is to use advanced magnetic resonance imaging (MRI), including diffusion tensor imaging (DTI), and resting-state and task-based functional magnetic resonance imaging (fMRI) to explore the link between brain structure and function in the setting of obesity.

Obesity is a growing health epidemic that is associated with an array of established cardiovascular and metabolic consequences. However, the effects of obesity on human brain structure and function are less well understood. Recent work demonstrates that elevated body mass and adiposity are linked to reductions in cognitive performance. Obesity at midlife is also associated with increased risk for dementia in later life. Obesity is also a risk factor for depression, however no structural correlate for this has been previously explored. This project will use advanced neuroimaging techniques, including functional magnetic resonance imaging (fMRI), structural MRI and diffusion tensor imaging (DTI), to map the neural circuitry abnormalities that are associated with obesity. The project will involve analysis of both prospective data and a large database containing MRI, EEG, cognition, genetics and clinical data from more than 1000 individuals.

In the Brain Dynamics Centre we focus on conditions of mental health that affect our young people and can persist into adulthood.

Our goals are to:

- find out what is causing conditions of mental health
- develop tests for early signs of illness, so that early intervention and prevention become a reality
- identify predictors of what treatment is best suited to each individual person.

This project has a number of possible directions that would depend on the background of the candidate - students with Psychology, Medical Science, Engineering, Computer Science and Medical backgrounds are encouraged to apply.

PhD students will be actively involved in assessment of human participants. They will be trained in acquisition of behavioural and brain imaging data, and the use of sophisticated statistical procedures. When based at the Brain Dynamics Centre, PhD students have a strong team-based support network. The BDC comprises a team of 60 members, including academic scientists, clinicians, PhD students and post-doctoral researchers.

Supervisors: Associate Professor Stuart Grieve and Dr Mayuresh Korgaonkar
Program type: Masters/PhD
Find more information at:
sydney.edu.au/research/opportunities/opportunities/1072
Ask a question at: sydney.edu.au/courses/ask_a_question